Manual Handling in Health and Social Care

Manual Handling in Health and Social Care

An A–Z of Law and Practice

Michael Mandelstam

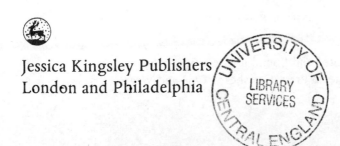

Jessica Kingsley Publishers
London and Philadelphia

First published in the United Kingdom in 2002
by Jessica Kingsley Publishers Ltd
116 Pentonville Road
London N1 9JB, England
and
325 Chestnut Street
Philadelphia, PA 19106, USA

www.jkp.com

Copyright © Michael Mandelstam 2002

Library of Congress Cataloging in Publication Data

A CIP catalog record for this book is available from the Library of Congress

British Library Cataloguing in Publication Data

A CIP catalogue record for this book is available from the British Library

ISBN 1 84310 041 X

Printed and Bound in Great Britain by
Athenaeum Press, Gateshead, Tyne and Wear

CONTENTS

Acknowledgements

This book has only been made possible by the numerous conversations the author has had with many people about manual handling issues.

Singling out names is therefore an invidious task; nevertheless I would like to mention in particular Howard Richmond at the Royal College of Nursing for making available to me details of a number of legal judgments I would otherwise not have been able to obtain, and also his colleague David Gardiner. Likewise, for tracking down the *Stainton* case, thanks to Anne Gaskell. For their insights, I should mention also Alison Cooke, Manual Handling Adviser for Surrey County Council; Norma Richardson, Manual Handling Adviser at Disabled Living in Manchester; and Jacqui Smith, editor of *The Column*. However, clearly, any errors, rash statements or other shortcomings are mine alone.

Disclaimer

Every effort has been made to ensure that the information contained in this book is correct, or at least is a reasonable interpretation. However, the reader should bear in mind that a book of this nature is likely to contain some errors; that the law changes and is anyway subject to inherent uncertainties; and that individual disputes possess their own unique set of circumstances and facts. The time of writing is January 2002.

INTRODUCTION

1. **Whom the book is for**
2. **Purpose of the book**
3. **Organisation and content of the book**
4. **Case law**
5. **Standards of manual handling and case law**
6. **Terminology and cross-referencing**

I. Whom the book is for

This is intended to be an easy-to-use book on manual handling law for staff and their managers working in the health and social care field – for instance, ambulance workers, care assistants, hospital porters, nurses, nursing auxiliaries, occupational therapists, physiotherapists, social workers, and staff working in NHS and social services equipment stores and delivering the equipment to people's homes. It will also be of interest to those working with children in schools, who might have to handle disabled children or other children whose behaviour is difficult to manage.

It is also aimed at disabled people and their representative organisations, various advisers, lawyers – and students taking higher education courses in health and social care, whether practice, policy or management related. Although the book is intended to be simple to use, it undoubtedly contains a substantial amount of detail; the reason for this is that many of the questions about manual handling asked both by professionals and sometimes by clients and patients relate to such detail. Equally, there are summaries at all levels of the book for quicker use – for instance, the Overview itself, the still more succinct summary contained in Section 1 of that Overview, the bold key words and introductory sentences at the head of legal cases in the A–Z List, and so on.

The book applies to England, Wales and Scotland. Indeed, a significant number of the legal cases included are Scottish. Northern Ireland is covered so far as health and safety at work legislation and related case law is concerned.

2. Purpose of the book

The overall purpose of the book is as an additional tool to assist manual handling decision-making at local level. Law is an obvious starting point, since it is legislation which underpins the very existence, and the powers and duties, of the NHS and of local authority social services departments – as well as the registration and inspection of care homes. More specifically of course it is the *Manual Handling Operations Regulations 1992*, which underlie manual handling policies and practices across the statutory, voluntary and independent sectors.

However, while much of the relevant law – at least the health and safety at work legislation and the common law of negligence – is relatively simple in principle, in practice manual handling issues sometimes resemble Gordian knots. The book does not claim that the law can straightforwardly cut such knots, but that it at least provides a framework within which to think through manual handling policy and practice. Where law is clear in both meaning and implications, it is obviously important to know what it states. But even where the law is less clear, it is nevertheless equally important to know that this is so, since either way there will be implications for local manual handling policies and practices.

Nevertheless, the reader should beware the adage (somewhat adapted here): 'To every complex problem there is an answer: simple, straightforward, logical and wrong.' For instance, even apparently logically constructed local policies and practices might rest on false or contentious premises – such as, for instance, a misunderstanding or narrow interpretation of what the relevant manual handling legislation or national guidance actually states and means.

3. Organisation and content of the book

Following this Introduction, the book provides an Overview of manual handling law and practice which stands alone, but which also anticipates and refers to entries in the A–Z List. The Overview is in effect the key to the book; and Section 1 therein provides a still more concentrated summary.

The A–Z List, the main body of the book, contains summaries and extracts of relevant legislation, case law and a range of words and phrases representing commonly asked questions. It is designed to give quick answers; at the same time, it allows the reader who has more time to follow cross-references, to read legal cases and so to build up a more detailed picture. In addition, three at-a-glance lists of terms, cases and legislation indicate what is in the A–Z List. The cases list itself comprises two parts, the first listing cases by the occupation of the claimant or legal case type; the second listing cases alphabetically.

As far as the author is aware, the approach of the book – particularly by considering the wider legal context of manual handling and including such an extensive collection of case law relevant to health and social care – is one not hitherto taken to this subject.

Legal context of manual handling

In terms of the overall legal context, the book considers not only the *Manual Handling Operations Regulations 1992*, but also other *health and safety at work legislation*, the common law of *negligence*, and the range of *welfare legislation* which ultimately underpins manual handling decision-making within the NHS and local authorities. Indeed, some of the problems affecting both employees and patients or clients in respect of manual handling policies and decisions, precisely stem from the implications of this legislation, rather than the 1992 Regulations themselves. For instance, matters such as assessment and meeting of patients' and clients' needs, lack of resources to meet needs, conflicts between what patients or clients want by way of manual handling (particularly in the community) and what the NHS or local authorities, or care agencies on their behalf, are prepared to offer – all flow ultimately from this welfare legislation.

Practical situations

The extensive legal case law and its detail included in the book are a reminder that manual handling is ultimately about individual people, and not rules and regulations. This is particularly so in the field of health and social care, where not only handlers, but also often the handled, are animate. No apology is therefore made for the inclusion of detailed case law, which precisely emphasises this point. In addition, many practitioners in the field find it easier to understand legal issues and principles when these are fully illustrated in practical situations – rather than presented only as dry and somewhat abstract rules. In a sense, the case law is also representative of the fact that everyday situations (manual handling or otherwise) in health and social care tend to be 'messy' with many blurred edges and beset by any number of variables – a fact well recognised by practitioners. This is in spite of the exhortations of senior managers, trainers, government departments and professional bodies who, quite properly, would like the world to run on straighter, more rational lines.

4. Case law

The legal case law included in the book covers a wide range of work situations, not just health and social care, where the factual situation or legal principle involved is relevant. For example, a council carpenter carrying doors upstairs (*Hawkes v Southwark London Borough Council*) could be equated with employees from a joint NHS/social services equipment store delivering manual handling or other equipment to people's homes. Likewise, important points about the *Manual Handling Operations Regulations 1992* were made in the *Hawkes* case concerning the nature of 'reasonable practicability' – and in the case of *Swain v Denso Martin* (a factory case) about the duty to reduce risk and to provide information.

Hierarchy of courts

The hierarchy of the courts for civil cases in England and Wales basically runs County Court, High Court, Court of Appeal, House of Lords – so that, for example, a

Court of Appeal decision is in principle weighty, whilst County Court decisions, most of which are anyway not reported, barely establish legal precedent. However, County Court decisions might have significant practical effect – for instance, in the form of awards of over £300,000 in manual handling cases (e.g. *Commons v Queen's Medical Centre*) – and sometimes discuss and highlight important legal issues. For instance, County Courts have considered manual handling injury arising from 'cumulative strain' rather than a one-off incident (e.g. *Commons v Queen's Medical Centre; Stone v Commissioner of Police for the Metropolis*), or the application of the *Manual Handling Operations Regulations (MHOR) 1992* to an injured person who is not strictly an employee (*Peck v Chief Constable of Avon*). Thus, some County Court decisions are included in the book.

For Scotland, the equivalent order of courts is Sheriff's Court, Court of Session (Outer House), Court of Session (Inner House), House of Lords.

A number of Australian cases involving manual handling in health and social care are also included because (a) they provide further illustration of practical situations which have been considered judicially; and (b) they are mostly negligence cases. The law of negligence in Australia is based on the same principles as in the United Kingdom, and judges sometimes look across the world to learn from each other's negligence case law when they are deciding difficult cases.

Identifying manual handling cases

Many manual handling cases are not reported in the published law reports and are tracked down only with some difficulty. The author is in no doubt that there are many which he has failed to identify and which, although technically publicly available, are in practice scarcely in the public domain. This overall difficulty is an additional reason why the author has included substantial summaries of the cases he has managed to obtain.

5. Standards of manual handling and case law

Manual handling cases over the last twenty years or so demonstrate that standards of legally acceptable practice – for instance, in manual handling techniques – in health and social care have changed over time, so that what a judge or expert witness stated was acceptable in 1989 might no longer be so in 2001 (e.g. *Brodie v Kent County Council*). Therefore, the reader who wishes to identify good practice in 2001 and beyond must refer to various national guidance on manual handling (which is listed under the entry *guidance* in the A–Z List). In this book, a fairly even mixture of successful and failed cases has been included, so as to represent both employer and employee point of view.

Indeed in some earlier negligence cases, the courts recognised (*Stewart v Highland Health Board*) that their approach would change and develop (*Bowfield v South Sefton (Merseyside) Health Authority*), and made statements almost of judicial intent – such as that it was time for staff such as student nurses properly to be protected, and that it was no longer acceptable to think of their serious injuries as simply the 'rub of the green' which had to be regarded as an inherent risk (*Clarke v Oxfordshire Health Authority*). In others, even where employer liability was overturned on appeal of the case, it was as though the judges at first instance were pointing the way forward to better protection of care staff, only to be pegged back by the more cautious appeal decisions of the time (e.g. *Bowfield v South Sefton (Merseyside) Health Authority; Lane v Capital Territory Health Commission*).

The reader should also note that sometimes court cases are heard many years after the date of the original accident and injury, but the judges will consider what constituted acceptable standards of practice at the time of the accident, not at the time of the hearing.

Notwithstanding generally changing standards, the book includes a significant number of older cases as well as new, since they are still relevant to understanding the approach of the courts. First, some of the older negligence cases in fact impose standards on employers as high as any likely to be imposed now anyway, even under the *MHOR 1992*. Second, some of these older cases that went against employees can be matched by more recent cases with a similar result. Lastly, some would almost certainly be decided differently now (and the author suggests this in the summaries of a few such cases); yet even these cases are of interest in showing how standards have changed.

Furthermore, it should be remembered that the outcome of cases is not always predictable, hinging as it does on a number of variables and the particular circumstances and facts of each case. Thus, there is no simple, all-embracing, system of precedent in manual handling cases, such that every aspect of certain older cases is no longer relevant; no doubt for this very reason, the courts seem sparingly to cite, let alone overrule, previous judgments in this field.

6. Terminology and cross-referencing

First, widespread, 'global' abbreviation has been avoided, with the exception of the *Manual Handling Operations Regulations 1992* which are referred to as the *MHOR 1992* throughout – and also the National Health Service which is shortened to NHS. Otherwise, abbreviation is introduced and used 'locally' in individual entries within the A–Z List or paragraphs in the Overview. Second, the terms 'council', 'local authority' and 'social services' are used, on the whole, interchangeably. Third, the reader should be aware that in *negligence* or other personal injury cases in England and Wales, the person bringing the case has in the past been known as the plaintiff, but is more recently known as the claimant. In Scotland he or she is referred to as the pursuer.

Lastly, selective cross-referencing, both from the Overview to the A–Z List, and between A–Z List entries, is achieved by means of italics.

LIST OF TERMS IN THE A–Z LIST

LIST OF CASES (BY OCCUPATION OF CLAIMANT AND BY TYPE OF CASE)

I. Personal injury civil compensation cases brought by employees: manual handling related

Ambulance workers. *Lang v Fife Health Board; Parkes v Smethwick Corporation; Stuthridge v Merseyside Metropolitan Ambulance Service.*

Care assistants. *Brodie v Kent County Council; Cantillon v London Nursing Homes; Fleming v Stirling Council; Gysen v St Luke's; Hopkinson v Kent County Council; Koonjul v Thameslink Healthcare NHS Trust; McIlgrew v Devon County Council; Miletic v Capital Territory Health Commission; Rowe v Swansea City Council; Schiliro v Peppercorn Child Care Centres*

Council and other public workers: various occupations, alphabetical by occupation. *Blacksmiths (Hall v Edinburgh City Council); caretakers (Hillhouse v South Ayrshire Council); carpenters (Hawkes v Southwark London Borough Council); electricians (McBeath v Halliday); fencers (Cullen v North Lanarkshire Council); firemen (Logan v Strathclyde Fire Board); gardeners (Mitchell v Inverclyde District Council); glass shop workers (Fotheringham v Dunfermline District Council); lifting buckets (Warren v Harlow District Council); police and related staff (Peck v Chief Constable of Avon and Somerset; Stone v Commissioner of Police for the Metropolis); post office workers (Rozario v Post Office; Stark v Post Office); roadworkers (Forsyth v Lothian Regional Council; Gilchrist v Strathclyde Regional Council; Skinner v Aberdeen City Council).*

District nurses. *Channon v East Sussex Area Health Authority; Doherty v Tunbridge Wells Health Authority; Hammond v Cornwall and Isles of Scilly Health Authority; Wardlaw v Fife Health Board.*

Foster carers. *Beasley v Buckinghamshire County Council.*

Hospital catering assistants. *Wakefield v Basildon and Thurrock Health Authority.*

Hospital craft ladies. *O'Neill v Boorowa District Hospital.*

Hospital laundry workers. *Anderson v Lothian Health Board; Boyd v Lanarkshire Health Board; Easson v Dundee Teaching Hospitals NHS Trust.*

Hospital porters. *McMenamin v Lambeth, Southwark and Lewisham Area Health Authority.*

Manual handling trainers. *Beattie v West Dorset Health Authority.*

Miscellaneous claimants and pursuers. *Airport workers (Gordon v British Airways);* **architectural masons** *(Kelly v Forticrete);* **bakery manageresses** *(Black v Carricks);* **crisp packers** *(Gissing v Walkers Smith);* **dancers** *(Woods v Barry Clayman Concerts);* **factory workers** *(Brown v Allied Ironfounders; Jude v Elliott Medway; Kinsella v Harris; Swain v Denso Martin);* **jeans factory workers** *(Black v Wrangler);* **lift engineers** *(Bunter v Liftwise);* **lorry drivers** *(Blanchflower v Chamberlain; Welsh v Matthew Clark Wholesale; Wild v United Parcel Services);* **maintenance engineers** *(King v Carron Phoenix);* **milkmen** *(Anderson v Associated Coop Creameries);* **rail workers** *(Wilson v British Railways Board);* **scrap metal yard workers** *(Chalk v Devizes Reclamation);* **steam cleaning operatives** *(King v RCO);* **telephone engineers and storekeepers** *(Divit v British Telecommunications; Watkinson v British Telecommunications).*

Midwives. *Wells v West Hertfordshire Health Authority.*

Nurses. *Bearman v Australian Capital Territory Community and Health Service;* **Blair** *v Lancaster Health Authority;* **Bowfield** *v South Sefton (Merseyside) Health Authority;* **Coad** *v Cornwall and Isles of Scilly Health Authority;* **Commons** *v Queen's Medical Centre;* **Dewing** *v St Luke's;* **Dickson** *v Lothian Health Board;* **Edwards** *v Waltham Forest Health Authority;* **Forder** *v Norfolk Area Health Authority;* **Halliday** *v Tayside Health Board;* **Kempsey District Hospital** *v Thackham;* **McCaffery** *v Datta;* **McGowan** *v Harrow Health Authority;* **McLean** *v Plymouth Health Authority;* **Moore** *v Norfolk Area Health Authority;* **Munrow** *v Plymouth Health Authority;* **Pacheco** *v Brent and Harrow Area Health Authority;* **Page** *v Enfield and Haringey Health Authority;* **Pollitt** *v Oxford Health Authority;* **Postle** *v Norfolk and Norwich Healthcare NHS Trust;* **Salvat** *v Basingstoke and North Hampshire Health Authority;* **Stewart** *v Highland Health Board;* **Williams** *v Gwent Health Authority;* **Woolgar** *v West Surrey and North East Hampshire Health Authority.*

Nursing auxiliaries. *Aitken v Board of Management of Aberdeen College;* **Bohitige** *v Barnet Healthcare NHS Trust;* **Brown** *v East Midlothian NHS Trust;* **Callaghan** *v Southern General Hospital;* **Charnock** *v Capital Territory Health Commission;* **Denton** *v South West Thames Regional Health Authority;* **Fitzsimmons** *v Northumberland Health Authority;* **Fraser** *v Greater Glasgow Health Board;* **Hadfield** *v Manchester Health Authority;* **Jones** *v South Glamorgan Health Authority;* **Laing** *v Tayside Health Board;* **Moran Health Care Services** *v Woods;* **Murray** *v Healthscope;* **Painter** *v Barnet Community Healthcare NHS Trust;* **Pearson** *v Eastbourne Area Health Authority;* **Seamner** *v North East Essex Health Authority;* **Shirley** *v Wirral Health Authority;* **Slater** *v Fife Primary Care NHS Trust;* **Sommerville** *v Lothian Health Board;* **Weston** *v South Coast Nursing Homes;* **Wright** *v Fife Health Board;*

Occupational therapists and assistants. *Stainton v Chorley and South Ribble NHS Trust.*

Physiotherapists and assistants. *Bruggemann v Ace Nominees Pty;* **Clarke** *v Adams;* **Stainton** *v Chorley and South Ribble NHS Trust.*

School staff. *Daws v Croydon London Borough Council;* **McLeod** *v Aberdeen City Council;* **Purvis** *v Buckinghamshire County Council;* **Taylor** *v Glasgow City Council.*

Social workers. *Colclough v Staffordshire County Council;* **Watkins** *v Strathclyde Regional Council;* **Wiles** *v Bedfordshire County Council.*

Student nurses. *Bayley v Bloomsbury Health Authority;* **Campbell** *v Dumfries and Galloway Health Board;* **Clarke** *v Oxfordshire Health Authority;* **Eaton** *v West Lothian NHS Trust;* **Gower** *v Berks;* **Lane** *v Capital Territory Health Commission;* **Young** *v Salford Health Authority.*

Swimming pool attendants. *Barnes v Stockton Borough Council;* **Paramerissios** *v Hammersmith and Fulham London Borough Council.*

2. Health and Safety Executive prosecutions

Health and Safety Executive v Barnet London Borough Council

Health and Safety Executive v Norfolk and Norwich Healthcare NHS Trust

3. Patient and client cases: civil compensation cases, judicial review cases

European Court of Human Rights. *D v United Kingdom;* **Price** *v United Kingdom;* **Z** *v United Kingdom.*

Health service ombudsman investigations. *Epsom and St Helier NHS Trust.*

Local government ombudsman investigations. *Barking and Dagenham London Borough Council;* **Bristol** *City Council;* **Camden** *London Borough Council;* **Islington** *London Borough Council;* **Redbridge** *London Borough Council;* **Rotherham** *Metropolitan Borough Council.*

NHS patients: judicial review cases. *R v Cambridgeshire Health Authority, ex p B;* **R** *v Central Birmingham Health Authority, ex p Collier;* **R** *v Central Birmingham Health Authority, ex p Walker;* **R** *v Hillingdon Area Health Authority, ex p Wyatt;* **R** *v North and East Devon Health Authority, ex p Coughlan;* **R** *v North West Lancashire Health Authority, ex p G, A and D.*

NHS patients: negligence cases. *A v National Blood Authority;* **Kent** *v Griffiths.*

Social services: adults, judicial review. *MacGregor v South Lanarkshire Council;* **R (Bodimeade)** *v Camden London Borough Council;* **R (Heather, Ward and Callin)** *v Leonard Cheshire Foundation;* **R (Khana)** *v Southwark London Borough Council;* **R (Rowe)** *v Walsall Metropolitan Borough Council;* **R** *v Avon County Council, ex p M;* **R** *v Birmingham City Council, ex p Killigrew;* **R** *v Cornwall County Council, ex p Goldsack;* **R** *v Gloucestershire County Council, ex p Barry;* **R** *v Haringey London Borough Council, ex p Norton;* **R** *v Kensington and Chelsea Royal Borough, ex p Kujtim;* **R** *v Lancashire County Council, ex p RADAR;* **R** *v North Yorkshire County Council, ex p Hargreaves;* **R** *v Secretary of State for Social Services, ex p Hincks.*

Social services: children, judicial review and other cases. *A v Lambeth London Borough Council;* ***R v Bexley*** *London Borough Council, ex p B;* ***R v Ealing*** *London Borough Council, ex p C;* ***Re O.***

Social services: negligence cases. *T (A Minor) v Surrey County Council;* ***Vicar of Writtle*** *v Essex County Council;* ***W*** *v Essex County Council;* ***Wyatt*** *v Hillingdon London Borough Council;* ***X*** *v Bedfordshire County Council.*

Special educational needs: judicial review. *Bradford Metropolitan District Council v A;* ***R v Brent and Harrow*** *Health Authority, ex p Harrow London Borough Council;* ***R v Harrow*** *London Borough Council, ex p M;* ***R v Lambeth*** *London Borough Council, ex p M.*

Special educational needs: negligence. *Phelps v Hillingdon London Borough Council.*

ALPHABETICAL LIST OF CASES (COURTS AND OMBUDSMAN) A–Z

A v Lambeth London Borough Council

A v National Blood Authority

Aitken v Board of Management of Aberdeen College

Anderson v Associated Coop Creameries Ltd

Anderson v Lothian Health Board

Barking and Dagenham London Borough Council

Barnes v Stockton Borough Council

Bayley v Bloomsbury Health Authority

Bearman v Australian Capital Territory Community and Health Service

Beasley v Buckinghamshire County Council

Beattie v West Dorset Health Authority

Black v Carricks

Black v Wrangler (UK) Limited

Blair v Lancaster Health Authority

Blanchflower v Chamberlain

Bohitige v Barnet Healthcare NHS Trust

Bolam v Friern Hospital Management Committee

Bolitho v City and Hackney Health Authority

Bowfield v South Sefton (Merseyside) Health Authority

Boyd v Lanarkshire Health Board

Bradford Metropolitan District Council v A

Bristol City Council

Brodie v Kent County Council

Brown v Allied Ironfounders

Brown v East Midlothian NHS Trust

Bruggemann v Ace Nominees Pty

Bunter v Liftwise

Callaghan v Southern General Hospital NHS Trust

Camden London Borough Council

Campbell v Dumfries and Galloway Health Board

Cantillon v London Nursing Homes Ltd

Chalk v Devizes Reclamation Company

Channon v East Sussex Area Health Authority

Charnock v Capital Territory Health Commission and Caroline Klefisch

Clarke v Adams

Clarke v Oxfordshire Health Authority

Coad v Cornwall and Isles of Scilly Health Authority

Colclough v Staffordshire County Council

Commons v Queen's Medical Centre Nottingham University Hospital NHS Trust

Cullen v North Lanarkshire Council

D v United Kingdom

Daws v Croydon London Borough Council

Denton v South West Thames Regional Health Authority

Dewing v St Luke's (Anglican Church in Australia) Association

Dickson v Lothian Health Board

Divit v British Telecommunications

Doherty v Tunbridge Wells Health Authority

Easson v Dundee Teaching Hospitals NHS Trust

Eaton v West Lothian NHS Trust

Edwards v National Coal Board

Edwards v Waltham Forest Health Authority

Epsom and St Helier NHS Trust

Fitzsimmons v Northumberland Health Authority

Fleming v Stirling Council

Forder v Norfolk Area Health Authority

Forsyth v Lothian Regional Council

Fotheringham v Dunfermline District Council

Fraser v Greater Glasgow Health Board

General Cleaning Contractors v Christmas

Gilchrist v Strathclyde Regional Council

Gissing v Walkers Smith Snack Foods Ltd

Gordon v British Airways PLC

Gower v Berks

Gysen v St Luke's (Anglican Church in Australia) Association

Hadfield v Manchester Health Authority

Hall v Edinburgh City Council

Halliday v Tayside Health Board

Hammond v Cornwall and Isles of Scilly Health Authority

Hawkes v Southwark London Borough Council

Health and Safety Executive v Barnet London Borough Council

Health and Safety Executive v Gloucestershire Ambulance Services NHS Trust

Health and Safety Executive v Norfolk and Norwich Healthcare NHS Trust

Health and Safety Executive v Trafford Health Authority

Hillhouse v South Ayrshire Council

Hopkinson v Kent County Council

Hunter v Hanley

Islington London Borough Council

Jones v South Glamorgan Health Authority

Jude v Elliott Medway Ltd

Kelly v Forticrete Ltd

Kempsey District Hospital v Thackham

Kent v Griffiths

King v Carron Phoenix Ltd

King v RCO Support Services and Another

Kinsella v Harris Lebus Ltd

Koonjul v Thameslink Healthcare NHS Trust

Laing v Tayside Health Board

Lane v Capital Territory Health Commission

Lane v Shire Roofing Co (Oxford) Ltd

Lang v Fife Health Board

Logan v Strathclyde Fire Board

MacGregor v South Lanarkshire Council

McBeath v Halliday

McCaffery v Datta

McGowan v Harrow Health Authority

McIlgrew v Devon County Council

McLean v Plymouth Health Authority

McLeod v Aberdeen City Council

McMenamin v Lambeth, Southwark and Lewisham Area Health Authority (Teaching)

Miletic v Capital Territory Health Commission

Mitchell v Inverclyde District Council

Moore v Norfolk Area Health Authority

Moran Health Care Services v Woods

Munrow v Plymouth Health Authority

Murray v Healthscope Limited trading as North West Private Hospital

O'Neill v Boorowa District Hospital

Pacheco v Brent and Harrow Area Health Authority

Page v Enfield and Haringey Health Authority

Painter v Barnet Community Healthcare NHS Trust

Paramerissios v Hammersmith and Fulham London Borough Council

Parkes v Smethwick Corporation

Pearson v Eastbourne Area Health Authority

Peck v Chief Constable of Avon and Somerset

Phelps v Hillingdon London Borough Council

Pollitt v Oxfordshire Health Authority

Postle v Norfolk and Norwich Healthcare NHS Trust

Price v United Kingdom

Purvis v Buckinghamshire County Council

R (Bodimeade) v Camden London Borough Council

R (Heather, Ward and Callin) v Leonard Cheshire Foundation

R (Khana) v Southwark London Borough Council

R (Rowe) v Walsall Metropolitan Borough Council

R v Avon County Council, ex parte M

R v Bexley London Borough Council, ex parte B

R v Birmingham City Council, ex parte Killigrew

R v Bouldstridge

R v Brent and Harrow Health Authority, ex parte Harrow London Borough Council

R v Cambridgeshire Health Authority, ex parte B

R v Central Birmingham Health Authority, ex parte Collier

R v Central Birmingham Health Authority, ex parte Walker

R v Cornwall County Council, ex parte Goldsack

R v Ealing London Borough Council, ex parte C

R v Gloucestershire County Council, ex parte Barry

R v Gloucestershire County Council, ex parte Mahfood

R v Haringey London Borough Council, ex parte Norton

R v Harrow London Borough Council, ex parte M

R v Hillingdon Area Health Authority, ex parte Wyatt

R v Kensington and Chelsea Royal Borough, ex parte Kujtim

R v Lambeth London Borough Council, ex parte M

R v Lancashire County Council, ex parte RADAR

R v North and East Devon Health Authority, ex parte Coughlan

R v North Derbyshire Health Authority, ex parte Fisher

R v North West Lancashire Health Authority, ex parte G, A and D

R v North Yorkshire County Council, ex parte Hargreaves

R v Secretary of State for Social Services, ex parte Hincks

Re O

Redbridge London Borough Council

Rotherham Metropolitan Borough Council

Rowe v Swansea City Council

Rozario v Post Office

Salvat v Basingstoke and North Hampshire Health Authority

Schiliro v Peppercorn Child Care Centres

Seamner v North East Essex Health Authority

Shirley v Wirral Health Authority

Skinner v Aberdeen City Council

Slater v Fife Primary Care NHS Trust

Smith v South Lanarkshire Council

Sommerville v Lothian Health Board

Stainton v Chorley and South Ribble NHS Trust

Stark v Post Office

Stewart v Highland Health Board

Stone v Commissioner of Police for the Metropolis

Stuthridge v Merseyside Metropolitan Ambulance Service

Swain v Denso Martin

T (A Minor) v Surrey County Council

Taylor v Glasgow City Council

Vicar of Writtle v Essex County Council

W v Essex County Council

Wakefield v Basildon and Thurrock Health Authority

Wardlaw v Fife Health Board

Warren v Harlow District Council

Watkinson v British Telecommunications PLC

Watkins v Strathclyde Regional Council

Wells v West Hertfordshire Health Authority

Welsh v Matthew Clark Wholesale ltd

LIST OF LEGISLATION

Care Standards Act 2000

Carers (Recognition and Services) Act 1995

Carers and Disabled Children Act 2000

Children Act 1989

Children (Scotland) Act 1995

Chronically Sick and Disabled Persons Act 1970

Chronically Sick and Disabled Persons (Scotland) Act 1972

Community Care (Direct Payments) Act 1996

Disability Discrimination Act 1995

Disabled Persons (Services, Consultation and Representation) Act 1986

Education Act 1996

Education (Scotland) Act 1980

European Convention on Human Rights

European directive on manual handling (90/269/EEC, Council directive on the minimum health and safety requirements for the manual handling of loads where there is a risk particularly of back injury to workers)

Factories Act 1961

Health and Safety at Work Act 1974

Health Services and Public Health Act 1968

Housing (Scotland) Act 1987

Housing Grants, Construction and Regeneration Act 1996

Human Rights Act 1998

Lifting Operations and Lifting Equipment Regulations 1998

Limitation Act 1980

Management of Health and Safety at Work Regulations 1999

Manual Handling Operations Regulations 1992

National Assistance Act 1948

NHS Act 1977

NHS (Scotland) Act 1978

NHS and Community Care Act 1990

Offices, Shops and Railway Premises Act 1963

Prescription and Limitation (Scotland) Act 1973

Provision and Use of Work Equipment Regulations 1998

Regulation of Care (Scotland) Act 2001

Social Work (Scotland) Act 1968

OVERVIEW

1. Summary

2. Background to manual handling

Prevalence of manual handling injury
Nature of manual handling injury
Vulnerability to injury of employees
Effect of manual handling policies on patients, clients and carers
Relevant law

3. Health and safety implications of the law for employees

Manual Handling Operations Regulations: basic duties
Inadequate application by employers of the law
Is manual handling with risk permitted?
Reasonable practicability in avoiding or reducing risk
Risk assessments (and organisation of services)
Blaming employees for their injuries
Manual Handling Operations Regulations and negligence compared
Other health and safety at work legislation
Employee safety and welfare legislation

4. Professional implications for employees

5. Patient and client safety

Patient and client safety: Manual Handling Operations
Regulations
Patient and client safety: Health and Safety at Work Act 1974
Patient and client safety: welfare legislation
Patient and client safety: bringing negligence cases
Patient and client safety: carers

6. Patient and clients: general welfare

Patient and client welfare: legal overview
Manual handling and detriment to patients or clients
Patient and client welfare under the Manual Handling Operations
Regulations
Patient and client welfare under NHS legislation
Patient and client welfare under social services legislation
Disagreements about manual handling
Withdrawal of services in case of disagreement?

7. Human rights and manual handling

1. Summary

The gist of the book is summarised in the following sixteen main points, which underpin the rest of this Overview and the *A–Z List.*

1. Significant risks of injury for employees

It would seem absolutely clear that in practice the manual handling of loads, particularly of people, in health and social care poses a significant risk of injury to employees.

For the prevention of such work related injury, there exists *health and safety at work legislation* such as the *Manual Handling Operations Regulations (MHOR 1992)*, together with other relevant provisions such as the *Health and Safety at Work Act 1974, Management of Health and Safety at Work Regulations 1999, Lifting Operations and Lifting Equipment Regulations 1998*, and *Provision and Use of Work Equipment Regulations 1998*. It is equally clear that both under the *MHOR 1992*, and under the common law of *negligence* (and even before the emergence of the *MHOR 1992)*, the courts have increasingly recognised the need to protect employees in health and social care (as well as other fields) from manual handling injury.

2. Needs of patients and clients

Clients and patients have needs in the manual handling context, the meeting of which might or might not – depending on the circumstances – be consonant with the provision of risk-free manual handling by employees. In terms of legislation, duties to meet client and patient needs are covered ultimately by various pieces of *welfare legislation* such as the *NHS Act 1977, NHS (Scotland) Act 1978, NHS and Community Care Act 1990, Social Work (Scotland) Act 1968, Care Standards Act 2000* and so on.

It is for the needs identified under this welfare legislation that manual handling solutions have to be found which do not pose unacceptable risks for employees (under *health and safety at work legislation*). However, the meeting of patient and client needs which are manual handling related is sometimes affected by matters other than such health and safety considerations. These include the manipulation by the NHS or local authorities of what is understood by patient or client 'need', the extent to which professionals respond to the views and wishes of patients and clients (and what happens in case of conflict), and the application of eligibility criteria and lack of resources. All typically limit what is available for patients and clients. Legally, these matters should be seen in the context of *welfare legislation*, and health and social care policies and rationing, rather than as simply flowing from the *MHOR 1992*.

In fact it is the identification of need under this welfare legislation which chronologically comes first; clearly, until this takes place, no health and safety issues arise for employees who might provide care or other services for individual patients and clients. Indeed, such welfare legislation is the whole reason for the existence and functions of public bodies such as the NHS and local authorities. For this reason, it is necessary to have some insight into the way in which this welfare legislation works and what the courts have to say about it in *judicial review* cases.

3. Manual handling policies and assessments

With the above two points in mind, competent manual handling assessments are required in order for health and social care agencies to arrive at informed manual handling decisions in particular situations – decisions that will take proper account of both the safety of employees, and of the needs and preferences of patients and clients.

4. Assessment: foreseeability of risk

For employees, the common law of negligence demands that employers assess manual handling risk of injury which is reasonably foreseeable; the *MHOR 1992* demand that foreseeable risk be assessed. This means that the *MHOR 1992* place the higher burden on employers (*Koonjul v Thameslink Healthcare NHS Trust*). For instance, the fact that an accident had not occurred for many years in the carrying out of a particular task might mean that the risk was not reasonably foreseeable; but this might not mean that it was not foreseeable, given the nature of the task (*Hall v Edinburgh City Council; Hawkes v Southwark London Borough Council*). However, the law does not demand that trivial risk be formally assessed (*Hillhouse v South Ayrshire Council*).

5. Risk assessments: general and specific

Manual handling risk assessments are sometimes referred to as either (a) generic or general, or (b) individual or specific. Indeed, as well as referring to suitable and sufficient assessments generally, both the *MHOR 1992* and the *Management of Health and Safety at Work Regulations 1999* refer specifically to *individual capability*.

6. General risk assessments

General risk assessments might, for example, be in terms of classes of employee (e.g. student nurses: *Clarke v Oxfordshire Health Authority*), of task and patient (e.g. bathing heavy patients on an intensive care unit: *Blair v Lancaster Health Authority*), of environment (e.g. district nurses working alone in the community: *Hammond v Cornwall and*

Isles of Scilly Health Authority), types of equipment used on a ward (e.g. the need for adjustable height beds: *Commons v Queen's Medical Centre*), and the maintenance of equipment (e.g. beds and castor units: *Denton v South West Thames Regional Health Authority*).

7. Individual risk assessments

Specific or individual assessments will be in terms both of an individual employee (e.g. with pre-existing back problems: *Wells v West Hertfordshire Health Authority*) or of an individual patient (e.g. in terms of a care plan, which takes account of a particular patient's needs and risks to staff: *Munrow v Plymouth Health Authority*). Such individual patient assessments might need to take account of the risk implications of changing needs, whether over a period of weeks (*Stainton v Chorley and South Ribble NHS Trust*) or perhaps even over the course of a day, when there is difference between a patient's or client's morning or evening ability to assist a nurse with manual handling (*Laing v Tayside Health Board*).

8. Avoiding or reducing risk

The law demands that risk be avoided or, failing this, reduced – so far as is reasonable in the common law of *negligence*, or so far as is reasonably practicable under the *MHOR 1992*. For instance, under the latter, it was held to be reasonably practicable to avoid risk in a hospital laundry (*Anderson v Lothian Health Board*).

In this context, reasonableness and reasonable practicability appear to amount in principle to much the same thing, both involving a weighing up of risk against the cost of removing it. Unless the cost is grossly disproportionate to the risk, a duty to avoid or reduce the risk will arise (*Hawkes v Southwark London Borough Council; Fitzsimmons v Northumberland Health Authority*). Depending on the outcome of this weighing up, the duty to avoid or reduce the risk may in effect be an absolute one, and arguments by employers about lack of resources will make little headway (and in fact seem seldom to be advanced in the case law).

Nevertheless, there remains a view that the *MHOR 1992* do not properly transpose the *European directive* on which they are meant to be based, and that the courts should take a stricter approach still to the meaning of reasonably practicable. To date, however, the courts have not done this.

9. Balanced decisions

Where there is apparently no consonance between employee safety and client or patient need, a careful decision is then clearly required, weighing up the relative risk to staff against patient or client welfare.

In such circumstances, consonance, or failing that, balanced decisions, will be achieved all the more often and readily, in proportion to the quality of policies and assessments, to the expertise of relevant professionals – and to the extent to which the needs, wishes and views of clients and patients are at least fully considered if not always acceded to. In particular, expert professionals in the form of manual handling advisers or others might be adept at finding solutions – otherwise elusive – which both safeguard employees in terms of avoided or reduced risk, whilst at the same time working out with patients and clients an acceptable way of meeting their needs. Thus, in principle and in an ideal world, conflict should be relatively rare (but see below for practical obstacles).

Not only are such balanced decisions required under the *health and safety at work legislation* and the *welfare legislation*, but they are also explicit under article 8 of the *European Convention of Human Rights*, which demands that any decisions interfering with people's privacy, home and family life should be necessary, in the sense of proportionate or balanced.

Nevertheless, in practice, such balanced decisions might be made more difficult where there are complicated medical conditions (e.g. *Redbridge London Borough Council*), rehabilitation needs in issue which carry a risk of injury to employees, and conflicts between the views of disabled people on safe lifting and those of professionals (the *Redbridge* case shows that it should not always be assumed that the disabled person's view is necessarily less expert than the organisation with whom he or she is disagreeing). In addition, such balanced decision-making might be hindered by factors such as those listed in Point 15 below.

10. Employee safety in relation to patient or client need

In negligence cases or in cases brought under the *MHOR 1992*, the courts as a matter of course recognise the need for sensitivity to patient and client need when manual handling solutions are decided upon. For example, the courts would not expect that patients should be caused pain (e.g. *Clarke v Oxfordshire Health Authority*). Likewise, the courts have recognised rehabilitation and independence as laudable aims (e.g. *Painter v Barnet Community Healthcare NHS Trust*); the need for patient mobility for basic health reasons such as obesity (*Stainton v Chorley and South Ribble NHS Trust*) or osteo-arthritis (*Sommerville v Lothian Health Board*); or the need for low beds to reduce the risk of injury for disabled children (*Koonjul v Thameslink Healthcare NHS Trust*).

Such patient or client needs will therefore limit the possible range of manual handling solutions which are sensitive to those needs. However, the law does not permit staff to be put at unacceptable levels of risk in order to further patient or client need. For instance, a wheelchair might be required to move a person, if adequately trained staff are not available for the manual handling required by the patient's condition (*Stainton v Chorley and South Ribble NHS Trust*).

Furthermore, local authorities and the NHS have statutory functions under different legislation – i.e. *welfare legislation* – to meet the needs of clients and patients. Nevertheless, under the welfare legislation too, the health and safety of employees has to be taken account of and might justify a local authority offering to meet a person's mobility need by means of a wheelchair rather than manual handling (*R v Cornwall County Council, ex p Goldsack*). It will be observed that this case, brought under welfare legislation by means of *judicial review*, reached the same type of conclusion (though in a different legal context) as the *Stainton* case, referred to immediately above, which was brought in *negligence.*

Although local authorities and the NHS are not obliged to meet people's preferences (and indeed not necessarily all of their needs either) under welfare legislation, it has nevertheless been pointed out, for example, that to neglect the views of residents in care homes about manual handling might mean that changes to systems of work might simply fail (RCN 2001, p.11).

11. Patient or client need not being met for reasons other than health and safety

Nevertheless, genuine health and safety concerns for employees aside, there are sometimes other reasons for patient or client detriment in the context of welfare legislation.

This might be the result of poor assessment, inappropriate or incompetent application of manual handling policies, an explicit breach of welfare legislation dealing with the assessment and meeting of people's needs, or breach of the common law principles of lawful decision-making which are looked for by the courts in *judicial review* cases (such as not fettering discretion, and taking account of relevant factors). Sometimes the reason given for not meeting people's needs is a shortage of *resources*; depending on the circumstances, this may or may not be a lawful defence. These considerations are not merely theoretical; in the case of *R v Birmingham City Council, ex p Killigrew,* which involved a manual handling assessment, the council's decision was struck down as unlawful, in effect on the suspicion that the decision to reduce services to the client was solely resource-led, without account taken of the client's need.

12. Systems of work, training, supervision, information, instructions, equipment

The tasks of identification, assessment, avoidance and reduction of risk will be carried out more or less competently depending on the degree to which an employer has a safe *system of work* (e.g. *Dickson v Lothian Health Board*) and provides adequate *training* (e.g. *Beasley v Buckinghamshire County Council*), *supervision* (e.g. *McGowan v Harrow Health Authority), instructions and information* (e.g. *Colclough v Staffordshire County Council*), appropriate *equipment* (e.g. *Commons v Queen's Medical Centre*), and competent staff undertaking appropriate tasks (such as drawing up care plans: *Munrow v Plymouth Health Authority*) in adequate numbers (*Forder v Norfolk Area Health Authority*).

Of course employees too have duties to take care of themselves and others, and to follow safe systems of work – as spelt out again both by the courts (*Woolgar v West Surrey and North East Hampshire Health Authority; Gordon v British Airways*) and in *health and safety at work legislation.*

13. National guidance on manual handling

In order to assure themselves, and courts of law, about their safe manual handling practices, employers might well refer to national *guidance*, of which there is a substantial amount in the manual handling field. Likewise employees might do so, in order to support their claim that the employer breached its duty.

The most comprehensive *guidance*, the best known and most frequently cited in court, is that published by the Royal College of Nursing and National Back Pain Association (now BackCare), entitled 'Guide to the handling of patients', currently in its fourth edition (RCN/NBPA 1997). Such guidance does not have the status of law, but has often (though not always) been accepted as indicating acceptable manual handling techniques – with the implication that an employer will have breached its duty if the guidance has not been heeded. Nevertheless, there are a number of important points to bear in mind about the role, nature and limitations of both this and other *guidance*, which are set out under the entry *guidance* in the A–Z List.

14. Potential difficulties in assessment and provision

The achievement of appropriate assessment and service provision as described above might appear straightforward in principle. However, in practice, difficulties for both employees and patients or clients sometimes arise owing to, for instance, situations of genuine conflict between patient or client need and employee safety; failure of employers to apply their minds to manual handling and staff safety; poor *systems of work* (including training, supervision, information, equipment etc.); ignorance of the law; lack of competent assessments of both risks for employees and of patient or client need; conflicting approaches and views between agencies and between professions; lack of appropriate staff to assess and deliver services; poor communication with patients or clients about safety matters; unreasonably rigid local manual handling policies; unreasonable patient and client demands; and the allocation generally of inadequate resources for implementation of appropriate manual handling solutions for staff, patients and clients alike.

Some of the above problems are pointed out in a Royal College of Nursing publication, which helpfully sets out a practical checklist for action in terms of an 'integrated back injury prevention programme' for care homes, but which also lists, realistically, barriers to implementation (RCN 2001).

15. Types of legal action

The general effect of how the law can be used formally – as opposed to informal use of it to raise awareness, improve practices and thereby avoid legal actions – in relation to manual handling issues is as follows.

Employees: Health and Safety Executive
In respect of the safety of employees, the Health and Safety Executive can take action against employers (including criminal prosecution) under *health and safety at work legislation* (including the *MHOR 1992*) either before or after accidents have occurred.

Employees: civil compensation cases
After an accident and injury have occurred, an employee could try to bring a civil compensation case under the *MHOR 1992*, any other relevant regulations (but not under the *Health and Safety at Work Act 1974* or the *Management of Health and Safety at Work Regulations 1999*), and in *negligence*.

Patients and clients: Health and Safety Executive
In relation to the safety of patients and clients, the Health and Safety Executive could take action against employers (including criminal prosecution) under some health and safety at work legislation either before or after an accident, probably on some aspect of a *system of work* not being safe.

Patients and clients: negligence cases
Following an accident, a patient or client could try to sue for compensation in *negligence* – but not under the *MHOR 1992* or any other *health and safety at work legislation*.

Patients and clients: judicial review cases
Patients and clients wishing to overturn a manual handling related decision made under *welfare legislation* by the NHS or a local authority could try to bring a *judicial review* case – this would normally be before, and in order to avoid, any accident or detriment. Unlike *negligence* cases, *judicial review* is not normally about seeking compensation for harm suffered.

2. Background to manual handling

The meaning and ramifications of the term 'manual handling' might not be immediately clear to the uninitiated. But to many they will be only too well known in terms of the sheer practical problems involved in manual handling, which can give rise to very considerable physical and mental stress – for example, to:

(a) **health and social care staff** – such as nurses, nursing auxiliaries, therapists, therapy assistants, care assistants – who through manual handling at work have suffered injury, major or minor, and which might terminate a career, or alternatively hinder permanently and to a various extent both work and home life;

(b) **managers in social and health care** charged with implementing manual handling policies, ensuring the health and safety of their staff, meeting the needs of patients and clients, and balancing their budgets;

(c) **parents** lifting and carrying a disabled child who by the day is becoming heavier;

(d) **carers** suddenly having to cope with partners, parents, children, friends or relatives who through illness or accident can no longer take their own weight;

(e)   **physically disabled people** who are arguing with the NHS or local authorities about what manual handling is appropriate in order for them to live independently and safely at home.

Prevalence of manual handling injury

The Health and Safety Executive states that within the health and social care sectors, manual handling underlies over 50 per cent of work-related injuries (HSE 1998, p.3). On this basis, it would seem clear that there is a strong case for stringent, appropriate application of health and safety at work legislation, policies and practices.

Of course, a significant proportion of the population has back problems anyway, further research is needed into the precise causes of back complaints, and not all pre-existing back conditions identified in manual handling cases will necessarily be due to previous work-related incidents. Further complicating factors include the existence of natural degeneration of the back as part of the ageing process, diverse and sometimes incompatible expert opinions on the causes and nature of back injuries (and the extent to which premature exacerbation of an existing back condition has been precipitated by such injuries), and psychological as well as physical effects of injury (and distinguishing these from genuine malingering).

Nevertheless, even allowing scope for all of this, it cannot be in serious doubt that manual handling in health and social care either initiates or exacerbates much back injury; and it should also be pointed out that in case of exacerbation, the original injury might well have arisen from manual handling at work – albeit over time and without the employee realising the potential seriousness of what was happening.

Whether the *MHOR 1992* have had an effect in reducing injuries in health and social care seems uncertain. Even now some of the judgments issued in the courts relate to injuries suffered prior to the implementation of the *MHOR 1992*. There are no statistics on the number of manual handling cases brought in all courts (in any case, as already mentioned, it is difficult to track many of the cases down) and anyway many are settled out of court. In any event, the level of court cases heard depends on a number of other factors, apart from the prevalence of injuries. Nevertheless, given the upsurge in manual handling policies and training over the last eight years or so, it would seem extraordinary if protection of employees in health and social care had not improved to some extent.

Even so, a Dr Dreena Kelly, writing an advice column in a Glasgow evening newspaper in September 2001, perhaps sums up what is so often still the case, and makes no reference at all to the *MHOR 1992*:

> In the 23 years I've been involved in the NHS, there is nothing more certain than the link between someone 'lifting for a living' and the incidence of back pain. For nurses and child care workers in particular, back pain is an occupational hazard. Only yesterday, as I was leaving my child's nursery, I saw a teacher struggling up the stairs obviously in pain. 'It's my back,' she said. The pain seemed to have aged her by about ten years. (Kelly 2001)

Nature of manual handling injury

The consequences of manual handling injury can be severe, affecting most aspects of work and home life. For this reason, some of the legal cases summarised in the book include a detailed breakdown of the disabling effects of injury, such as effects on sport, dancing, washing clothes, making beds, driving, sexual intercourse, and the turning of a happy nurse into a sufferer of chronic pain attended by depression (*Gower v Berks*); the effect on pregnancies, childcare, and handling of children (*McGowan v Harrow Health Authority; McIlgrew v Devon County Council*); the wrecked careers of competent, ambitious and enthusiastic – as opposed to 'lackadaisical' – professionals (*Munrow v Plymouth Health Authority*); and the sheer pain of the injury which might be constant and necessitate numerous unsuccessful treatments (*Jones v South Glamorgan Health Authority*), or involve operations, physical sickness, and morphine, with no improvement expected (*Laing v Tayside Health Board*).

Vulnerability to injury of employees

Typically demonstrated in health and social care manual handling cases reaching the courts is the vulnerability of either young, or older but perhaps still untrained, employees (often women) to injury which can be severely disabling and suddenly ruin both work and home life. Even when an initial injury does not immediately have such a drastic effect, the injury might endure, restricting work and home activity to a certain extent, and liable to be exacerbated at a later date. Typically, the injured person might 'soldier on', not realising the seriousness and real consequences of the injury (e.g. *Coad v Cornwall and Isles of Scilly Health Authority; Kempsey District Hospital v Thackham; Wells v West Hertfordshire Health Authority*).

However, it is often too late to make a claim for earlier injury (when a final exacerbating incident occurs), not just because of legal time limits (since the courts seem to be sympathetic to waiving these limits in case of back injury, in one case allowing a writ to be served after 10 years, which would normally be seven years out of time: *Coad v Cornwall and Isles of Scilly Health Authority*) – but because of the difficulty of proving the earlier injury or string of injuries and the *cumulative strain* they gave rise to (e.g. *Channon v East Sussex Area Health Authority*). These difficulties have left employers relatively free to argue that the previous injuries caused a degenerative condition, and either totally to deny liability, or at least to seek to reduce drastically any damages awarded, on the basis that the most recent injury has merely accelerated a problem which would have terminated the employee's career in any event. Given that the employee might have incurred these previous injuries during long years of dedicated work in the public service such as the NHS, the employer is in effect heaping insult upon injury by arguing in this way (but for examples of recent cases argued on the basis of cumulative strain, see e.g. *Commons v Queen's Medical Centre; Stone v Commissioner of Police for the Metropolis; Wells v West Hertfordshire Health Authority; Welsh v Matthew Clark Wholesale*; and also *Black v Wrangler*).

Effect of manual handling policies on patients, clients and carers

Notwithstanding the above, concern has grown over the last few years that manual handling policies in health and social care are sometimes detrimental to patients, clients and carers (Henwood 2001, p.67; Jones and Lenehan 2000) and that this can be due to over-restrictive and inappropriate application of policies (Cunningham 2000). There is also considerable uncertainty about how to balance properly the *rehabilitation* needs of patients with the reasonable safety of staff

However, it is also the case sometimes that manual handling policies are inappropriately blamed for detriment suffered by patients, clients and carers – when in fact the real culprit is inadequate resources made available by the NHS or local authorities in terms of numbers or competence of staff, equipment, or the money to pay for these. For instance, in one case involving a manual handling assessment, a local authority took account of employee safety and its resources, but not apparently the client's need. Therefore, the unlawfulness and inappropriateness of the decision did not lie with the manual handling policy or assessment, but with the failure to adhere to community care legislation in relation to that assessment of need (*R v Birmingham City Council, ex p Killigrew*).

Overall, it is fair to say that manual handling issues excite substantial divisions of opinion amongst professionals, patients, clients and disability organisations. Indeed it is such divisions that probably account for the delay in publishing Health and Safety Executive guidance on manual handling in people's homes; at the time of writing, the final version was still unavailable (HSE 2001).

Relevant law

In seeking to identify the balance identified immediately above – between employee safety, client or patient need, and resources – it is necessary to consider the relevant law. This is because organisations within health and social care are of course subject to it – namely (a) *health and safety at work legislation* which affects all organisations; (b) *welfare legislation* as it underlies both the existence, and powers and duties of, local authorities and the NHS; and (c) regulatory legislation, such as the *Care Standards Act 2000* or the *Regulation of Care (Scotland) Act 2001*, as it affects care providers whether statutory, private or voluntary.

Specifically, *health and safety at work legislation*, in the form of the *MHOR 1992*, has given a significant impetus to manual handling policies, practices and indeed court cases. However, there is also a much wider legal context which underlies decision-making about manual handling in health and social care; and a failure to understand this may lead to inadequate decision-making both legally and professionally (*R v Birmingham City Council, ex p Killigrew* appears to illustrate not only unlawful decision-making but also, at least on the basis of the reported facts of the case, arguably flawed professional decision-making as well, in that assessment of the client's needs did not appear to be thought out or well documented):

(a) **European directive**. Underlying the *MHOR 1992* is a *European directive* and, ultimately, any interpretation of the regulations must be informed by, and be within the meaning of, the original wording of this directive (e.g. *Cullen v North Lanarkshire Council*, in which the court referred to the directive when considering the breadth of manual handling tasks and type of injury covered by the *MHOR 1992*).

(b) **Health and safety at work legislation framework**. In United Kingdom legislation, the *MHOR 1992* do not operate in isolation but sit within a framework of health and safety at work legislation including (i) the *Health and Safety at Work Act 1974* (containing duties of employers towards employees, and also a general duty towards non-employees, such as patients, clients and carers); (ii) the *Management of Health and Safety at Work Regulations 1999* (including risk assessments of both employees and non-employees); (iii) the *Lifting Operations and Lifting Equipment Regulations 1998*; and (iv) the *Provision and Use of Work Equipment Regulations 1998*.

(c) **Statutory duties under welfare legislation**. Local authority social services departments and the NHS are subject to a range of duties and powers under *welfare legislation* (including associated directions and guidance issued by central government) concerning the assessment of people's needs and provision of services. Although some of these duties are stronger than others, particularly on the social services side, at the very least it must be recognised that any manual handling decision taken in respect of a patient or client is, overall, within the context of this *welfare legislation*, and not simply *health and safety at work legislation*.

This *welfare legislation* includes the *NHS Act 1977, NHS (Scotland) Act 1978, NHS and Community Care Act 1990, Social Work (Scotland) Act 1968, Chronically Sick and Disabled Persons Act 1970*, and so on. It is this legislation that underlies the balancing act described above, between patient or client need, staff safety and available resources.

(d) **Judicial review**. Patients and clients can challenge decisions made under welfare legislation by way of judicial review, which is about overturning such decisions, not about seeking compensation for harm suffered (for which, see under *negligence* below). The courts apply certain common law principles in order to test the lawfulness of decisions, such as whether all relevant factors were taken account of, there was a fettering of discretion (i.e. a rigid policy), or illegality (blatant contravention of legislation).

(e) **Regulatory legislation**. From April 2002, implementation will take place in England and Wales of the *Care Standards Act 2000* and in Scotland of the *Regulation of Care (Scotland) Act 2001*, dealing with the regulation of care across the local authority, voluntary and private sectors – including manual handling, related equipment and individual care plans – provided by, for example, care homes, domiciliary care providers, and independent health providers.

(f) **Common law of negligence**. The common law of *negligence* remains highly relevant since it is frequently used when both employees and non-employees seek compensation for harm suffered in manual handling accidents. The rules, developed and continually modified by the law courts, pose a threefold test of whether there was a duty of care owed, whether it was breached and whether the breach caused injury. *Negligence* cases still form a substantial part of the case law involving employees seeking compensation for manual handling injury. Non-employees cannot use *health and safety at work legislation* (such as the *MHOR 1992*) to bring compensation claims anyway and so must sue in *negligence*.

(g)   **Human rights**. The *Human Rights Act 1998* came into force in the United Kingdom in October 2000, and is expected (whether or not erroneously) by some people to affect manual handling decisions – in particular perhaps in relation to (i) the right to respect for privacy, home and family life; and (ii) the right not to be subjected to degrading treatment (under articles 8 and 3 respectively of the *European Convention on Human Rights*).

3. Health and safety implications of the law for employees

This section considers the health and safety implications for employees involved in manual handling of the *MHOR 1992*, other *health and safety at work legislation*, the common law of *negligence*, and *welfare legislation*.

Manual Handling Operations Regulations: basic duties

The *MHOR 1992* demand in essence that employers should avoid, so far as is reasonably practicable, the need for employees to undertake manual handling which involves a risk of injury. Failing this, the duty is at least to take appropriate steps to reduce the risk of injury to the lowest level reasonably practicable, and to provide information and indications about the task and load. Underlying these duties is the duty to carry out suitable and sufficient risk assessments. The *MHOR 1992* do not create any explicit obligations on the part of employers toward non-employees.

Inadequate application by employers of the law

The *MHOR 1992* – in common with much other *health and safety at work legislation* – are sometimes, in practice, applied either ineffectively or not at all, in which case employees suffer injury and employers are vulnerable to civil compensation claims in the courts brought under the regulations. By the same token, employers might fail to take reasonable care in the manual handling context for the purpose of the common law of *negligence*, and so be subject to liability on that count also. Manual handling cases continue to be brought by employees across the work spectrum, from health care to factory work. In addition, failure to comply with the *MHOR 1992* also leaves employers vulnerable to *improvement notices* served by the Health and Safety Executive or even criminal prosecution – for instance, where an ambulance service NHS Trust has not been carrying out manual handling risk assessments (*Health and Safety Executive v Gloucestershire Ambulance Service NHS Trust*).

Repeatedly arising in many personal injury cases is the question of whether the employer had in place a safe *system of work*. In addition, there are many other key, recurring themes as follows (the italicised headings are expanded in the A–Z List with reference to illustrative case law):

(a) *employers* applying their mind to risk (sometimes the court asks whether a 'senior mind' in the organisation did so);

(b) *custom and practice* (the dangers of tolerating unsafe practices);

(c) *employee responsibilities* (in terms of asking for assistance, taking their own decisions, contributory negligence);

(d) *employee protection* (afforded by the courts in relation to the consequences of e.g. altruistic instinct to help patients or clients, inexperience, lack of training, reliance on more senior staff, misjudgements);

(e) *under-staffing*;

(f) *everyday tasks* (as viewed by the courts, for instance, bed-making, filling a children's sandpit or routine heavy work by labourers);

(g) *individual capability* of employees;

(h) *emergency situations*;

(i) *patient and client need* (risk assessment, individual care plans, competence of such care plans, need for mobility, risk to staff, finding the balance between need and risk);

(j) *MHOR 1992: case law* (points considered by the courts and particularly relating to the regulations, e.g. risk assessment, foreseeability of risk, avoidance of risk, reduction of risk, cumulative strain, scope in terms of injury, treating manual handling operations as a whole, credibility of witnesses);

(k) *guidance* on manual handling (and its legal significance);

(l) *instructions and information* (whether they are supplied at all or are adequate);

(m) *training* (whether it is provided at all or is adequate);

(n) *equipment* (e.g. its absence, failure, non-use, misuse, mispositioning – including hoists, beds, cot sides, lifting straps, chairs, wheelchairs and so on);

(o) *supervision*;

(p) *cumulative strain*;

(q) *manual handling techniques*;

(r) *evidence* (importance of *documentation*, reliability, credibility, specificity);

(s) *time limits* for bringing legal cases;

(t) *restraint*;

(u) *causation of injury* (i.e. breach of duty might not always mean liability for the injury claimed for; in addition is the question of the extent to which the disability claimed for flows from the accident).

The above themes are enduring both in cases under the *MHOR 1992* and in *negligence*, and also in cases involving other *health and safety at work legislation* (including some which was superseded by the *MHOR 1992*; a few cases involving this older legislation are covered in this book).

Is manual handling with risk permitted?

A frequent question asked is whether the *MHOR 1992* permit manual handling either with some degree of risk attached to it, or even at all.

First, duties under the *MHOR 1992* are not triggered by manual handling tasks which do not carry a risk other than trivial, and risk assessments will not be required where the risk is negligible (see e.g. HSE 1998a, p.42, and a case such as *Hillhouse v South Ayrshire Council*).

Second, the *MHOR 1992* refer to avoidance of manual handling with risk of injury if this is reasonably practicable; otherwise to a reduction of risk to the lowest level reasonably practicable. They clearly do not state baldly that it is unlawful in all circumstances for lifting or manual handling with risk to take place. However, the implication is that in some situations it might, in law, be reasonably practicable to avoid altogether manual handling with risk – for instance, in a modern hospital laundry (e.g. *Anderson v Lothian Health Board*) – and in many others to reduce the risk to an acceptable level, through *risk assessment* which is then followed by a modifying of the task or situation in some way. All of this might typically need to be supported by the provision of appropriate training, supervision, competent staff, equipment, information, and so on.

Removal of all risk?

In some situations, the removal of all risk is not going to be reasonably practicable since otherwise, as both guidance and the courts have pointed out, there would be, for example, no adequate fire brigade (HSE 1998, p.8 – but this does not mean, of course, that risk must not be reduced: *Logan v Strathclyde Fire Board*); much reduced *rehabilitation* or *therapeutic handling* for NHS patients (HSE 1998a, p.43); no saving of patients or clients in emergency lifesaving situations (BackCare 1999, p.12); and, in another context, even no public dancing (*Woods v Barry Clayman Concerts*). Thus, in one case, the court indicated that a certain level of risk in walking an obese patient would have been acceptable if carried out by two properly trained therapists, but not when one of them was inadequately trained (*Stainton v Chorley and South Ribble NHS Trust*). This was a *negligence* case, but even had it been considered under the *MHOR 1992*, the court would not necessarily have decided this particular point any differently.

Other cases in both *negligence* and under the *MHOR 1992* have involved acceptance by the courts that some risk in health care, whether handling patients or making beds, was inevitable if it stemmed from *patient need* (e.g. *Brown v East Midlothian NHS Trust; Fitzsimmons v Northumberland Health Authority; Koonjul v Thameslink Healthcare NHS Trust*) – although a court might consider very carefully whether, for

example, a patient care plan was drawn up competently – if it involved manual handling posing a higher risk to staff, albeit with the patient's last chance of rehabilitation and independence in mind (instead of being consigned to bed) (*Bayley v
Bloomsbury Health Authority*).

National guidance on manual handling risk.
Where a local policy states that under no circumstances should any manual handling
with risk take place, it is not –contrary to the apparent belief of many staff – simply
repeating what the *MHOR 1992* state, because they state no such thing.

It should also be noted that national *guidance* also does not go so far. For example,
the guidance issued by the Royal College of Nursing and National Back Pain Association (RCN/NBPA 1997), 'Guide to the handling of patients', is often referred to as
the rationale for local policies prohibiting altogether any lifting or manual handling
with risk. What has perhaps been less well-observed is that even this guidance in fact
states that (a) no lifting does not mean no manual handling, but refers to lifting only
as the taking of full body weight; (b) therefore it does not preclude an employee from
'giving a patient some assistance, or using pushing, pulling, upward or downward
forces' so long as these 'forces are as low as is reasonably practicable' (p.23); and (c) it
advocates careful assessment and minimising risk, but 'without compromising the
patient's rehabilitation' (p.4).

The guidance also states that if the patient's needs are:

> ...genuinely so complicated that there is a true conflict of interest, a formal
> risk assessment must be undertaken with great care. When deciding what is
> reasonably practicable, the risk to the patient from how elements of care are
> given or withheld, and his needs, must be taken into account as well as the
> risks to the nurse. A balance must be found where one party's benefit does not
> significantly increase the other party's risk. (RCA/NBPA 1997, pp. 23–24)

However, the guidance points out that such conflict is often avoidable. For instance,
assisting a patient to stand might potentially carry a high risk; but this is reduced to a
low one if a good assessment has been undertaken and the employees position themselves properly or use the appropriate equipment (p.23). This last point is well made
and in principle is straightforward enough; in practice problems sometimes arise precisely because of the difficulty in obtaining a competent assessment, competent staff
and the appropriate equipment, all of which might mean that in practice conflict exists where it need not.

Further national guidance
Similarly, guidance on 'Manual handling in the health services', issued by the Health
and Safety Commission (HSC 1998), explicitly states that when patients have rehabilitation and mobility needs, manual handling with some risk might be required, albeit after careful assessment and reduction of the risk (p.43). Other guidance, 'Safer
handling of people in the community' (BackCare 1999, p.12), points out that poli-

cies in the form of catchphrases such as 'no lifting' or 'minimal lifting' might cause 'division and cause misinterpretation which is unhelpful and can even jeopardise the provision of safe and effective care' (BackCare 1999, p.12). For instance, one set of guidance for physiotherapists working with children states in bold the principle: 'wherever possible avoid manual handling' (APCP, p.8). Taken literally and out of context, this could be taken to mean that children must not be handled at all, even where there is little or no risk.

However, importantly, yet more guidance, 'Guidance on manual handling for chartered physiotherapists' (CSP 2002), issued by the Chartered Society of Physiotherapy, a professional body in the rehabilitation field, states firmly in its 'position statement' the importance of rehabilitation of patients, and that manual handling is an integral part of physiotherapy. It states that a risk assessment must always be undertaken and steps taken to minimise risk - but thereby clearly envisages that manual handling attended by risk will be necessary in some circumstances, if the rehabilitation of patients is not to be abandoned (p.4).

Reduction of risk
If the above suggests that in some limited circumstances, manual handling with some degree of risk will be both practically necessary and sanctioned under the *MHOR 1992*, nevertheless it should not be taken to mean that health and social care staff should therefore be routinely subjected to unacceptable risks. As already stated, in many situations risk can be significantly reduced, if not avoided altogether, through adequate risk assessments which take account of the needs of patients and clients, different ways of meeting that need, the nature of the activities or tasks involved, equipment that will reduce the risk, adjusting the environment, and so on.

It is one thing to find an acceptable manual handling solution shaped around the patient's or client's need, but quite another to put staff at unacceptable risk in meeting that need. The law does not sanction or demand the latter. So, for instance, whilst care plans involving a certain amount of risk may be acceptable, they need to be kept up to date, so that when the patient's or client's condition deteriorates staff are not put at risk (*Hammond v Cornwall and Isles of Scilly Health Authority; Stainton v Chorley and South Ribble NHS Trust*) and staff need to be trained so as to deal with those risks (*Bayley v Bloomsbury Health Authority*).

Reasonable practicability in avoiding or reducing risk
The practical implications of the *MHOR 1992* hinge much on the meaning and application of the term 'reasonably practicable', which qualifies both the duty to avoid manual handling with risk or alternatively the duty to reduce the risk.

Traditionally, the courts have interpreted this term as meaning that the employer must weigh up the risk involved in a particular operation against the operation's cost – in terms of the money, staff, time – involved in the removal or reduction of that risk (*Edwards v National Coal Board*). Unless the cost is grossly disproportionate to the risk, then it will be reasonably practicable to do something about the latter. Thus, if the cost is low, it will be reasonably practicable to do something about either a high or low risk (e.g. *Hawkes v Southwark LBC*); and likewise, in principle, if the cost is high but the risk is also high. However, if the cost is high but the risk low or trivial, the courts may accept that it is not reasonably practicable to reduce or remove the risk.

There is a cogent view that the costs, both obvious and hidden, of manual handling injury – for instance, in NHS establishments – are so high that on any view it is reasonably practicable for NHS Trusts to take substantial steps (and incur significant expenditure) to reduce manual handling risk (since such steps would be cheaper than doing nothing). The costs of employee injury to the NHS include, for instance, contractual and statutory sick pay, treating injured employees or injured patients, paying temporary staff, recruitment of permanent replacement staff, training and induction of replacement staff, the wasted training of the injured staff who retire prematurely, defending legal actions, effects on morale, and the time and effort spent by management on all these issues (RCN/NBPA 1997, p.17). Certainly, the costs of failing to take reasonably simple steps can be very high in manual handling compensation payments; for instance, a flat wheelchair tyre (together with a failure over some years to introduce adjustable height beds) ultimately cost one NHS Trust £330,000 (*Commons v Queen's Medical Centre*); and failing to provide at least some basic information about manual handling for a social worker meant that a local authority had to pay compensation of £204,000 (*Colclough v Staffordshire County Council*). An out-of-court settlement of £800,000 was reported in relation to a 36-year-old male nurse who was trying to move a 12-stone patient who was paralysed, sedated and ventilated in an intensive care unit. The nurse was using two blue plastic sheets, because the appropriate equipment (costing £3500) was not on the ward (Ellis 2000).

The courts have not considered reasonable practicability solely in terms of cost to the employer, but have looked also at potential detriment to patients and clients. For instance, in one case the courts accepted that it was not reasonably practicable to remove any potential risk posed to bed-making staff by the low beds which lay against walls, since both their height and position were to protect disabled children from injury (*Koonjul v Thameslink Healthcare NHS Trust*). Guidance for physiotherapists puts it another way, namely that in its view it is not always reasonably practicable to avoid manual handling in physiotherapy - and that the utility to the patient of the proposed manual handling is an important consideration in the decision about reasonable practicability (CSP 2002, pp.4,12).

(One sidelight on an interpretation of 'reasonably practicable' and the question of foreseeability of risk arose in the Crown Court in a Health and Safety Executive prosecution. The duty under s.3 of the *Health and Safety at Work Act 1974*, subject to reasonable practicability, not to expose non-employees to risk was breached through the non-checking of equipment which led to a patient's death – even though the particular procedure had been performed without incident (and without such checking) 30,000 times previously: *Health and Safety Executive v Norfolk and Norwich Healthcare NHS Trust*.)

Risk assessments (and organisation of services)

Under the *MHOR 1992* and indeed the *Management of Health and Safety at Work Regulations 1999*, employers have a duty to carry out suitable and sufficient *risk assessments*. The *risk assessment* under the 1999 Regulations is required to identify manual handling tasks carrying a risk of injury in the first place; where that injury cannot be avoided, then the *risk assessment* duty contained in the *MHOR 1992* is triggered, with a view at least to reducing the risk (HSE 1998, p.7). In *negligence* cases, the courts have long looked for adequate *risk assessments*.

Both sets of regulations also refer to *individual capability*. In *negligence* cases, the importance of assessing individual employee capability has also been recognised. Thus employers are required to make not just so-called general or 'generic' risk assessments of classes of employees (e.g. student nurses: *Clarke v Oxfordshire Health Authority*), of patients and clients (e.g. heavy patients on an intensive care unit: *Blair v Lancaster Health Authority*), of situations, tasks and environments (e.g. the making of low beds for children in a residential unit: *Koonjul v Thameslink Healthcare NHS Trust*); but also assessment of the ability of individual employees (e.g. one with back trouble which she has previously reported: *Wells v West Hertfordshire Health Authority*). By the same token, risk assessment will clearly have to take account of *patient and client needs* on an individual basis, something long since considered by the courts in negligence cases (e.g. *Laing v Tayside Health Board; Munrow v Plymouth Health Authority; Stainton v Chorley and South Ribble NHS Trust*), and under the *MHOR 1992* (*Brown v East Midlothian NHS Trust*).

Failure to carry out risk assessment

The courts look beyond failure to carry out a risk assessment under the *MHOR 1992* (and in *negligence*) in order to see whether the employer nonetheless took steps to avoid or reduce risk. The virtue of doing this (a) assists the employer who is alive to the risk and has acted appropriately, albeit without an identified risk assessment; but(b) penalises the employer who fails to carry out a risk assessment, and claims that therefore the duty to reduce risk never arose at all (*Swain v Denso Martin*).

However, it has been pointed out that it might be difficult for the courts to decide after the event about foreseeable risk and what avoidance or reduction was reasonably practicable at the time (Zindani 1998, p.57). Indeed, in one case the Court of Appeal recognised the difficulty which the judge at first instance had got into, in deciding what the hypothetical (it had never taken place) risk assessment would have concluded (*Hawkes v Southwark London Borough Council*). Nevertheless, in a significant number of cases, the courts have simply concluded on the evidence presented to them (but not by the employer) that it was indeed reasonably practicable for the risk to have been avoided or reduced (e.g. *Anderson v Lothian Health Board; Logan v Strathclyde Fire Board*). Equally, it is true, the courts have sometimes concluded the opposite – that a risk assessment would have not have resulted in any particular steps being taken by the employer (*Hillhouse v South Ayrshire Council; Postle v Norfolk and Norwich Healthcare NHS Trust; Purvis v Buckinghamshire County Council*).

Quality and nature of risk assessment

Nevertheless, a practical problem affecting manual handling decisions is the quality and varying nature of these risk assessments. For instance, (a) a wide variety of different professionals might carry out what are called risk assessments, and some will simply be more competent than others; (b) the nature and form of risk assessments might vary; (c) final decisions might be affected by blanket policies on manual handling that do not properly take account of individual patient and client needs; and (d) where more than one party is involved, and each carries out an assessment, risk assessments might conflict, leading to significant difficulties for both clients and organisations. For instance:

(a)   **Residential home, conflicting risk assessments**. A residential home brings in a manual handling adviser who concludes that continued manual handling of a resident, placed by social services in the home, constitutes too great a risk and that a hoist will have to be used. The resident disagrees and uses a different manual handling adviser who concludes the opposite. Nevertheless the home ceases to provide manual handling which (i) distresses the client who claims that the hoist is hastening a deterioration in his specialist medical condition; (ii) means that the home, which was receiving extra payment from social services for the special personal assistance and manual handling received hitherto, is in breach of contract; and (iii) means that social services, which had assessed the need for this extra assistance and manual handling, is now potentially in breach of its community care obligations to meet its client's needs, and is also paying public money (i.e. the extra payment) for a service no longer being provided (see *Redbridge London Borough Council*).

(b)   **Residential home, hospital, conflicting risk assessments**. A hospital assesses that a patient is fit to return to the residential home in which he was living prior to a chest infection and hospital admission. The assistant manager of the residential home, reported to have no formal qualifications for assessing patients, refuses to have him back, on the basis of his inadequate mobility (with its attendant manual handling implications) – despite an opposite conclusion drawn by the NHS physiotherapist concerned. This decision has the effect of blocking a hospital bed and possibly putting the residential home in breach of its contract with the local authority purchaser of the man's place in the home (as reported in *Therapy Weekly* 2001).

(c)   **Community care direct payments; conflicting views of risk**. A person is receiving community care direct payments from a local authority social services department, so that she can buy her own services and assistance. She wishes to use the money to purchase personal assistance including manual handling. The local authority, however, as part of its assessment, looks at the manual handling risks and states that they are not acceptable. However, the client challenges this conclusion, arguing that the manual handling risk assessment applied by the social services department was of the type applied to nursing home staff, who have to deal all day long with a wide variety of residents under both physical and mental disability; in contrast her situation was different in that she was one client, who could teach her personal assistants safe manual handling in a limited, stable and predictable context.

(More generally, disabled people have sometimes maintained that there are safe manual handling techniques capable of protecting both disabled people and care assistants; it has been reported that one survey, conducted by the National Centre for Independent Living, of 124 assistants working for disabled people over a period of three years, found that none had sustained a back injury (Henwood 2001, p.68).)

(d) **Social services, domiciliary care agency, conflicting risk assessments.** A local authority social services department assesses a person, concludes that certain manual handling is safe (e.g. raising an obese person's fluid-ridden legs on to a foot stool) and contracts with a personal care agency to deliver a range of services including this manual handling task. A few days into the care package, the care agency rings up the local authority on a Friday morning, stating that on the basis of its own risk assessment, it will withdraw its carers with immediate effect – unless equipment for leg-raising is delivered to the client's home by the afternoon. This situation gives rise to the following difficulties for: (i) the client as to whether her needs will be met; (ii) the local authority in practically responding to the ultimatum and in ensuring the client's needs are met; and (iii) the care agency which is concerned about the safety of its staff, possible litigation in case they are injured, and a possible breach of its contract with the local authority.

(e) **Respite care for disabled children; risk assessments; varied background and competence of assessors.** The organisers of schemes for respite care for disabled children were given the task of carrying out risk assessments, but were concerned both that they were not qualified to do this and that they would be vulnerable to legal action. Many of the social workers involved felt that occupational therapists would be better suited to conducting the assessments.

Overall, in a survey carried out of the 66 schemes conducting such risk assessments, 40 per cent were carried out by social workers, 29 per cent by occupational therapists, 11 per cent by social workers and therapists together, and the rest variously by a children's social worker, back care coordinator, care manager, care manager and risk assessor, adult placement officer, district social worker, freelance risk assessor, family link carer with moving and handling assessor and an independent physiotherapist (Jones and Lenehan 2000). This illustrates the hotch-potch of personnel who might be called on to make manual handling decisions, and the potentially highly diverse expertise they apply – some adequate, some perhaps not.

(f) **Sidestepping restrictive policies.** A family link scheme based within a local authority sidestepped the authority's corporate policy prohibiting the lifting of children – a policy allegedly based on 'Guide to the handling of patients' (RCN/NBPA 1997) – by purchasing occupational therapy assessments from an independent agency which did not have such an exclusionary policy (Jones and Lenehan 2000).

(g) **Conflicting risk assessments and staff's disregard of policy**. A man with severe physical and learning disabilities in hospital has been manually handled by carers for many years. A risk assessment is carried out by a physiotherapist involved with his treatment, who feels that such manual handling can continue to be undertaken without undue risk. Furthermore when in a hoist he becomes most distressed and this in itself constitutes a risk both to himself and staff. However, the overall nurse manager for the hospital states that it is absolutely clear, according to the Royal College of Nursing's guidance, that her nurses should not be handling him manually. However, the nurses quietly tell the physiotherapist that they have no intention of using a hoist, since (i) they have managed him quite safely for many years; and (ii) they are concerned about the greater risks to everybody of his being distressed in the hoist.

Clear arrangements for risk assessment

The above examples illustrate difficulties affecting risk assessment of manual handling situations. Some of them underline the point made firmly in guidance issued by the Health and Safety Commission that where contracting arrangements are in place between agencies, there need to be clear arrangements for competent risk assessment, cooperation and coordination, so that all concerned follow a common care plan for a client or patient (HSC 1998, pp.39–40). Such clear arrangements covered in contracts between agencies might cover, for instance, risk assessment, avoidance of conflict, and a procedure for resolving such conflict where it does arise. They might also go beyond the risk assessment issue to deal with, for instance, the level of competence to be expected of care agency staff, responsibility for supply and maintenance of manual handling equipment (such as hoists), contractual penalty clauses, and so on.

Competency of risk assessment

Some of the examples also raise the question of just who is competent to carry out risk assessments, a question not answered by the legislation itself. Clearly, there must be an assumption that legal duties can only be carried out if performed competently; and the courts have accordingly to come to conclusions on the individual facts of cases.

For instance, in one case the courts were of the view that a senior, rather than a more junior, employee should have actively drawn up a patient's care plan (*Munrow v Plymouth Health Authority*); and in another case, oral evidence, but no documentation, about a purported risk assessment by a man called 'Harry' with no surname produced, clearly would not serve (*Wells v West Hertfordshire Health Authority*). In a third, the Court of Appeal felt that it would have been 'natural' for the firm's health and safety officer, rather than the injured employee, to have carried out a risk assessment in relation to a task of unknown quantity and risk (*Swain v Denso Martin*). And in a case involving a patient's care plan that involved her walking with one stick and one nurse assisting (rather than two nurses) in order to promote her independence and rehabilitation, the judge considered most carefully whether the care plan was competently drawn up in the sense of balancing patient need with staff safety. He was satisfied that it was, since it was the result of careful and 'anxious consultation' between the ward sister, nurses and physiotherapist (*Bayley v Bloomsbury Health Authority*).

Blaming employees for their injuries

Unsurprisingly, employers in many manual handling cases attempt to lay the blame for accidents at the door of employees – and vice versa.

Indeed, employees do have responsibilities. They must take reasonable care of themselves (*Health and Safety at Work Act 1974*, s.7), use equipment in accordance with instructions and training given, as well as inform the employer about health and safety concerns generally (*Management of Health and Safety at Work Regulations 1999*, r.14), and make full and proper use of any system of work involving manual handling (*MHOR 1992*, r.4). For example, in *Gordon v British Airways*, the court found no liability, given that the employee had failed to follow a system of work which avoided the need for manual handling. The common law of *negligence* also recognises that an employee might be wholly to blame for an accident, or at least partially so in the form of *contributory negligence* – a concept which is also applied by the courts in compensation cases brought by employees under the *MHOR 1992*.

Generally speaking, in relation to work injury (not just manual handling) the courts take the approach that employees sometimes do 'silly' things (*Kelly v Forticrete*) whether through boredom, tedium and repetitive work causing the mind to wander (e.g. *King v RCO*), or through altruism in health care work (e.g. *Wells v West Hertfordshire Health Authority*). There is consequently a burden on the employer by means of a safe *system of work, training* and *supervision* etc. to take *reasonably practicable* steps to avoid this happening. In manual handling cases in particular, this judicial approach is pronounced in the health care context, where on a number of occasions the courts have emphasised that the responsibility for a safe *system of work* lies within the higher reaches of the organisation, and should not be left to individuals lower down – for example, ward sisters – to work out such systems (e.g. *Clarke v Oxfordshire Health Authority*). However, this does not preclude the courts sometimes finding that in all the circumstances, an employee was responsible for her own decision and that the employer is not liable (e.g. a nurse as in *Woolgar v West Surrey and North East Hampshire Health Authority*).

Manual Handling Operations Regulations and negligence compared

This book covers a substantial number of manual handling personal injury claims, considered judicially under the *MHOR 1992*, the common law of *negligence* or both. The following paragraphs consider the relationship between these two areas of law and the implications for understanding the cases heard under them. (Cases considered specifically under the *MHOR 1992* are summarised under the entry in the A–Z List: *Manual Handling Operations Regulations 1992: case law*.)

Stronger duties

The *MHOR 1992* in principle impose more stringent duties on employers than the common law of negligence. They also place an added deterrent on employers, since the Health and Safety Executive can through *improvement notices* and criminal prosecution seek to enforce the regulations, whether before or after injuries to employees have been suffered.

Foreseeability of risk

The higher burden placed on employers by the *MHOR 1992* is mainly as follows. In the law of *negligence*, a frequent question asked by the court is whether the risk of the injury actually incurred was reasonably foreseeable; and, if so, whether the employer took reasonable steps to do something about it. So, for example, in the absence of previous accidents of the same type, the courts might accept that an accident was not reasonably foreseeable (*Hall v Edinburgh City Council*).

However, the *MHOR 1992* effectively force employers to apply their minds to a greater extent. Employers must identify manual handling tasks involving a risk of injury, and avoid them if reasonably practicable – or at least reduce the risk to the lowest level reasonably practicable. The risk of injury referred to here need only be foreseeable, not reasonably foreseeable, thus making greater demands of employers (*Anderson v Lothian Health Board; Cullen v North Lanarkshire Council; Hillhouse v South Ayrshire Council*), since although the risk must be real it need not be probable (*Koonjul v Thameslink Healthcare NHS Trust*).

In one case, a question appears also to have been raised by the claimant, but not answered by the Court of Appeal, as to whether the *MHOR 1992* demand a still stricter interpretation (*King v RCO*). There is some precedent for this question; for instance, under the manual handling provisions of the *Factories Act 1961* (superseded by the *MHOR 1992*), it was held that foreseeability was not a requirement for liability to be established (*Fotheringham v Dunfermline District Council*). However, the unanswered argument in the *King* case was based not on this Act, but on the European directive underlying the *MHOR 1992* (see further under *European directive on manual handling* in the A–Z List).

Avoiding or reducing risk so far as is reasonably practicable or as is reasonable

Once risk assessment has been carried out, the *MHOR 1992* then demand that employers do what is reasonably practicable; the law of negligence demands that employers do what is reasonable. At this stage – in effect once risk has indeed been identified under either area of law – it is not totally clear how great the difference is between them.

This is because reasonable practicability under the *MHOR 1992*, and reasonableness in negligence, appear in principle indistinguishable, since both entail a balancing of level of risk against the cost of doing something about it. This seems apparent from the case of *Edwards v National Coal Board*, as applied in *Hawkes v Southwark London Borough Council*, a case involving the *MHOR 1992*; and also from the negligence case of *Fitzsimmons v Northumberland Health Authority* (at the Court of Appeal stage). Another way of putting it would be that a slight manual handling risk would not justify a draconian measure (*Wakefield v Basildon and Thurrock Health Authority*). In principle, a lack of resources under either area of law will not be a defence if a significant risk has been neglected by the employer (e.g. *Denton v South West Thames Regional Health Authority*), although the courts will of course be aware of the limited resources available (*Moore v Norfolk Area Health Authority*; see also *resources* entry in the A–Z List).

Implications for understanding negligence cases
The implications of all of this for understanding manual handling cases decided in negligence are roughly as follows. First, in a substantial number of negligence cases, the courts have anyway imposed demanding obligations on employers, such that it is doubtful whether the *MHOR 1992* would add a great deal (e.g. consider *Bayley v Bloomsbury Health Authority*, for the court's analysis of training requirements). Second, in those negligence cases – particularly older ones – where the courts did not impose such demanding obligations, then either the *MHOR 1992* or simply the lapse of time (and changed standards in relation to manual handling, even in negligence cases) mean that liability might now be decided otherwise.

Third, not all failed negligence cases would be – or are – decided otherwise under the *MHOR 1992*, since sometimes the employer's actions satisfy both areas of law (e.g. *Brown v East Midlothian NHS Trust*), or employees' cases are simply weak on the evidence, however considered.

Lastly, given that judges and lawyers are human and that law is an art rather than a science, it would not be too surprising if some cases depart from the general points made immediately above – such as in the case of *Fraser v Greater Glasgow Health Board* in which the court contrived (perhaps dubiously) to find liability in negligence but not under the *MHOR 1992*.

Other health and safety at work legislation
Other health and safety at work legislation is directly relevant to manual handling and the safety of employees.

Health and Safety at Work Act 1974
The *Health and Safety at Work Act 1974* refers to a safe *system of work, information, training, instruction, supervision*, and to the safe use, handling, storage and transport of *equipment* (s.2).

Management of Health and Safety at Work Regulations 1999
The *Management of Health and Safety at Work Regulations 1999* refer to matters such as risk assessment of both employees and non-employees, review of risk assessment,

taking into account *individual capabilities*, information, training, cooperation and co-ordination in a shared workplace, and so on.

Lifting Operations and Lifting Equipment Regulations 1998
The *Lifting Operations and Lifting Equipment Regulations 1998*, often referred to as *LOLER 1998*, impose a range of duties in relation to lifting equipment used at work including strength and stability, positioning and installation, marking of safe work-ing load, organisation of lifting operations, examination and inspection.

Provision and Use of Work Equipment Regulations 1998
The *Provision and Use of Work Equipment Regulations 1998*, often referred to as *PUWER 1998*, impose duties concerning matters such as the initial state of the equipment, purpose and suitability of the equipment, working conditions, maintenance, infor-mation, instructions and training – and cover both lifting equipment and other equipment used at work.

Scattergun approach
The case of *Mitchell v Inverclyde District Council* demonstrates the 'scattergun' ap-proach that so much legislation allows in some manual handling-type situations. In-volving a grass-cutting operation, the injured employee argued his case under the *MHOR 1992, PUWER 1998*, the Personal Protective Equipment at Work Regula-tions 1992, and the common law of *negligence*.

Employee safety and welfare legislation
The courts have recognised in *judicial review* cases that in carrying out their statutory duties under *welfare legislation*, local authorities and the NHS can take account of the health and safety of employees or other service providers when offering, or with-drawing, a service. For instance, the court readily accepted that manual handling considerations were material to the decision whether to provide human walking as-sistance or a wheelchair at a local authority day centre (*R v Cornwall County Council, ex p Goldsack*); that the NHS could withdraw a service when district nurses were threat-ened and abused (*R v Hillingdon Area Health Authority, ex p Wyatt*); and that likewise in certain circumstances a local authority could withdraw a service in case of violent be-haviour (*R v Kensington and Chelsea Royal Borough, ex p Kujtim*).

4. Professional implications for employees
The obvious professional implications of the points already made above are that (a) an employee, sensibly protected from injury by a local manual handling policy, is likely to have a longer professional career; but (b) an excessively restrictive local pol-icy might prevent an employee, such as a physiotherapist, from applying his or her rehabilitation skills which involve manual handling – to the detriment of patients.

Rehabilitation

This latter factor could in some circumstances lead to rehabilitation professionals sometimes resenting and feeling threatened by restrictive manual handling policies which interfere with their job as they see it. This is understandable, particularly if policies designed to deal with basic 'care handling' by the generality of nurses are inappropriately applied to rehabilitation and 'therapeutic' handling (CSP 2002, p.11). Equally, however, statistics apparently revealing high levels of work-related back injury amongst, for example, physiotherapists, should give such professionals pause for thought – and cause to question constructively their own expertise, a point made by guidance for physiotherapists working in the neurology field (ACPIN 2001, p.6).

✶ Implications for managers

Patterns of manual handling injury raise not only legal questions, but also professional questions in terms of the role of at least some managers in health and social care in protecting their staff from injury. It would appear that they sometimes have allowed – particularly through inadequate supervision and systems of work – their fellow, albeit inexperienced staff, to suffer serious injury perhaps early in their career. It is almost as though an attitude has sometimes prevailed that such injury is an occupational hazard; that what was good enough for those managers when they trained is good enough for others twenty years later.

In the past, indications of this sort of attitude have emerged in some of the legal cases – perhaps where ward sisters simply did not apply thought, care and decision to the risk run by student nurses, and did not intervene if the latter were 'quite happy' when lifting highly dependent patients (*Clarke v Oxfordshire Health Authority*); or where the views of practising nurses giving evidence showed a lack of understanding of basic mechanics and were totally at odds with expert evidence (*Dickson v Lothian Health Board*). Similarly, in another case, an experienced nurse and clinical teacher was sceptical about the expert evidence on a safer type of lift, did not stress lifting techniques in her teaching, and felt that most of the responsibility 'lay on the girls to look after their patients and to look after themselves when they undertook lifting' (*Fitzsimmons v Northumberland Health Authority*).

Even if a new generation of senior staff, more aware of manual handling issues than their predecessors, might tend to take a different approach, nevertheless avoidable injury to care and rehabilitation staff might still occur for other reasons, such as the effect of lack of resources on matters such as training, supervision, or staffing levels; the pressure to which staff are subjected by workloads; or lack of support from higher management (for this last point, see *Painter v Barnet Community NHS Healthcare Trust*).

Rationing of services

Consideration of what manual handling policies allow in principle – and also what the *MHOR 1992* allow in law – is only half the picture. This is because although manual handling policies might set out what an employee can or can't do, in practice they will not determine how many patients or clients can actually benefit from any manual handling, equipment and rehabilitation which is in principle permitted.

For instance, the number of patients and clients benefiting from nursing and therapy services in hospital or the community will be a function of factors such as local levels of staffing, resources for equipment, eligibility criteria for services, and competence of management. In law, issues such as these do not ultimately come under *health and safety at work legislation* but rather *welfare legislation*, which underlies health and social care rationing. See section 6 below and also *patient and client need*.

5. Patient and client safety

This section considers how client and patient safety – in the narrow sense of avoidance of specific accidents rather than general welfare (see section 6 below) – is covered by manual handling related law, under both *health and safety at work legislation*, the common law of *negligence* and *welfare legislation*.

Patient and client safety: Manual Handling Operations Regulations

Adherence to the *MHOR 1992* – and the taking of reasonable care (with negligence actions in mind) – will not only serve to protect employees from injury but might also incidentally, though not necessarily, sometimes protect patients and clients from manual handling accident.

Nevertheless, as already explained, the *MHOR 1992* do not apply explicitly to non-employees, and this accounts for the observation that application of the regulations seems more often to be about protection of employees than of patients or clients (Cunningham 2001). However, this does not mean that patient and client safety is not, at least to some extent, implicit in the *MHOR 1992*. As explained above, the courts sometimes consider the safety of patients or clients when ruling on what was or wasn't reasonably practicable in terms of risk avoidance or reduction (e.g. *Koonjul v Thameslink Healthcare NHS Trust*).

Patient and client safety: Health and Safety at Work Act 1974

Unlike the *MHOR 1992*, s.3 of the *Health and Safety at Work Act 1974* does contain an explicit duty in respect of the health and safety of non-employees – including patients, clients, carers, and staff of other organisations. In addition, risk assessment under r.3 of the *Management of Health and Safety at Work Regulations 1999* covers non-employees as well as employees. These legal provisions are in some circumstances used by the Health and Safety Executive (HSE) to take action, particularly where an unsafe *system of work*, rather than an individual clinical decision, has already caused – or is at least putting patients or clients at risk of – accident and injury.

For instance, under s.3 of the 1974 Act, the HSE has prosecuted the NHS for causing the death of a patient when equipment was not properly checked (*HSE v Norfolk and Norwich Healthcare NHS Trust*), and when patients fall out of bed and are scalded on hot pipes (e.g. *HSE v Trafford Health Authority*). Likewise, the HSE might serve an *improvement notice* if the NHS and the local authority social services department are not maintaining their equipment (including manual handling items) loaned to people at home. It could also consider a breach of s.3 where, for instance, there is poor communication between a local authority social services department and a private care agency, with whom the authority has contracted to deliver services, of essential information about a client's needs and situation – so putting perhaps both client and agency staff at obvious risk. Such information might cover, for instance, particular manual handling issues, an aggressive pet or aggressive tendencies of a client (see HSE NIGM 7/F1998/2).

It should be noted, however, that clients and patients cannot use this health and safety at work legislation to pursue civil actions for compensation.

Patient and client safety: welfare legislation

When local authority social services departments and the NHS decide under *welfare legislation* (see further below) about people's needs and what services to provide, it is clear that in practice the safety of patients and clients is taken into account at least twofold. First, the eligibility or priority of patients and clients for services will often hinge on the degree of risk they are facing (see e.g. DH 2001c). Second, once an individual professional is carrying out an assessment and considering an appropriate solution, he or she will as a matter of course wish to avoid alighting on an unsafe solution for fear of injuring the client, making a bad professional decision and even being sued in negligence at a later date.

Safety explicit in welfare legislation

Furthermore, in law, safety is explicit in at least four key pieces of social services legislation relevant to manual handling related decisions. Under s.2 of the *Chronically Sick and Disabled Persons Act 1970*, there is a specific – i.e. in respect of each individual client – potential duty to arrange the provision of home adaptations and additional facilities for a person's greater safety, comfort and convenience; and for older people under s.45 of the *Health Services and Public Health Act 1968* there is a general power to arrange the same. Under s.17 of the *Children Act 1989*, there is a general duty to safeguard and promote the welfare of children in need, including disabled children. And under s.23 of the *Housing Grants, Construction and Regeneration Act 1996*, there is in certain circumstances a duty to approve a grant application for an adaptation to make a dwelling safe for a disabled occupant.

Of course, even where the word 'safe' or 'safety' does not occur in social services and health care legislation, it is surely implicit, since it is difficult to see how needs can genuinely be met if service provision ignores or compromises safety. For instance, in one manual handling related case the judge found a local authority's assessment legally flawed in various respects, including the fact that it had not explained how the reduced service now on offer would meet the client's needs in case of emergency (*R v Birmingham City Council, ex p Killigrew*).

For *judicial review* challenges to decision-making under such legislation, see section 6 in this Overview.

Patient and client safety: bringing negligence cases

As already explained, patients and clients cannot use *health and safety at work legislation* to bring compensation claims in the court; they must use the common law of *negligence*. Ironically but inevitably, it is easier in principle for patients and clients to bring a *negligence* case after harm has occurred – if they can show that it was caused by a carelessly taken or implemented manual handling decision – than to bring a *judicial review* case to prevent the harm occurring in the first place, by challenging the assessment at the outset (but see *R v Birmingham City Council, ex p Killigrew* for just such a successful challenge). This is because professional competence is examined closely in *negligence* cases, whereas *judicial review* concerns itself primarily with administrative decision-making by public bodies and with points of law.

Causation of harm

Causation of harm in negligence might anyway not be easy to prove. For instance, it might be one thing for a person to bring a negligence case against the NHS or social services based on harm suffered in a straightforward manual handling accident when he or she is dropped by two obviously ill-trained care staff (see e.g. comments in *Wyatt v Hillingdon London Borough Council*); but quite another to demonstrate whether a deterioration in a medical condition or functional ability was caused by use of a hoist (instead of manual handling) or whether it would have occurred in any event. And even if causation of harm can be shown, it has further to be proved that the cause was a careless or incompetent decision or action – also not necessarily straightforward, since the courts do not demand of professionals that they should have made the perfect or best decision in the circumstances, but merely a reasonably competent one.

Lack of resources and other defences

In negligence cases brought by patients or clients, the courts will tend to shy away from imposing liability on the NHS or on local authorities, if the issue is fundamentally and overall one of resources (e.g. *Kent v Griffiths*) or one of policy, priorities or sensitive decision-making in a difficult statutory context such as child protection legislation (e.g. *X v Bedfordshire County Council*).

Patient and client safety: carers

It is accepted that informal *carers* of disabled and chronically or terminally ill people are subject to very considerable stress, both physical and mental, and suffer injury from manual handling (Henwood 1998, p.25). Local authority carers' legislation, involving assessment and possibly service provision for carers, should mean in principle at least that safety issues are considered for carers (see *carers*, and related entries, in the A–Z List). No equivalent legislation exists for the NHS.

Notwithstanding such legislation, a local authority in one *judicial review* case unlawfully reduced personal assistance services for a woman with multiple sclerosis – shortly after informing her husband (who was also her carer) that, if he continued to manually handle his wife, he might suffer serious injury which would prevent him caring for her in the future (*R v Birmingham City Council, ex p Killigrew*). The plight of carers was also illustrated in a *negligence* case, when the court was unimpressed with the health board's denial that two nursing staff were needed for a particular patient – on the grounds that until recently, the patient's wife had managed him alone – since the reason for the health board's intervention in providing home care was precisely because his wife had injured herself assisting the husband out of the bath (*Laing v Tayside Health Board*). In addition, local government ombudsman investigations into delay in the provision of home adaptations and other services sometimes reveal the manual handling plight of informal carers (see cases in this book: *Barking and Dagenham London Borough Council; Bristol City Council; Camden London Borough Council; Islington London Borough Council; Rotherham Metropolitan Borough Council*).

Carers and legal cases
Informal carers are of course non-employees and will be covered in principle by both s.3 of the *Health and Safety at Work Act 1974* and also r.3 of the *Management of Health and Safety at Work Regulations 1999*, under which the Health and Safety Executive can in principle take action. Alternatively, were informal carers themselves to attempt to bring negligence cases alleging injury suffered through the advice, actions or omissions of NHS and local authority staff, it is not clear overall how the courts might react. There might be considerable obstacles in the way of identifying a relevant standard of care and also causation of harm, and the courts anyway might fear opening the floodgates to a new type of case involving such litigants (RCN/NBPA 1997, p.20).

6. Patient and clients: general welfare

Taking health and welfare more generally – as opposed to safety in a narrow sense of conventional accident (see section 5 above) – concern is sometimes expressed that manual handling decisions do not always benefit, and in some respects are to the detriment of, patients and clients. Such concerns relate sometimes to services being denied altogether, and sometimes to the nature, amount or quality of services and equipment being provided. The legal situation is that people's welfare is protected in law to a certain extent, at least in principle, but certainly not to the point where every need or preference must be met.

Patient and client welfare: legal overview
The following paragraphs consider frequently asked questions about the meeting of needs and preferences of patients and clients, whether or not manual handling related.

Varying competence of manual handling assessments

The observation that some manual handling assessments are better than others is un-remarkable; such a comment could in principle be applied to all NHS and social ser-vices, i.e. some are above average and some below. This is simply a truism; by the nature of an average, some practice will come above it and some below. Despite cen-tral government's enthusiasm for the concept of 'best practice', it should be remem-bered that it is a logical impossibility for all, or even most, service providers to attain such practice at the same time; were they to do so, this comparative term would lose its very meaning.

Nevertheless, if manual handling assessments and the decisions arising from them are seriously flawed, it might be possible to challenge certain aspects of them legally in *judicial review* proceedings – particularly in the social services context. In the NHS context, it is generally much more difficult to bring a judicial review case to challenge the adequacy of assessment. Otherwise, professionally flawed assessments can more easily be challenged – but only retrospectively and if they have given rise to harm – by means of *negligence* cases which do analyse in detail professional compe-tence. But even then, if a particular decision is deemed by the court to come within the band of reasonably competent decisions (but not necessarily the most compe-tent), the negligence case will fail.

Alternative to the courts, the *local government ombudsman* is unable directly to question professional judgement, although he or she can consider whether a local authority has acted properly to obtain and act on such judgement (e.g. *Redbridge Lon-don Borough Council*). The *health service ombudsman*, on the other hand, does have the power to investigate professional judgement.

People's manual handling preferences

NHS and social services legislation ultimately does not demand that people's manual handling preferences be acceded to, but only that in some circumstances (and at least taking account of those preferences) people's needs should be met. In other words preference is relevant to, but not decisive of, the outcome of an assessment. Of course, where preferences and assessed need happily coincide, then the satisfying of one will satisfy the other as well.

Nevertheless, the concept of need is flexible and relatively easily manipulable by the NHS and by local authority social services departments. Clearly the more restric-tive the definition of need, so the greater part of a person's concerns will be relegated to the status of mere preference.

Meeting all assessed manual handling needs?

However, even when need – as opposed to preference – is assessed, neither the NHS nor local authority social services departments must always meet it. Local authorities apply eligibility criteria, such that certain levels of need will not necessarily trigger services (although once criteria are met, then a duty to provide services may arise). However, the NHS can lawfully argue lack of resources, even if a person apparently meets such eligibility criteria as may exist. So, even when it is accepted that a manual handling need is present, it does not follow that in law it has always to be met.

Manual handling needs and preferences overriding employee health and safety?
There is nothing in any of the legislation (including human rights legislation) implying that the wishes and needs of disabled people about manual handling should simply override genuine health and safety concerns in respect of employees; conversely, it is equally clear that safe manual handling solutions should be sensitive to the identified needs of patients and clients.

Choosing a cheaper or safer manual handling option to meet need
Generally speaking, where more than one option is available for meeting a person's need, then the NHS or local authority is free to choose the option which is cheaper or safer, even if it does not accord with a person's wishes, so long as it can be reasonably argued that the option chosen does genuinely meet the need.

Failing to make adequate provision for manual handling because of lack of resources
In some limited circumstances, it is possible to challenge local authority social services departments for failure to provide what has been assessed as required, whether or not the failure is attributable to a lack of resources. However, outside these limited circumstances, resources play the decisive role in determining what is provided in health and social care – and the effect of limited resources is difficult, sometimes apparently impossible, to challenge legally.

Manual handling and detriment to patients or clients
Apparent adverse consequences of manual handling decisions for clients and patients are reported to include pain, discomfort, inappropriate and unsafe use of hoists, deterioration in medical condition or physical function, lack of dignity and privacy, inability of disabled children to participate in school activities or attend respite care, restrictions in outings and social activities, and so on.

Depending on exact circumstances, the degree of detriment (or even abuse) and the eventual practical consequences (including accidents) of some of the examples given below, there might in principle sometimes be a legal protection and remedy, but sometimes not. However, it does also seem clear that in practice at least some of the problems which occur are likely to decrease in proportion to the sufficiency of competent staff carrying out assessments and delivering services, and to the adequacy of the available resources for implementing manual handling policies and decisions.

In particular, expert manual handling advisers, sensitive both to staff safety and to client and patient needs and feelings – and also good at talking to people – are likely to be crucial in resolving many situations to the relative satisfaction of all concerned, and in training others in the organisation to think in the same way.

(a) **Pain or deterioration of medical condition or functional ability.** Hoisting, as opposed to manual handling, might cause people physical pain, cause deterioration in a medical condition and hasten functional deterioration (and even make any residual manual handling less safe, because the person has become less able).

(b) **Safety and dignity.** Hoisting might be regarded as an indignity, if people feel they are being moved around like objects rather than people, perhaps also exposed to embarrassing and undignified view whether in their own home or in an institution.

(c) **Accessing public places.** Disabled people might be unable to go out and access certain public places because of the manual handling assistance – which their personal assistants are no longer allowed to perform – required for the person to use certain otherwise inaccessible facilities (such as toilets).

(d) **Inappropriate equipment supplied.** Equipment might in some circumstances be the right solution, but inappropriate products might be supplied instead because of a lack of resources in the NHS or social services.

(e) **Equipment inappropriately supplied.** Alternatively, equipment might not be the best solution but is nevertheless supplied because it is cheaper than supplying two or more assistants to handle the person manually.

(f) **Blanket policies and rehabilitation.** The imposition of blanket 'no lifting' policies might impede or prevent essential rehabilitation (for the above examples (a) to (f), see generally Cunningham 2000).

(g) **Staff convenience.** Nurses on a ward might use a hoist to get a person out of bed and back to bed, because despite the fact that the person can take her own weight and the handling risks to staff are minimal, it takes too much time to do this. Short-staffed as they are, the nurses simply use the hoist because it is quicker – even though this will probably over time lessen the person's physical abilities.

(h) **Ability of carers to use equipment.** Patients or clients might detect feelings of insecurity in carers who are not confident about using equipment such as hoists, and themselves feel unsafe, or perhaps in the past have suffered injury from inexpert use of slings (RCN/NBPA 1997, p.24).

(i) **Disabled children unable to attend short break schemes.** It was reported in a survey of 102 short break services for disabled children that children were in some cases unable to continue attending, because the services had identified manual handling risks and equipment required to deal with them, but had no money to buy the equipment (Jones and Lenehan 2000).

(j) **Small child hoisted at nursery.** A relatively light child, who mostly takes his own weight albeit with assistance, has to be hoisted at nursery as a result of a risk assessment. A visiting therapist is concerned that this is in neither his physical nor his social interests.

(k) **Children at school**. It is sometimes alleged that, because of concerns about manual handling, children are not handled adequately at school – for example, they might be left in their wheelchairs all day or for lengthy periods. This can result in risk of pressure sores and urinary infection, stiffness, or worsening of muscle contractures, and can even lead to rationing of fluids so as to minimise trips to the toilet. Similar issues might arise in respect of older people in hospitals or care homes.

(l) **Implications at school of manual handling concerns: a parent's reported view**. One example – reported from a parent's point of view – concerned an 8-year-old child with fairly severe athetoid cerebral palsy whose place in a mainstream school might be jeopardised by manual handling concerns. For instance, his learning support assistant was told that she should not support him and should instead push him in a wheelchair – even though this would mean he could not practice weight-bearing or walking with support – with the consequence that he would lose such ability altogether. He would not be allowed to go on a school trip to an inaccessible museum because staff would not be allowed to carry his wheelchair. He would not be able to attend respite care in a carer's house unless he slept downstairs, had no baths and used a commode. He didn't like sleeping downstairs by himself. His mother lifted him singlehanded when he was at home and was concerned about her son's self-esteem and right to privacy. She believed that the health and safety rules imposed locally were about avoiding compensation cases in the mistaken belief that absolute safety was achievable; and that the zealousness of the manual handling team in ensuring safety for staff was at the expense of consideration of her son's individual needs (Parkinson 1999).

(m) **Rigid manual handling policies in school**. Teachers in a school are unclear about the manual handling of pupils.

However, competent assessment of the children's needs (physical and psychological), and the actual risk posed to staff, subsequently identifies (i) which children should be manually handled and when (it might be safer in some situations than in others); (ii) which should be hoisted and when; and (iii) how the manual handling and hoisting should be carried out, with not just employee risk of injury in mind, but also, crucially, the children's physical and psychological well-being. For instance, it is pointed out that young children quite naturally expect human contact, and that hoisting need not preclude this – and that it need not necessarily be 'degrading', since some children actually enjoy it and think it exciting.

(n) **Wrong equipment for the carer**. A man in the later stages of cancer has suddenly lost his ability to walk because of the spread of the tumour to his spine. His wife is facing the problem of what to do over the next week or so, when social services is due to assess, about getting him in and out of bed to the lavatory. She rings up the district nurse who arranges for a commode with detachable armrests to be delivered. However, it is completely the wrong height for the bed. She rings up again and another commode, this time of the right height, is delivered, but the wife subsequently discovers that it has no detachable arms which in the circumstances would make the manual handling significantly easier and safer. However, she now has to make do.

(o)   **Moving a patient two inches**. A woman on a hospital ward in a wheelchair regularly complains that her back is hurting her. A physiotherapist realises that she needs moving about two inches back in her wheelchair from time to time. The woman does not have the ability to do this herself. Even with a non-slip pad underneath her, she keeps on slipping forward slightly. The nurses are not allowed to shift her position manually, and must in principle use a hoist. They point out that the reason for this is that although this one handling task in isolation would not pose a risk, nevertheless if they were to repeat it for patients all day long, they would be at significant risk of injury. However, continually to use the hoist for such handling takes considerable time; and even with the hoist they sometimes get the woman's position wrong anyway.

(p)   **Using the wrong hoist out of convenience**. Home care staff insist on using 'open', rather than fully enclosed, slings for clients, because it makes taking them to the lavatory much easier, and involves fewer transfers and less handling of the residents in and out of hoists. They also encourage clients to say that they prefer this type of hoist. However, a manual handling risk assessment is to the effect that such slings are not safe for some of these clients.

(Unless otherwise attributed, the above are anecdotal but representative of the type of situation typically described to the author in a range of personal communications from practitioners who are involved with patients and clients with manual handling needs.)

Patient and client welfare under the Manual Handling Operations Regulations

As already stated, the *MHOR 1992* do not refer to non-employees. Nevertheless, it might be thought that the test of what is 'reasonably practicable' for an employer to avoid, or reduce the risk of, must bear some relation to the employer's activity. In other words, in the health and social care context, it would seem in principle a nonsense to suggest that something could be reasonably practicable if it would clearly and substantially undermine the very purpose for which the NHS or social services exist – namely, the basic meeting of *patient and client need*. This has already been covered in section 3 above.

Patient and client welfare under NHS legislation

The NHS is under a very general duty to provide services to its patients in England and Wales under ss.1 and 3 of the *NHS Act 1977*, and in Scotland under ss.1, 36 and 37 of the *NHS (Scotland) Act 1978*. The duty is so general that it can be very difficult for patients to enforce in law the provision of services (manual handling related or otherwise), even when it is accepted clinically that a service is required – and still more difficult to challenge the adequacy of assessment at the outset. See under *patient and client need*, where arguments based on lack of resources, fettering of discretion (rigid NHS policies), and taking account of all relevant factors are considered.

Patient and client welfare under social services legislation

Local authority social services departments come under very much more specific duties in legislation than does the NHS, to assess needs and decide about services. As a result, the courts tend to see social services decision-making as more administrative than clinical, as significantly more circumscribed legally than NHS decision-making, and as a result more amenable to judicial interference by the courts in *judicial review* cases. See under *patient and client need*, where arguments based on lack of resources, fettering of discretion (rigid social services policies), and taking account of all relevant factors are considered.

Relevant legislation includes the *NHS and Community Care Act 1990, National Assistance Act 1948, Chronically Sick and Disabled Persons Act 1970, Chronically Sick and Disabled Persons (Scotland) Act 1972, Social Work (Scotland) Act 1968*, Health and Social Care Act 2001, *Carers (Recognition and Services) Act 1995, Carers and Disabled Children Act 2000, Children Act 1989, Children (Scotland) Act 1995*, and so on. Given the impact of manual handling on informal *carers*, the importance of the social services carers' legislation should be particularly borne in mind, namely local authorities' specific duties to assess carers, and their power to provide services for them (See under *carers* and related entries in the A–Z List).

Disagreements about manual handling

In practice, manual handling decisions sometimes become complicated and lead to disagreements between patient or client and the service provider. Disabled people, or their representatives, might say that they should 'come first' (Hasler 2000); equally a local authority might feel that its staff should come first on the basis that injured staff serve nobody.

Presumably the answer is that there should be a compromise in the case of a true conflict of interest, just as the Royal College of Nursing and National Back Pain Association guidance suggests (RCN/NBPA 1997, p.24). After all, it would be an irony were disabled people seen to be indifferent to disability suffered by their carers; just as indifference by statutory agencies to the needs of disabled people would be equally unacceptable. Two examples of complexity are as follows:

(a) **Dispute in residential home**. In a local government ombudsman investigation concerning a disabled resident of a residential home, placed there by a local authority, the complications included (i) medical opinion about the detrimental effect on the resident of use of a hoist; (ii) conflicting risk assessments about whether he could be handled safely without a hoist; (iii) the man's wish to choose his own carers and to be handled only by women; (iv) the care home's refusal to carry out any more manual handling, with the result that the man's elderly parents attended the residential home to carry out personal care tasks for him; and (v) the local authority's statement at one point that he would simply have to stay in bed, despite the view of the general practitioner that this could have adverse medical consequences (*Redbridge London Borough Council*).

(b)   **Dispute in a person's own home**. Another reported example of complexity concerned a severely disabled man being cared for by his wife at home; he was becoming incontinent, had no effective mobility and was unable to communicate (although he could hear). Two care assistants visited twice daily. He physically resisted the carers, although it was not clear whether he felt unsafe, simply wanted not to be handled, or whether these were involuntary actions. In the event, his wife was asked to administer a muscle relaxant prior to the arrival of the carers.

A risk assessment was commissioned by the local authority. This identified the need for an electric hoist, suitable bed, removal of furniture from the bedroom to allow safe transfer to a wheelchair, and for a third carer, in the light of the man's physical resistance. In addition, neither the wife nor the three sons living there wanted incontinence supplies in the house and tried to insist that the care assistants take the heavy commode to the bottom of the garden when emptying it – which activity would itself constitute a manual handling risk. The social worker involved was also concerned that if a care assistant became sick, the care package could not be sustained (George 2001).

Withdrawal of services in case of disagreement?

If disagreement persists between patient or client and service provider in the context of manual handling, there comes a point when the question arises as to whether local authorities or the NHS can simply 'walk away' on the basis of a person's unreasonable refusal to accept the service offered (for instance a hoist, instead of the manual handling preferred by the person).

Avoidance of impasse

The first, obvious and practical point to make, is that in many cases careful negotiation, explanation and compromise will resolve the impasse, which should be avoided if possible. Second, guidance from the Health and Safety Commission states that the refusal of patients or clients to use equipment or rearrange furniture might mean that the duties of care staff will have to be restricted in order to ensure their safety (HSC 1998, p.41). A similar point – for instance, restricting nursing care to bed – is made by Royal College of Nursing guidance (RCN/NBPA 1997, p.24). This of course does not represent a complete withdrawal of service, but an alternative avenue of provision.

Nevertheless, there is understandably unease about such situations: on the one hand, nobody wants to see employee welfare threatened; on the other, there is concern sometimes about the implications for the client or patient of service withdrawal, how their needs will otherwise be met, or indeed their reaction to that withdrawal. In one instance, after the local authority social services department had proposed to withdraw care after a man refused to have a hoist in the home for his wife, the man attempted (unsuccessfully) to kill both himself and his wife – and was prosecuted for attempted murder (*R v Bouldstridge*).

Competent assessment

Such tensions or conflict about manual handling inevitably raise the question about when services can be withdrawn lawfully by local authorities or by the NHS from clients or patients who unreasonably refuse to accept what is offered.

The NHS Trust or local authority would wish to be sure that it has carried out at the very least a sound assessment, considering all relevant aspects of need, the various options for meeting it, and the extent of any health and safety risks to staff. For instance, there is a great difference between an individual-based assessment carried out by a competent person and with full participation of the patient or client, and a so-called assessment which consists only of the imposition of a blanket policy, with no account taken of individual need and circumstances, and carried out by a less than competent person. Although there is clearly room for differing professional judgements and also varying skills, the courts might judicially review grossly inadequate assessments, at least in the social services context (*R v Ealing London Borough Council, ex p C*).

Compromises, and the meeting of need in an alternative manner, should be fully explored, since this is quite different from simply withdrawing services altogether. As already stated, the courts have quite readily accepted that there may be different ways of meeting a person's need, and that the health and safety of employees is a relevant factor in the local authority's decision as to which option it will offer a client (*R v Cornwall County Council, ex p Goldsack*).

Unreasonable refusals by NHS patients

The courts have ruled in the NHS context in a *judicial review* case that, when a patient's husband was being consistently abusive and aggressive to the district nurses who were visiting his wife (who had disseminated sclerosis), the health authority was quite entitled to withdraw the service after due warning (*R v Hillingdon Area Health Authority, ex p Wyatt*). In other words, the behaviour constituted a refusal to accept the service on the conditions on which it was reasonably being offered, with the safety of the nurses in mind. In another type of case, this time brought in *negligence*, the judge similarly stated that in the light of the high risk presented by one particular patient, the nurses would have been entitled to say to the patient that he must use a hoist, if he wanted continued care (*Munrow v Plymouth Health Authority*).

Unreasonable refusals by social services clients

Likewise in the social services context, the courts have ruled that in the face of aggressive conduct – which in effect would be a refusal to accept a service on the reasonable terms on which it is offered – the duty to meet a person's community care needs is not absolute; and that there comes a point at which the local authority can withdraw. However, before taking such an extreme step, the authority must have carried out a reasonably thorough assessment and be satisfied that the client's conduct is not caused by the very community care need – such as a mental health problem – which the local authority is under a duty to meet (*R v Kensington and Chelsea Royal Borough, ex p Kujtim*).

In another case also, the courts indicated that services should not lightly be wholly removed. It concerned an elderly couple who had requested of the local authority under s.21 of the *National Assistance Act 1948* one type of accommodation (dwelling in the community), but were instead offered another (residential care) which they refused. The court held that this refusal under s.21 of the 1948 Act did not absolve the local authority of its obligation to continue to provide a number of non-residential services for the couple under s.29 of the same Act (*R (Khana) v Southwark London Borough Council*).

Thus, even if there is a justification of last resort in withdrawing services from those patients and clients who, one way or another, unreasonably refuse a service on the terms on which it is offered, it is clear that such withdrawal should be considered and implemented cautiously.

7. Human rights and manual handling

The *Human Rights Act 1998* incorporated the *European Convention on Human Rights* into United Kingdom law in October 1998. The effect of the 1998 Act is that United Kingdom courts are now able to consider claims in relation to the rights contained in the Convention, rather than claimants having to take their case to the European Court of Human Rights (although resort to the European Court continues to be available).

Inevitably, there has been speculation about how the implementation of the Act will affect health and social care provision, including manual handling. In summary, it is likely that (a) the effect will not be dramatic in terms of radical interference with health and social care generally (and manual handling in particular), in terms of policies and resources; (b) that nevertheless human rights will no doubt be found to be breached in some, and maybe more extreme, situations (which might involve manual handling issues); (c) that the 1998 Act will heighten judicial scrutiny of some health and social care decision-making; (d) that such heightened scrutiny might consider whether balanced decisions are being made (including, for instance, a weighing up of patient or client wish or need, against a local authority's or NHS Trust's limited resources and its concern about the health and safety of its staff). Even so, it should be emphasised that with such recent implementation of the 1998 Act, and thus paucity of case law in the United Kingdom courts, this summary must be taken as provisional.

With manual handling in mind, these general points are expanded upon under the entry *European Convention on Human Rights*, with respect to article 3 (concerning degrading treatment) and article 8 (concerning the right to respect for privacy, home and family life). In addition, there is a brief explanation about how the courts approach human rights matters.

A–Z LIST

A v LAMBETH LONDON BOROUGH COUNCIL
Children in need; welfare legislation; s.17 of the Children Act 1989; no enforceable duty

A case concerning s.17 of the *Children Act 1989*, which is in principle at least broad enough to cover a wide range of services and equipment for children in need, including manual handling related services and equipment.

The actual case involved a family with three children, two of whom were autistic; they clearly needed alternative accommodation, since their present dwelling was overcrowded, damp, unhygienic and dangerous. In considering the local authority's general duty to safeguard and promote the welfare of children in need under s.17 of the *Children Act 1989*, the court concluded that the identification of need under s.17 did not mean that the local authority had to meet that need, since there was no enforceable duty in respect of individuals ([2001] EWHC Admin 376, High Court). This decision was subsequently upheld by the Court of Appeal ([2001] EWCA (Civ 1624)).

A v NATIONAL BLOOD AUTHORITY
Product liability; infected blood; Consumer Protection Act; reliance on original directive

A case illustrating that the courts might choose to look at the original wording of a *European directive* (which is what the *MHOR 1992* are based on), rather than the wording of the United Kingdom legislation transposing the directive. It involved personal injury compensation sought under Part 1 of the Consumer Protection Act 1987, in respect of patients who had received blood infected by hepatitis. Just like the *MHOR 1992*, Part 1 of this Act is based on a European directive; and the court chose wholly to consider the original wording of the directive, rather than wording in the 1987 Act ([2001] 3 All ER 289, High Court).

AITKEN v BOARD OF MANAGEMENT OF ABERDEEN COLLEGE
Nursing auxiliary; credibility as witness; MHOR 1992

A nursing auxiliary sought damages under the *MHOR 1992* for an injury allegedly sustained in 1995 when she was assisting a patient to the lavatory from his wheelchair. The case failed, since the court found that the pursuer was not a credible or reliable witness, and that most of the evidence did not support her version of events either in relation to causation (i.e. a link between the alleged accident and her prolapsed disc) or to what actually happened, since lifting this patient was not normal practice (he suffered from cerebral palsy and did not need to be lifted) ([2000] GWD 2–74, Sheriff Court, Scotland).

ANDERSON v ASSOCIATED COOP CREAMERIES LTD
Milkman; time limits for bringing case; manual handling injury

A case illustrating that the courts are prepared to allow the exceeding of the legal *time limit* for bringing some manual handling cases.

A milkman alleged injury suffered in 1992 at the age of 24, through aggravation and acceleration of a pre-existing degenerative prolapsed disc suffered earlier in this employment. He complained about the system of work and the requirement to lift and handle excessively heavy and awkward loads, in particular crates and cages of dairy products. The question arose over whether the *Limitation Act 1980* precluded his bringing the case at all, since his claim had been eleven months out of the normal prescribed time of three years for bringing a personal injury case.

First, under s.14 of the *Limitation Act 1980*, the Court of Appeal agreed with what the judge at the first hearing had said: namely that the chance remark of a chiropractor made in the loosest and most general terms did not serve to impute to the plaintiff the requisite knowledge, such that the three-year time period would begin to run. Second, and independently, as to the judge's preparedness to use, under s.33 of the 1980 Act, the discretion to waive the time limit once it had expired, the Court of Appeal agreed with the judge as well, given that the extra eleven months did not disadvantage the defendants whatsoever (1997, Court of Appeal, unreported).

ANDERSON v LOTHIAN HEALTH BOARD
Hospital laundry worker; case; avoiding risk; reducing risk; adequacy of instructions; MHOR 1992

A hospital laundry worker was injured in 1994 lifting a 44lb load of laundry. Before the accident, the occupational health doctor had recommended a system involving the lifting of no more than 40lb loads. Information about this was passed to operators by word of mouth.

Avoiding the need for manual handling. The court, sitting in 1996, found a contravention of r.4(1)(a) of the *MHOR 1992* (duty to avoid, so far as reasonably practicable, the need for manual handling operations involving risk of physical injury). It reasoned as follows. First, the risk of injury need not be probable, but merely a foreseeable possibility. In the present case there clearly had been both a manual handling operation, and one that involved a risk of injury. It was for the employers to show that it was an operation that it was not reasonably practicable to avoid. In fact, first, the employer had not invoked such a defence; and second, if it had done so, it would still have failed, since the judge was not satisfied on the evidence that it was not reasonably practicable to avoid the handling of the laundry. Liability was therefore established on this ground.

Reducing the risk of injury. Liability being thus established, the case brought under r.4(1)(b) (risk assessment and taking of appropriate steps to reduce risk of injury) did not arise. However, had it done so – in circumstances in which it was decided that it was not reasonably practicable to avoid altogether the manual handling with risk – then liability would still have been established. This was because measures taken under r.4(1)(b) had to reduce the risk of injury to the lowest level reasonably practicable. The employer had in fact passed down instructions by word of mouth that loads were not to exceed 40lbs, but not posted up written notices – until after the accident. Yet clearly if it was reasonably practicable to place such notices after the accident, it would have been reasonably practicable beforehand ((1996) SCLR 1068, Outer House, Court of Session, Scotland).

BARKING AND DAGENHAM LONDON BOROUGH COUNCIL 1998
Local government ombudsman investigation; delay in assessment for home adaptations; manual handling implications; maladministration

This was an investigation by the *local government ombudsman* illustrating, amongst other things, the manual handling implications for clients and *carers* of delay in dealing with applications for *home adaptations.*

The complainant claimed that the council had delayed unreasonably in meeting the need for home adaptations and day care for her husband who was disabled. They lived in a council house with bedrooms, bathroom and WC upstairs. The husband had chronic arthritis and Steele Richardson Syndrome, a progressive form of Parkinson's disease.

Priority allocation and date given to application. In September 1993, they requested a ground-floor toilet, so that the husband could remain downstairs permanently. A care worker visited, noted that the husband did not want a commode and warned that there might be a delay of six to eight weeks in assessment. The husband was classified as medium priority, despite having had several falls, slipped in the bath and had trouble getting up the stairs. In September 1994, he was given a high priority (but was probably given a new date – i.e. September 1994, rather than October 1993 – which meant he went to the end of the high priority waiting list). Both the failure initially to allocate a high priority, and then to stick to the original date of application (after the priority had been raised) was maladministration. Had this not occurred, the need for adaptations would probably have been considered before a huge influx of work in May 1995.

Assessment and further delay because of workload. By March 1995 the man had fallen backwards down the stairs on several occasions, at which point his wife visited the council office. In May 1995, he was assessed by an occupational therapist from an external agency used by the council to clear the backlog of cases. Adaptations were recommended but a survey of the property did not take place until June 1996; though this was distressing, the ombudsman accepted on balance that this was because of a huge increase in workload rather than maladministration. However, in October 1995 when an extension was first mentioned, no check was made by social services with the housing department to see whether the house was on its list for future adaptations; referral did not take place until February 1997. This was maladministration.

Failure to record meeting. There was then a conflict of evidence about what took place at a meeting in September 1996. The council maintained that the couple were asked to consider moving into housing association accommodation, but that they had refused. The couple denied that this option was ever mentioned. However, the council did not write to the couple after the meeting to give them a record of what had occurred and an outline of the options. This was maladministration.

The ombudsman stated that had the couple received a clear explanation, they would have accepted the housing association option immediately, as they did in fact at a later date in February 1997. At the meeting, the council officers had explained that neither social services nor the housing department had the money to carry out the adaptations. The ombudsman concluded that the principal injustice lay in the prioritising of the occupational therapy assessment; absent this, and it was likely that the shower and toilet would have been installed before the husband's condition had deteriorated. The ombudsman accepted that by July 1996, this deterioration meant that the council considered that conversion of a cupboard downstairs was no longer a suitable option – but this did not remove the injustice, since the husband had been denied a downstairs toilet and shower for several years.

Demands on carer, including manual handling. All this had caused 'a great deal of distress, worry and inconvenience. The demands made on [the wife] have been enormous and I can only guess at the embarrassment and frustration' of the husband. For example, by 1996, the wife was usually alone with her husband all day, having to get him up, dress him, and help him on the stairs. His prostate problems meant that she needed to help him up and down more often – and when he fell, he often pulled her down with him.

Recommendations. The ombudsman recommended that £3,000 compensation be paid in recognition of the suffering caused, and an apology be given to the son-in-law to whom the council had not explained its complaints procedure in terms of how to make a formal complaint (1998, case 97/A/0337).

BARNES v STOCKTON BOROUGH COUNCIL
Swimming pool attendant; inflatable slide; system of work; instructions; contributory negligence

A negligence case involving swimming pool equipment, illustrating the courts' typical concern about *system of work* and *instructions*.

A swimming pool attendant, 28 years old, was in 1994 engaged in pulling on two ropes in order to fold up an inflatable slide, which was hanging over the side of the pool. He stepped on the slide, tripped over the air hose which was under it, fell and injured his back. The slide had been put away in the same manner for years; there had been no formal instructions.

The Court of Appeal found the council negligent in that there should have been some *system of work* laid down for dealing with the slide, and at the least instructions should have been given to employees not to remove it by standing on the slippery surface without first removing the air hose. The fact that the employees, if they had thought about it, would have realised the hazard did not serve to alleviate the duty on the employer. However, the injured employee was 50 per cent contributorily negligent since he had carried out the task for many years, knew the slide was slippery and that the hose was under it, and could have waited for assistance from another member of staff, but chose not to. Thus the damages of £6,500 would be halved (1997, Court of Appeal, unreported).

BAYLEY v BLOOMSBURY HEALTH AUTHORITY
Student nurse; walking a patient; adequacy, specificity and relevance of training; negligence case

In 1983, a student nurse aged 20 was injured when walking a 79-year-old woman. She was halfway through her training. The court examined the patient's care plan, of which walking was a part, as well as the training which had been given; in respect of the latter the health authority was found to be liable in negligence.

Accident when walking the patient. The patient in question weighed about 9.5 stone, had been on the ward some three or four weeks, and was known to be unsteady on her feet. She had a care plan which required her, when moving about, to have a walking stick and be accompanied by one nurse. She was a bit confused or demented. When being walked back to her bed from a chair, she decided to sit down, although she was nowhere near the bed. At this point, the nurse was holding on the patient's left arm, one arm on her wrist, the other under her elbow. This was not the way she wanted to hold on, but the patient would not allow her (because she felt she was being attacked) to put one arm round her waist (which would have been more in accordance with her training). The nurse said that she had observed the grip that she was using being employed by other staff. As the patient went down, the nurse tried to hold her up unsuccessfully; the nurse was wrenched forward and injured.

Care plan with risks for staff nevertheless acceptable. The original nursing plan arranged by the nursing sister, other nurses and a physiotherapist had been that two nurses were required to walk with her. But this plan was something of a 'counsel of despair', because with two nurses her rehabilitation would have been hindered or prevented. A walking frame was then tried, but soon she was carrying it; this led to the present plan of a walking stick and one nurse, a month before the accident. However, between this time and the accident, she had suffered a series of falls. Nevertheless the judge accepted that the care plan was a proper one, hearing evidence from the sister at the time (now director of nursing services at another hospital) that falls were the price to be paid for attempting to give people their independence back, whereas 25 years earlier they would have been consigned to bed. The judge considered that this was a 'laudable' aim, was satisfied that the care plan was alighted on only after 'anxious consultation', and that it was the patient's last chance of an independent life. However, such a care plan with its 'built-in and deliberately accepted risks, impinged on the overall safety of the nurses, particularly of student nurses... That being so, it was encumbent on those who brought that plan into effect to make perfectly sure that the student nurses in particular were capable of dealing with the additional problems that the plan presented'.

Inadequate training on particular risk. The judge then considered whether adequate training had been provided, and concluded that (a) it had taught how to move the patient; (b) holds and positioning were taught; (c) the emphasis was on prevention but not on the dangers to the nurse and in particular her back; (d) there was insufficient practice to overcome the nurse's instinct to catch, or try to save, the patient at any stage; (e) there was insufficient emphasis given – immediately before exposure to the ward – on the added dangers of patients falling; (f) when an individual care plan called for a calculated risk to be taken, insufficient steps were taken to ensure that all nurses and student nurses were prepared to cope with the additional dangers that the patient posed in the particular circumstances.

The judge felt that such steps should have been taken in order to protect the student nurse not only against her instinct when faced with totally unexpected behaviour by the patient, but also against momentary inattention to technique, or simple misjudgement of the patient's mood and what she was likely to do on that day. Damages were awarded of £20,000 (1987, High Court, unreported).

BEARMAN v AUSTRALIAN CAPITAL TERRITORY COMMUNITY AND HEALTH SERVICE
Enrolled nurse; nursing home; heavy lifting; adequate beds; chairs; absence of lifting equipment; insufficient wardsmen; system of work; negligence case; liability established

An enrolled nurse alleged that when lifting a resident, she suffered a severe injury in 1978 (when she was aged 29). The resident was described as about ten to eleven stone in weight, had suffered a stroke, could not walk, and was a gentle man but difficult to move because one of his legs was locked in the 'foetal position' against his chest, and because he had a will of his own and could be awkward with staff. The manager of the nursing home in fact described him more colloquially as a 'cantankerous old bugger who threw himself around a lot'. The nurse had to transfer him from his armchair to his bed, which had high guard rails around it which could be moved up and down. During the lift – made more difficult because of the winged, high armchair, and carried out with assistance from another member of staff – she was pushed down onto the rail with the resident on top of her, and was injured.

Beds and rails. The beds in the nursing home varied in height but were not adjustable. They tended to be very low which made it difficult for nurses to lift patients in and out of bed. The beds were fitted with guard rails for patient safety; however, when lowered, they tended to hinder the nurses, whose legs came into contact with them beneath mattress level. This meant that they had to bend over more than they otherwise would have.

Lifting equipment and wardsmen. Lifting equipment was provided for the first time in the nursing home in 1977, in the form of a 'Henry lifter' – a hoist with canvas sling, operated hydraulically with chains. It was seldom used by staff because in their general opinion it was impractical to use and actually dangerous, since the chain was so heavy that it would cause injury if it hit a patient. A second piece of lifting equipment was introduced before the plaintiff's accident, but it was not for transfers into bed. Because of persistent staff complaints about heavy lifting, two wardsmen were employed in 1977; however, their rotas meant there would be no wardsman for some evening shifts. Overall the court was satisfied that the nursing staff were constantly complaining about the heavy lifting, the unsatisfactory beds, the unsuitable chairs provided by relatives, the absence of lifting equipment, and the insufficiency of male wardsmen.

Nature of the lift. The employer argued that the chair had nothing to do with the injury; and that in any case the lift was complete when the patient grabbed the rail and the nurse was injured by being pushed against it. The judge rejected this, finding that the lift was a very awkward one, given the patient's posture, the shape and height of the chair, and the patient's pulling and jamming of the rail.

Liability. The court found the employer liable for failure to provide a safe system of work:

> This embraced a number of factors. There was a failure to lift a patient who was known to be a 'heavy' lift. I am prepared to assume that a male wardsman would have been physically stronger than the nurses on duty, including the plaintiff. The very reason wardsmen were employed at [the nursing home] was to assist in the nursing care of the aged, which involved helping the nurses in lifting patients. I find that those failures amounted to a breach of the duty of care in all the circumstances, including the awkwardness of the lift out of [the patient's] high, wing-backed armchair, the height of the bed to which he was to be transferred, the obstruction which the guard rail of the bed presented and all the other facts relating to the awkwardness of the lift to which I have already referred.

Contributory negligence. As to contributory negligence, the court found none, stating:

She was working under pressure, and to some extent urgency. There were only three nurses to look after some 46–48 patients, many of whom were non-ambulatory and there was a great deal of work to be done. A fact-finding tribunal should not fail to appreciate the concomitant features of the nurses' duties in relation to geriatric non-ambulatory patients. The plaintiff did not do anything contrary to instructions. She may have failed to request assistance but there was no assistance available anyway. I can find no failure on her part to take reasonable or adequate care for her own safety. Nor was the use of such mechanical aids as were available a practical course in all the circumstances. ([1990] ACTSC 3, Supreme Court of the Australian Capital Territory)

BEASLEY v BUCKINGHAMSHIRE COUNTY COUNCIL
Foster parent paid by local authority; manual handling injury; whether duty of care owed; negligence case

The plaintiff had been acting as a paid *foster carer* to a handicapped teenage boy, placed with her by the council. She claimed that on five occasions between 1991 and 1993 she had suffered back injury when trying to catch, lift, save or restrain him.

She argued that she should have been provided with a hoist or other lifting equipment earlier than she was; that the defendant failed properly to assess the placement; and that had it done so, it would not have placed such a heavy and disabled child with her. This was in the light of her complete lack of experience in caring for children with such a disability. She also claimed that she should have been trained in lifting techniques and should have been warned of the risks of the work. The local authority attempted to have the case struck out on grounds of public policy, namely that it was not in the public interest that local authorities should owe a duty of care in such circumstances, even had it acted negligently.

The court found that the case should not automatically be struck out. First, it concerned the practical manner in which the local authority was proceeding, not policy; and the judge could not see why the imposition of a duty of care was inconsistent with, or would discourage, the due performance of the authority in carrying out its statutory duties in respect of children. Furthermore, on the public policy question, it would surely be 'poor public policy' to impose a heavy burden on charitable, lowly paid volunteer foster parents, but for those parents to have no recourse if the authority behaved carelessly. The judge referred to the foster parent as a 'quasi-employee' of the authority and pointed out that it would be odd if a nurse could sue a health authority but a foster parent could not sue a local authority ([1997] PIQR P473, High Court).

BEATTIE v WEST DORSET HEALTH AUTHORITY
Manual handling training; height matching; supervision of trainees; negligence of trainer

The plaintiff was a state enrolled nurse attending in 1985 a lifting and moving session of training. The trainees were divided into groups of three, with each group practising lifting. Two trainees would lift the third. The plaintiff, who was four foot eleven inches high, was matched with another trainee who was five feet seven inches tall. As they lifted the third trainee from chair to bed, the second trainee came up quickly and straightened her legs; the weight of the lifted trainee shifted to the plaintiff's left side and she felt a knife-like sensation down her left leg.

The court found that the lift being practised was a cradle lift, which the plaintiff said she would not have used in that situation normally, and which the trainer (although she denied this) had in effect invited the teams to practise. The trainer, even though she was looking at the trainees, did not stop this lift. Further, she:

> gave no proper instructions to the trainees as to how they should cope with differentials in height. In fact she gave none at all but relied on their common sense interpretation of the general principles. She ignored the fact that beginners need both instruction and supervision… I have no hesitation in concluding that the plaintiff was injured as a result of a lack of proper instruction of inexperienced trainees; of a failure to pair, within reasonable limits of height, those engaged in training to lift, and in failing properly to supervise the practical exercise.

Damages of £43,000 were awarded (1990, High Court, unreported).

BLACK v CARRICKS
Bakery manageress; lifting trays; responsibility of employee/manageress; Offices, Shops and Railway Premises Act 1963; negligence case

An older case brought under a piece of now obsolete health and safety at work legislation, in which the court ruled that the employee was responsible for the decision that led to her injury.

The manageress of a bakery had staff off sick in March 1973; she was injured when lifting trays weighing 24lb. She had informed her employer, whose response on the telephone was that she should manage the best she could and perhaps get a customer to help. She decided to do it alone; the Court of Appeal agreed with the judge at first instance that she had not been 'required' to lift; she could have decided not to do so under the *Offices, Shops and Railway Premises Act 1963* (s.23, now obsolete). Nor, under the common law of negligence, had the injury been reasonably foreseeable ([1980] IRLR 448, Court of Appeal).

BLACK v WRANGLER (UK) LIMITED
Clothing worker; cumulative strain; keeping abreast of relevant information; MHOR 1992; negligence case

A negligence concerning alleged injury suffered cumulatively over many years, including the question of what sort of information an employer should be aware of.

The pursuer sought damages for back injury caused – over a long period of time (she was employed between 1976 and 1995) in a jeans factory – by her daily pushing and pulling of trucks loaded with garments, and the lifting of the garments out for inspection. The claim was under the common law of *negligence* and the *MHOR 1992*. It was not based on one particular incident but on the daily manual handling operations which had allegedly caused a progressive deterioration of her back. The employer sought dismissal of the action without full probation (i.e. without a full hearing).

The court held that the case should proceed because (a) a relevant research paper produced by a university was not on the face of it the sort of document an average employer could have been expected to retain and read; nevertheless, this one (published in 1980) had been referred to in a consultation document published through Her Majesty's Stationery Office in 1982; (b) the pursuer had offered to prove that she had made complaints, thus suggesting that she was not solely relying on the 1980 paper; (c) there was specificity in that she had named managers and supervisors to whom she had complained; and (d) causation of injury was a matter of proof which required inquiry ([2000] GWD 12–441, Outer House, Court of Session, Scotland).

BLAIR v LANCASTER HEALTH AUTHORITY
Nurse; lifting obese patient unnecessarily; custom and practice; cumulative stress; negligence case

A state enrolled nurse aged 37 was injured in 1980 when carrying out a 'total lift' on an 'enormously obese' patient of some 16 or 17 stone with three other nurses during a night shift on the intensive care unit. She would have borne a quarter of the weight, some 55–60lb; she felt something go in her back. Earlier on that shift, she had also been turning another patient of about 15 stone and very ill.

The judge agreed with the view of the plaintiff's expert that the method of turning the patients involved extraordinarily unnecessary effort and risk, in that they were lifted vertically, whereas the correct method would have been to slide patients to the side of the bed and roll them over. The judge did not find it necessary to make a finding on staffing levels or the availability of assistance from other wards, because for 'two nurses regularly to carry out total lifts of 15 stone, let alone "exceptionally obese" patients, was, on the evidence, a breach of the defendants' duty of care'. There was no evidence of how this practice had become established, but had anyone looked at it critically, it would have been stopped immediately because of the high risk of back injury in a situation of cumulative stress brought about by repeated lifts during a work shift. Damages of £77,000 were awarded (1987, High Court, unreported).

BLANCHFLOWER v CHAMBERLAIN
Lorry driver; instructions; system of work; contributory negligence; negligence case

A negligence case, in which the Court of Appeal balanced the employer's failure to give a warning against the employee's responsibility to take reasonable steps.

The employer failed to give specific warning to an experienced lorry driver about handling an unusually large tarpaulin on a lorry with a poor foothold. The driver had picked up a load of soya animal feed in a tractor and trailer unit. The sheet rucked up in the middle; he stood on top of the load to pull the sheet free and fell over the back. Despite the driver's experience the employer had a duty to give some instruction on operating the tarpaulin, since it was bigger and heavier than a normal sheet of tarpaulin and there were protruding hinges. There was thus no safe *system of work*; however, there was 50 per cent contributory negligence since the risk was obvious and could have been avoided. On this basis the damages of £151,900 were halved ([1996] CL 96/2997, Court of Appeal).

BOHITIGE v BARNET HEALTHCARE NHS TRUST
Nursing auxiliary; cuddle lift; common sense failure to pull up trousers of patient in a different way; lack of training irrelevant; negligence case

A case where the court effectively found the plaintiff to blame for failing to use her common sense, given that the lift being employed was acceptable and proper, and one that she understood. She was an auxiliary nurse injured in 1990 when attending a patient at home, who weighed 7.5 stone and was slightly built. She had lost her claim in the County Court, and now appealed to the Court of Appeal.

Cuddle lift; pulling up trousers from ankles. The patient could take weight on her legs, and could put her arms around the shoulders or neck of a nurse if required; she had been adamant that she would not have a hoist in her bedroom or in the house at all; so the nurses had to undertake lifts from bed to pushchair, and from pushchair to electric wheelchair. On the particular day in question, the plaintiff was injured when the patient made a movement with her arms, or with arm and body, which damaged the nerve roots in her right shoulder. She was injured at the point at which she was holding the patient in a standing position and attempting to pull up her trousers from around her ankles. The lift being used by the nurse was the 'cuddle lift', which all the nurses used with this particular patient.

Failure of employee to apply common sense; irrelevance of lack of additional training. The judge at first instance preferred the expert evidence put forward for the employer, concluding that for this particular patient, the cuddle lift was acceptable and proper practice. In agreeing with the judge's conclusion, the Court of Appeal stated that it was of the view that the plaintiff:

...correctly understood and used the cuddle lift and knew the importance, for her own protection, of keeping her back straight. The cuddle lift was appropriate and in accordance with good nursing practice for use with this patient. The plaintiff and the other nurses concerned used the cuddle lift without assistance both before and after the plaintiff's accident. The cause of the plaintiff's accident was her failure to pull up the patient's trousers before lifting her from the WC or in not sitting her down again before dealing with her trousers, that so to do was a matter of obvious common sense and that, accordingly, the judge was right to accept the correctness of...evidence that it did not appear that any additional training in safe manual lifting would have contributed to the prevention of this accident (1997, Court of Appeal, unreported).

BOLAM v FRIERN HOSPITAL MANAGEMENT COMMITTEE
Test of professional carelessness; negligence

A famous case (involving electro-convulsive therapy) setting out the test for establishing professional carelessness in *negligence* cases:

How do you test whether this act of failure is negligent? In an ordinary sense it is generally said you judge it by the action of the man in the street. He is the ordinary man. In one case it has been said you judge it by the conduct of the man on the top of a Clapham omnibus. He is the ordinary man. But where you get a situation which involves the use of some special skill or competence, then the test as to whether there has been negligence or not is not the test of the man on the top of the Clapham omnibus, because he has not got this special skill. The test is the standard of the ordinary skilled man exercising and professing to have that special skill. A man need not possess the highest expert skill; it is well established law that it is sufficient if he exercises the ordinary skill of an ordinary competent man exercising that particular art...[he] is not negligent, if he is acting in accordance with a practice accepted as proper by a responsible body of medical men skilled in that particular art... It is not essential...to decide which of two practices is the better practice, as long as you accept that what the defendants did was in accordance with a practice accepted by responsible persons ([1957] 2 All ER 118, High Court).

BOLITHO v CITY AND HACKNEY HEALTH AUTHORITY

A case (involving bronchial blockage and the question of intubation for a two-year old boy) elaborating upon the traditional test (see *Bolam v Friern Hospital*) for carelessness in *negligence* cases – and emphasising that the court must satisfy itself of the logic, reasonableness and responsible nature of a body of professional, expert opinion before accepting it as valid:

In the vast majority of cases the fact that distinguished experts in the field are of a particular opinion will demonstrate the reasonableness of that opinion... But if in a rare case it can be demonstrated that the professional opinion is not capable of withstanding logical analysis, the judge is entitled to hold that the body of opinion is not reasonable or responsible ([1997] 4 All ER 771, House of Lords).

BOWFIELD v SOUTH SEFTON (MERSEYSIDE) HEALTH AUTHORITY
State enrolled nurse; Bobath method; experienced nurse; recent assessment of patient; previous back trouble; negligence case

The Court of Appeal overturned a decision in favour of the plaintiff at first instance, on the grounds that there was no evidence that a recent assessment of the patient was lacking, and that the plaintiff was sufficiently experienced to take her own decision. However, prophetically, the court looked ahead to the law changing and perhaps becoming more stringent in the protection, in the public interest, of nurses. It might be therefore that this case would be decided differently in 2001.

Accident: Bobath technique. A state enrolled nurse (SEN) began work as a student nurse in 1972 at the age of seventeen; in 1974 she became a state enrolled nurse. In 1978 she was appointed as a senior nurse on a stroke rehabilitation unit. By the time of the accident in 1980, she had a history of back trouble which had included some time off from work. The accident occurred when she was adopting the Bobath technique for assisting patients from their beds to chairs. This involved the nurse placing her legs on either side of the patient's bad leg, then instructing him to put his arms around her waist while she put her arms around the back or shoulders of the patient; he would then be instructed to stand up with his weight on his good leg. The judge stated that if properly performed this would not be lifting in the ordinary sense of the word, because of the patient bearing his own weight. During the operation, the patient jumped and his full weight was transferred to the nurse, causing injury.

Liability at first instance (assessment and nurse's experience). At first instance, the judge found in favour of the plaintiff on the grounds that 'in the absence of a careful and up to date assessment of the condition of a patient, who has suffered a stroke, as to his ability to concentrate, there remains a foreseeable risk that he may suddenly lose his powers of concentration, even though for the preceding three months he has reacted satisfactorily to instructions'. Yet there was no evidence of such an assessment. In addition, the man weighed fifteen stone which was potentially a heavy load in the absence of cooperation; and although the nurse was a senior SEN she was not sufficiently experienced to make a decision about the patient's ability to cooperate; this would need to have been decided by a physiotherapist.

Appeal: no liability (assessment and nurse's experience). On appeal, the Court of Appeal now overturned this decision on the following grounds. First, there was no evidence to suggest that a recent assessment had not been carried out. Second, it was reasonable for the nurse to make her own assessment of the patient to cooperate. Third, an alternative argument, that the employer should have ensured that the nurse did not carry out heavy lifting because of her previous back problems, was also rejected. This was on the basis of the fact that the employer knew she had a 'vulnerable back' when she applied to the stroke rehabilitation unit for a job did not in itself mean the employer should not have employed her for such work. Even after an incident in 1979 when she had been off work for 16 days after lifting a patient, the employer was not obliged to remove her from such work since (a) the nurse was herself experienced enough to consider whether she should continue with such work; and (b) the employer was

> entitled to pay heed to this factor and…entitled to rely on the certificate which was supplied by her own GP that she was fit to return to work. A reference for assessment by the occupational health department, to which it seems she had herself reported in March 1979, would in fact have been carried out by a general practitioner. In my view, therefore, it was not negligent to continue to employ her in this department. Further there was no obligation to warn a person, who had the training and experience of the plaintiff, of risks so far as they existed of which she must herself have been fully aware.

Future development of the law and liability. The court also added:

> We have been urged…in powerful submissions to the court, to hold that in the public interest the court should assist the nursing profession to eliminate or reduce the very high incidence of back injuries which are known to exist in that profession. Nothing I have said in this judgment should be taken to imply that I have no regard to this important factor. But to my mind that important principle is not advanced by enlarging the scope of a duty in situations where such enlargement is not justified. That does not mean, of course, that the law in respect of the existence or nature of a duty cannot from time to time be enlarged. Of course it can, as occurs in multiple similar circumstances of injury case (1991, Court of Appeal, unreported).

BOYD v LANARKSHIRE HEALTH BOARD
Hospital laundry worker; breach of MHOR 1992 but no liability; credibility of evidence

A hospital laundry assistant aged 63 sought damages, claiming injury to his right arm in 1994, when he was lifting a laundry bag into a cage for storage. The judge found a breach of the *MHOR 1992*, but that this breach did not cause the accident.

    The court found that (a) although the bags arrived on trolleys, they needed manually sorting into yellow and white piles; (b) therefore there was a risk of injury under r.4 of the *MHOR 1992*; (c) although the laundry training manual contained instructions not to lift bags that were too heavy, some were very heavy and their weight could only be ascertained when they were taken out of the trolley; (d) the employer had put forward neither arguments that it was not reasonably practicable to avoid the need for the lifting, nor evidence about any risk assessments undertaken; and (e) there was no evidence of assessment relating to the factors listed in schedule 1 to the *MHOR 1992* being undertaken by someone with appropriate expertise. The court was therefore of the view that the employer was in breach of the *MHOR 1992*.

However, the pursuer's account was neither credible nor reliable. There was conflicting evidence, and it was up to the pursuer to define the circumstances in which the injury occurred in precise enough terms to allow the court to decide what happened. The pursuer's alternative argument, that it was enough to establish that an injury had occurred arising from some sort of manual handling, was not enough. There was no liability ([2000] GWD 9–341, Outer House, Court of Session, Scotland).

BRADFORD METROPOLITAN DISTRICT COUNCIL v A
Education; defining special educational needs; nursing at school; Education Act 1993

With the meeting of disabled children's needs in mind – including manual handling related needs – this case illustrates that some services will be deemed in law to be incapable of being special educational provision, and so not easily amenable to enforcement. See *Education Act 1996* and *Education (Scotland) Act 1980*.

The case established that nursing care required at school by a child could not in law be deemed to be a special educational need under the Education Act 1993 (now the *Education Act 1996*); unlike, for instance, speech and language therapy, the provision of nursing was not on the borderline between educational and non-educational provision ([1997] ELR 417, High Court).

BRISTOL CITY COUNCIL
Local government ombudsman investigation; need for rehousing; severely disabled son; manual handling; appalling catalogue of neglect by council; maladministration

This was an investigation by the *local government ombudsman* illustrating, amongst other things, the manual handling implications for clients and *carers* of a local authority's application of a blanket policy, which prevented the authority from responding to client need.

Manual handling. The complainants were council tenants and the parents of a teenage boy who required twenty-four-hour care. He had cerebral palsy, microcephaly, developmental delays, spastic quadriplegia, chest problems, he was unable to walk or talk and used a wheelchair. His parents had always carried him up and down the stairs, but as he grew older, bigger and heavier this became increasingly difficult.

Fettering of discretion: blanket policy. In the light of this, the family's need for rehousing was 'severe and going to worsen' as the son got older; yet the council gave inadequate consideration to these exceptional needs when applying its policy of not arranging a move in case of rent arrears. This was a fettering of discretion and maladministration. In addition, the lumping together of rent and housing benefit when considering the amount of rent in arrears was unlawful under housing benefit legislation; therefore the council's failure to differentiate rent arrears from overpayment of housing benefit was maladministration.

Disabled facilities grants: no information given. The parents were told several times that the council did not have the money to fund adaptations but were not told about disabled facilities grants; in fact some of the council's officers were not even sure whether council tenants were legally entitled to such grants (which they clearly were); this was maladministration.

Appalling neglect. For the above, and other, reasons, the ombudsman found an:

> appalling catalogue of neglect by the Council. It seems to me to have disregarded its obligations to this family trying to cope with the needs of one of its members who is suffering from severe disability. To whom should such a family turn if not to the Council, especially when, as in this case, the Council is also its landlord? Yet at every approach the family has been spurned. They have been the victim of a too-rigid adherence to policy; they have suffered from poor communication between social services and housing officers which has meant that those officers who were attempting to help were rendered helpless by other officers presumably responding to their own priorities; they have been told that a lack of resources has meant they cannot be helped with aids and adaptations yet officers have failed to point them in the direction of other resources within the Council's control.

Recommendations. This was 'very substantial' injustice; the ombudsman did not conclude that the father's heart attack 'derived specifically' from the council's maladministration, 'but the toll on [the family's] health and well-being must have been enormous'. He recommended that the council apologise, make an ex gratia payment of £20,000 (but in such a way that benefit entitlement was not affected), review its arrangements for dealing with the housing needs of disabled people, and ensure that its housing officers were adequately trained (1998: cases 96/B/4035 and 96/B/4143).

BRODIE v KENT COUNTY COUNCIL
Care assistant; lifting resident from the floor; whether hoist should have been used; negligence case

A negligence case in which the Court of Appeal found in favour of the employer, in respect of an injury incurred by a care assistant when lifting a resident back into bed from the floor. The reference to use of hoists not being common practice illustrates how times have changed in the manual handling field, and the case might be decided differently today.

Resident falling onto floor. The plaintiff was a woman in her fifties with a long history of back trouble, some of which was known to the council when it employed her as a care attendant in a residential home for older people. The accident in question occurred in 1980. A resident had fallen out of bed into a small space between the bed and a wall. The system in the home was that when this occurred, the resident was not to be moved until approved by either the matron or assistant matron. On this occasion, the emergency bell was rung, three members of staff were present to lift the resident, but the space allowed only two of them to act. The plaintiff took the top end of the resident, while the assistant matron placed her hands under her knee and thigh. The plaintiff was injured in the ensuing lift.

Liability at first instance: no use of hoist. The judge at first instance found the employer liable for not generally having a system of work involving use of a hoist and also specifically in respect of the assistant matron not calling for the hoist in the specific circumstances. It appeared that there was a hoist available in the bathroom, but that it was not in practice used, because it was cumbersome and time-consuming to use.

Appeal: no liability on basis of hoists not being in common use. The Court of Appeal overturned this decision, finding that there was nothing to suggest that common practice demanded that a hoist be used to lift a resident off the floor in such circumstances; and that furthermore it would not have been to the benefit of the resident to have waited for the hoist to be brought and operated. No evidence was given to the court that hoists of any sort were in common use or indeed used at all in hospitals or nursing homes throughout the country (1986, Court of Appeal, unreported).

BROWN v ALLIED IRONFOUNDERS
Factory workers; moving paint stillages; established practice; Factories Act 1961; custom and practice

An older manual handling case, brought under now obsolete health and safety at work legislation, s.72 of the *Factories Act 1961*. The House of Lords found liability, insofar as the toleration of unsafe custom and practice by an employer was in effect a requirement on employees to undertake unsafe lifting.

The plaintiff was employed in a factory; her normal work had ceased temporarily, so she was asked to help in another department, where she had to paint stillages (wire mesh cages) weighing 1.25 hundredweight (140lb) each. In order to paint the bottom of the stillages, they had to be turned on their side. The normal practice was for two women to turn the stillages; however, the chargehand knew that some women did this on their own. The plaintiff turned them on her own, although she could have obtained assistance.

The court found that the chargehand knew that, having sent the plaintiff to paint the stillages alone, she might be one of those women who moved the stillages alone. She was therefore in effect employed to turn the stillages, which amounted to a breach of statutory duty under s.72; the question of whether assistance was potentially available was irrelevant. The plaintiff won her appeal ([1974] 2 All ER 135, House of Lords, appealed from the Court of Session, Scotland).

BROWN v EAST MIDLOTHIAN NHS TRUST
Auxiliary nurse; falling patient; negligence case; employer fulfilling obligations; MHOR 1992

An auxiliary nurse on a rehabilitation assessment ward for elderly people sought damages for a back injury suffered in 1997 when she tried to stop a patient falling. She claimed a breach of duty of care in negligence, in relation to a safe *system of work* including adequate staffing and *training*; and also a breach of the *MHOR 1992* given that this was an operation carrying risk.

Negligence: training and staffing. As far as the negligence case went, the court held that it was not established that the training was inadequate and that in any case it could see no causal connection between any possible failure in training and the accident. Also the nurse had received assistance quickly when she called for it; there was no proof that absence of staff caused the accident.

MHOR 1992: general and particular risk assessment. Likewise, the *MHOR 1992* were satisfied in various respects. The need for manual handling by nursing staff could not be avoided. The training course satisfied the requirement of suitable and sufficient assessment generally. The care plan satisfied the requirement of such an assessment for this patient in particular; indeed there was 'no need for the assessment to take any particular form', so long as it was suitable and sufficient – which meant it had to be related to the manual handling operations which might be required for each individual patient.

Pursuer's fault. The pursuer, together with other nursing staff, was aware of the contents and significance of the care plan, and of the risks associated with the patient. It was the pursuer's own actions that led to reasonably foreseeable injury in that she could have gone over to the patient to stop him standing up unescorted, and at the same time called for assistance. Her failure to do this led to an emergency situation in which she was injured. Even if the *MHOR 1992* had been breached, the court was not satisfied that the breach caused the accident ([2000] SLT 342, Outer House, Court of Session, Scotland).

BRUGGEMANN v ACE NOMINEES PTY
Physiotherapist aide; moving table; negligence case

A physiotherapist aide, 48 years old, was injured in 1981 when moving unassisted a heavy traction table – which was in an abnormal position on Monday morning because it had been moved by contractors over the weekend. She had had two successful laminectomies for a lower back complaint some years before. Her duties each morning included tidying up the cubicles of a busy sports medicine clinic but not moving the traction table. At first instance, the judge had found the employer liable, although he had found also 25 per cent contributory negligence.

In a two-to-one split decision, the Supreme Court now overturned this decision, essentially on the grounds that it 'may have been correct to conclude that there was a foreseeable risk of injury, but that was a risk extremely unlikely to occur. Its magnitude and the degree of probability that it would occur was so slight that the failure to warn or to do anything is not properly characterised as a breach of the duty owed'. In other words, even if it the employer had foreseen that the contractors would move and not replace the table – and that then the employee would try to move it unassisted – there was no obligation to have taken steps to warn ([1986] 41 SASR 25, South Australian Supreme Court).

BUNTER v LIFTWISE
Lift engineer; asking for help; Construction (General Provisions) Regulations 1961; negligence case

A manual handling case, brought in negligence and under r.55 of the Construction (General Provisions) Regulations 1961 (now obsolete), illustrating that employers cannot simply leave everything for employees to decide.

A lift engineer, together with another employee, was in 1991 installing heavy lift gates weighing 320lb each; it was common ground that they were too heavy for two men to move. The plaintiff telephoned for lifting equipment, but this request was refused and he was told to get help from building site labourers. In the event the two of them did it by themselves. The judge at first instance had found no liability, on the basis that the employee should have asked for help. Citing *Brown v Allied Ironfounders*, the Court of Appeal now overturned this decision and allowed the appeal; the man had asked for help, and the employer should have specified whether it was a 2,3 or 4-man job. Instead it was left up to the men to decide. However, the plaintiff was 25 per cent contributorily negligent since he was experienced and failed to take sufficient care of himself, so the £5,500 damages would be reduced by a quarter (1997, Court of Appeal, unreported).

CALLAGHAN v SOUTHERN GENERAL HOSPITAL NHS TRUST
Auxiliary nurse; unconvincing evidence; MHOR 1992; negligence case

An auxiliary nurse claimed that in 1996 she was injured when leaning across a 23-stone patient – described as strong, confused, restless and aggressive – in bed to restrain her in order to allow intubation.

The court found on the evidence that the size and width of the patient and the height of the bed would have made reaching across the patient and holding both her hands difficult to achieve (the employer's manual handling adviser stated that it was hard to envisage); that the pursuer anyway would only have had to hold one of the patient's hands, not both; and that the patient did not on this occasion, as alleged, struggle or resist so as to cause injury. The judge accepted that the pursuer's back condition did exist (and rejected the suggestion that she was malingering) but concluded that it had not arisen from the incident complained of ((2000) SLT 1059, Outer House, Court of Session, Scotland).

CAMDEN LONDON BOROUGH COUNCIL
Local government ombudsman investigation; manual handling; home adaptations; delay; maladministration

This was an investigation by the local government ombudsman illustrating, amongst other things, the manual handling implications for clients and *carers* of delay in dealing with applications for *home adaptations*.

A woman who was a council tenant requested a special chair. An occupational therapist visited in March 1990 to assess for this and other potential needs. The woman walked with Fischer sticks, had limited knee movement and had very limited strength and movement in her hands. The living room and kitchen were on the first floor, and on the second were the bedroom, bathroom and WC. The occupational therapist suggested the installation of a stairlift between the first and second floors.

Long delay between assessment and placing of order. The occupational therapist then first approached the housing department in April 1990. A joint visit which should have been made within seven days was not made for six weeks. The specification required by the procedure was never supplied; and an order which should have been placed within 14 days took 22 months – even though the installation was not complex and required only removal of a radiator and confirmation that the bannisters did not need altering. Adaptations for disabled council tenants had been paid for out of the repairs budget; in October 1991, the council imposed a moratorium on expenditure because the financial position was worse than had been anticipated. Thus ordering of the lift was put off and contributed to the overall delay.

Star and Starlet Chambers. In this financial difficulty, decisions on whether works could be approved were taken by a central 'Star Chamber' (for works over £10,000) or by a 'Starlet Chamber' at district level (under £10,000).

Ineffective liaison, missing records, insufficient resources. There was no effective liaison between departments, crucial records were missing and the council could not explain the delays. Under s.2 of the *Chronically Sick and Disabled Persons Act 1970*, insufficient resources were no justification for delay. Indeed, once

> the Council became aware of their financial position they should have instituted procedures to ensure that adaptation works were prioritised on a borough-wide basis. Instead it appears that whether a need was met depended on competing demands on the local repairs budget for a particular week. I cannot therefore be certain that people with similar needs were dealt with in a similar way.

The overall wait was nearly two years between the assessment visit and placing of the order, during which time the woman's condition worsened.

Worsening condition of woman during wait: manual handling on stairs. The woman took water tablets to reduce swelling, but this meant that she had to go to the lavatory several times a day. Her hand and elbow suffered from gripping the stair rail. Her knees got worse. Her husband had to push her up the stairs from behind. She had to go down the stairs backwards, stop halfway up, and stay upstairs once there because it was too painful to come down. She took a lot of painkillers and wore hand splints to protect her joints (which the occupational therapist explained would not recover their function once lost). She got depressed about all of this.

Staff's unfamiliarity with procedures and inconsistent adoption. It also became apparent that some key staff had never been aware of the council's written procedures for adaptations, and that the procedures were not adopted uniformly by different housing area teams.

Conclusions and recommendations. The delays, non-following of and ignorance about procedures, lack of liaison, and missing records, all amounted to maladministration. The ombudsman recommended that the council pay £1,000 to the couple and review procedures, so that in future it could act on a corporate basis and ensure that priority would be dealt with on a borough-wide basis, rather than be dependent on the state of the local repairs budget in any particular week (1993, case 91/Λ/1481).

CAMPBELL v DUMFRIES AND GALLOWAY HEALTH BOARD
Student nurse; lifting patient out of bed; instructions and training about lifting equipment; breach of duty but no liability; negligence case

The pursuer was a student nurse seeking damages for a back injury allegedly sustained in 1983, when as a student nurse she lifted a patient out of bed. She claimed that she had never been instructed that an 'Ambulift' lifting aid kept in the ward bathroom could have been used instead of a manual lift. Breach of duty was established but no liability.

Breach of duty. The court found on the basis of 'one way' expert evidence that in 1983, such lifting aids were used mainly in bathrooms. National guidance issued in 1981 by the Royal College of Nursing and Back Pain Association was referred to. Therefore the plaintiff's case was that while the proper method of lifting a patient was in any given case a matter for judgement for the nurses, there was always a risk of back injury in manual lifting and by 1983 it had become obviously necessary that in exercising their judgement nurses should be instructed to have regard to the possible option of using mechanical aids such as the Ambulift. The judge agreed, finding that by 1983, the pursuer should have been instructed or trained in the possible bedside use of the Ambulift.

No liability. However, the court did not find liability because (a) it did not accept the nurse's version of events as to what actually happened, in terms of the lift that she claimed caused the accident and the role of a chair which fell over during the operation; and (b) it was not satisfied that, even had an Ambulift been available, it would have been used by the pursuer, since the patient was a dead weight of nearly 12 stone, and the court accepted that to use a hoist would have required more physical lifting than a manual lift and would have been too stressful for both patient and nurse ((1991) SLT 624, Outer House, Court of Session, Scotland).

CANTILLON v LONDON NURSING HOMES LTD
Nursing home assistant; reaching in and falling into freezer; injuries sustained; negligence case

In 1980, a nursing home employee, aged 55, reached into the bottom of a chest-type deep freezer, overbalanced, managed to get herself out in a few seconds but claimed to have sustained enduring injuries. This had occurred by reason of her height (five foot two inches) and perhaps weight (over thirteen stone); she had stood on tiptoe and overbalanced. The judge found this was a 'pure accident'; that there was nothing wrong in installing the particular freezer, and in failing to give specific instructions about its use; and thus nothing wrong that had caused the accident. It was 'just one of those things' (1983, High Court, unreported).

CARE AGENCIES
Domiciliary care agencies have duties under health and safety at work legislation generally, and under the *MHOR 1992* in particular, to take steps to identify and avoid or reduce risk for their employees. Even where a care agency is under contract to social services or the NHS, this responsibility continues. During 2002, it is expected that such care agencies will be registered and inspected under the *Care Standards Act 2000* and the *Regulation of Care (Scotland) Act 2001*. Draft national standards for England on domiciliary care refer specifically to manual handling within the standard on risk assessment (DH 2001d, standard 12).

Duty of local authorities or the NHS to supply care agencies with relevant information. The Health and Safety Executive has in the past pointed out, in the context of manual handling, that a failure by the statutory agency (e.g. social services) in such a situation to supply the care agency promptly with relevant details about a client's needs or about other relevant aspects of the home situation, might prevent the care agency from properly carrying out its own risk assessment and discharging its obligations towards its employees and towards non-employees (i.e. clients). Such information might be about the weight and mobility of clients, whether they are continent or not, aggressive or have violent tendencies or aggressive pets (HSE NIGM 7/F/1998/2). The local authority in such a situation could be in breach of its duty under s.3 of the *Health and Safety at Work Act 1974* towards non-employees (who are in this context the employees of the care agency and the client); just as it might if it takes too little care in the tendering out and monitoring of a contract with the independent sector (*Health and Safety Executive v Barnet London Borough Council*).

Agency responsibilities to those on its books. Care agencies sometimes attempt to avoid their responsibilities as employers by treating staff on their books as self-employed persons rather than employees. However, even where the courts sometimes accept for tax purposes that a person is self-employed, for health and safety work purposes they sometimes conclude the opposite – by applying a test as to who is really controlling the work – and treat the person as an employee and thus covered by relevant law such as the *MHOR 1992* (see e.g. *Lane v Shire Roofing* and the manual handling case of *Peck v Chief Constable of Avon and Somerset*). But even where the person is viewed as a genuine non-employee of the agency for all purposes, s.3 of the *Health and Safety at Work Act 1974* would still apply (see HSE 1998, p.3).

CARE ASSISTANTS

Care assistants working within the NHS, social services, residential homes, nursing homes or domiciliary care agencies, might well find themselves carrying out manual handling tasks. Their employer has duties in *health and safety at work legislation* generally, and under the *MHOR 1992* in particular, to take steps to identify and avoid or reduce risk to care assistants. Care assistants might be put at risk by poor manual handling policies, training and supervision; equally, the same factors might sometimes lead them – understandably in such circumstances – to react over-cautiously and defensively in what manual handling they are prepared to undertake.

Where the employer of a care assistant is a disabled person in his or her own home, then *health and safety work legislation* is thought not to apply by virtue of s.51 of the *Health and Safety at Work Act 1974*. However, the disabled person would still owe duties as an employer under the employment contract, and a duty of care under the common law of *negligence*. Certainly care assistants employed in such situations might be concerned about both their own safety and that of their disabled employer (Glendinning *et al.* 2000, p.26; Henwood 2001, p.67).

Where care assistants are employed through a *community care direct payment* the case (brought by a care assistant) of *Smith v South Lanarkshire Council* is relevant, in which an employment appeal tribunal upheld a decision that, in all the circumstances of the situation, her apparent employers were two disabled people – but that in reality the employer was the local authority.

Cases involving care assistants include: *Brodie v Kent County Council; Cantillon v London Nursing Homes; Fleming v Stirling Council; Gysen v St Luke's; Hopkinson v Kent County Council; Koonjul v Thameslink Healthcare NHS Trust; McIlgrew v Devon County Council; Miletic v Capital Territory Health Commission; Rowe v Swansea City Council; Schiliro v Peppercorn Child Care Centres.*

CARE HOMES

Under the *Care Standards Act 2000* (for England and Wales) and the *Regulation of Care (Scotland) Act 2001* (both due to come into force during 2002), care homes have to provide adequate facilities, services and equipment – including those related to manual handling – to a basic minimum standard, appropriate to the level of care for which the home is registered. (By way of specific contract with a local authority or NHS Trust, homes might of course have to provide more than this minimum – but this would be a contractual duty rather than a statutory duty under the regulatory legislation.) The Royal College of Nursing has produced a publication specifically for care homes on an integrated back injury prevention programme (RCN 2001).

Equipment provision in care homes. Beyond this, where equipment additional to that expected to be provided by care homes within their fee levels is required by individual residents, then if it is social care equipment, it should be arranged separately by the local authority social services department. If it is specialist nursing or medical equipment, it should be supplied by the NHS (for England and Wales, see guidance on continuing care: HSC 2001/15, and on 'free nursing home care': HSC 2001/17).

National standards. Nevertheless there is uncertainty about when services and equipment (including those related to manual handling) will come under the minimum expected of care homes, as set out in national standards – the application of which will guide registration and inspection of homes – and when the NHS and social services will be expected to provide, or at least pay for, extra services and equipment to meet special, individual needs of residents.

By way of example, standards applying to care homes for older people in England are vague on manual handling; for instance, they mention the provision of 'aids, hoists and assisted toilets and baths…which are capable of meeting the assessed needs of service users' (DH 2001b, standard 8). In terms of meeting residents' health care needs, the standards mention pressure care and continence but not manual handling (standard 22). However, they do make reference to the *MHOR 1992*, in respect of the employer's obligations toward staff (standard 38), since of course *health and safety at work legislation* applies to care homes just as to other organisations. For instance, in the past inspection and registration conditions imposed on nursing homes have usually included induction training on manual handling (SSI 2001, p.14).

CARE STANDARDS ACT 2000

During 2002, this Act will come into force and underpin in England and Wales the regulation of care provided by local authorities and the independent sector – including manual handling related services and equipment – in respect of, for example, care homes, domiciliary care providers, and independent health providers. For more detail, see *care homes* and *care agencies*; for Scotland, see the *Regulation of Care (Scotland) Act 2001*.

CARERS

Local authorities in England and Wales have explicit duties to assess the ability of certain carers to care, under the *Carers (Recognition and Services) Act 1995* and the *Carers and Disabled Children Act 2000* – and also, under the latter Act, to consider whether their needs call for services. In Scotland, the equivalent duties under the 1995 Act are to be found in s.12A(3A) of the *Social Work (Scotland) Act 1968* and s.24 of the *Children (Scotland) Act 1995*. At the time of writing, there is no equivalent to the 2000 Act in Scottish law.

Under these Acts, the carer must be providing substantial care on a regular basis. This condition is interpreted variably by local authorities (CNA 1997, p.36), although the most recent Department of Health guidance on the 2000 Act urges that an enlightened approach be taken, and in particular that the situation of the carer – and the impact of the caring, both physical and psychological, on the carer – be fully taken into account (DH 2001a, p.6). In addition, under these Acts, the assessment must be requested by the carer. Where the carer does not wish for an assessment and so does not request it, a local authority still has a duty to have regard to the person's ability to care for a disabled person under s.8 of the *Disabled Persons (Services, Consultation and Representation) Act 1986* when deciding what services to arrange for the disabled person (s.8 of the 1986 Act applies to both England and Scotland).

Clearly, manual handling considerations will be a key part of some carers' assessments, since carers might experience considerable physical and mental stress in handling the person they are caring for. Equipment, adaptations, personal assistance for manual handling, advice and information are all potentially relevant. By the same token, a failure by local authorities to think through and act promptly on the manual handling implications for carers will have a detrimental effect on the latter, as the *local government ombudsman* has pointed out many times in findings of maladministration (e.g. *Barking and Dagenham London Borough Council; Bristol City Council; Camden London Borough Council; Islington London Borough Council; Rotherham Metropolitan Borough Council*).

It is notable that no explicit parallel duties apply to the NHS, notwithstanding the fact that it is thought substantial numbers of informal carers of NHS patients suffer manual handling injuries (Henwood 1998, p.25).

CARERS (RECOGNITION AND SERVICES) ACT 1995

Under this 1995 Act, applying to England and Wales, local authorities have a duty to assess the ability of carers to provide care. Equivalent Scottish provisions are contained in s.12A(3A) of the *Social Work (Scotland) Act 1968*, and s.24 of the *Children (Scotland) Act 1995*. (For the importance of carers generally in the manual handling context, see under *carers*).

The circumstances are that the carer must be providing or intending to provide a substantial amount of care on a regular basis, and must request an assessment; also that an assessment is being or has been carried out of the person being cared for. Services cannot be provided for the carer, but the carer's assessment must be taken into account when the decision is being made as to what should be provided for the person being cared for. Paid carers or volunteer carers working for a voluntary organisation do not count as carers for the purposes of this Act.

The Act applies both to carers (of any age) caring for people aged eighteen or over (who must have had or be having a community care assessment) and to carers of disabled children under part 3 of the *Children Act 1989* and s.2 of the *Chronically Sick and Disabled Persons Act 1970*.

CARERS AND DISABLED CHILDREN ACT 2000

Under this 2000 Act, applying to England and Wales (at the time of writing, there is no equivalent for Scotland), local authorities have in some circumstances a duty to assess the ability of a *carer* to provide care. (For the importance of carers generally in the manual handling context, see under *carers*).

The circumstances are that the carer must be aged at least 16 years, must be providing or intending to provide a substantial amount of care on a regular basis, and must request an assessment. An assessment of the person being cared for is not a requisite (unlike under the *Carers (Recognition and Services) Act 1995*), but in that case the local authority must be satisfied that the person being cared for would potentially be eligible for community care services (and therefore be at least eighteen years old), were he or she to be assessed.

Services may be provided for the carer directly (again unlike under the 1995 Act), but (a) there is no duty to provide them and (b) they cannot be provided for the carer if they would be in effect intimate services for the person being cared for. In other words, even if a carer would benefit from such an intimate service, it would have to be provided directly for the person being cared for (i.e. under s.47 of the *NHS and Community Care Act 1990*, or s.12A of the *Social Work (Scotland) Act 1968*). Thus personal assistance and equipment for manual handling of the person being cared for would presumably be classed as intimate services and could not be provided under the 2000 Act; whereas the provision of training, information and advice on manual handling for the carer would not be intimate in relation to the person being cared for.

In addition, there is a duty to assess, on request, a person with parental responsibility for a disabled child who is providing or intending to provide substantial and regular care, if the local authority is satisfied that the child and his or her family are potentially eligible for services under s.17 of the *Children Act 1989*.

Paid carers, or volunteer carers working for voluntary organisations, do not come within the Act.

CAUSATION OF INJURY

Causation of injury bears twofold on the outcome of manual handling legal cases. First, even if a breach of duty under the *MHOR 1992* or in the common law of *negligence* can be shown, the court still has to be satisfied that the breach caused the injury (*Boyd v Lanarkshire Health Board*). For instance, proving a failure to carry out a risk assessment (*Hawkes v Southwark London Borough Council*) or to provide training (*Purvis v Buckinghamshire County Council*) will not be enough to establish employer liability, if the court is of the view that the accident would probably have happened anyway.

Second, even where liability is established, the employer might contest whether the extent of the injury claimed for can be accounted for by the particular accident in question, and so try to reduce the amount of damages payable. Such questions often involve detailed expert evidence as to matters such as a pre-existing back condition and how far it has been exacerbated and 'accelerated'; unrelated incidents subsequent to the accident; exaggeration by the employee; psychological considerations; alleged malingering; future employment prospects; witness credibility and so on. It is beyond the scope of this book to deal with these, but some manual handling cases are concerned substantially, and sometimes wholly, with such matters (e.g. *Colclough v Staffordshire County Council; Jones v South Glamorgan Health Authority; Pollitt v Oxfordshire Health Authority*).

CHALK v DEVIZES RECLAMATION COMPANY
Scrap metal yard; moving lump of lead under truck; efficacy of instructions; negligence case

A negligence case illustrating a tendency of the courts sometimes not to find liability in the context of what they consider to be everyday, commonsense tasks.

The plaintiff was employed as a labourer in a scrap metal yard. In 1991, a lump of lead fell off a pallet, and the plaintiff bent down to 'slew' (this word was distinguished from 'lift') it round and felt a pain in his back. He alleged that his employer had failed to provide either any, or proper, training. At first instance, the judge (recorder) had found that no instruction was given and so found in his favour. But the Court of Appeal now could not see, in this 'one-off incident…how any advice or training could be given in relation to it…The task was a relatively simple one and the piece of lead, as appears from the passages in the evidence…moved quite easily'. On the facts it was:

> quite impossible to make a finding that a system of work was unsafe in relation to training or instruction without evidence and a finding as to what the instruction and training should be… The plaintiff could not have been instructed as to how to carry out this particular operation and there is no reason why he should have been instructed not to do it. If one endeavours to envisage general instructions in relation to either the lifting or the moving of heavy objects, then such instructions would not in my view have had any effect at all on what the plaintiff actually did on this occasion, because the plaintiff, as he said himself, exercised his own common sense and judgement and it is easier for him to rotate or slew the piece of metal in the way in which he did and it was his misfortune that in doing so he sustained his injury to his back. No instruction would have prevented this particular accident from occurring ((1999) Times Law Reports, 2 April 1999, Court of Appeal).

CHANNON v EAST SUSSEX AREA HEALTH AUTHORITY
District nurse; lifting terminally ill patient for injection; under-staffing; over-work; cumulative strain argued; specificity of evidence; negligence case

The plaintiff was a district nurse claiming damages for an injury allegedly suffered in 1978 (at which time she was 37 years old) when she attended an elderly woman, whose terminal illness was being nursed at home. The woman was very heavy, unable to move herself and comatose or at least semi-comatose. The nurse had partially to lift and turn the patient and administer an injection; the woman's daughter assisted her. On this occasion she felt her back 'snap'. The nurse now claimed that the district nursing team was generally understaffed; that in the few weeks leading up to the accident, there was an even greater load on the plaintiff and team in general; and this had led to her injury.

Understaffing and overwork. The judge at first instance rejected these claims. The Court of Appeal upheld this decision. On the first question, the judge heard conflicting evidence as to whether three-and-half district nurses to cover a population of about 17,000 represented under-staffing; he concluded not, and the appeal court did not now disturb this finding. On the more specific allegation concerning the weeks up to the accident, when staff holidays meant that there was short-staffing in one particular week owing to staff on holiday, the Court of Appeal found no negligence. It went on to say that even had this been negligent, the plaintiff's evidence linking her injury with any overwork was not strong enough. Part of this evidence referred to the general fact that muscle tone, fatigue and repetitive jobs could lead to back problems, but had not specifically applied this to the plaintiff – who had argued that longer hours and heavier work had predisposed her to, or directly caused, a disc lesion (1989, Court of Appeal, unreported).

CHARNOCK v CAPITAL TERRITORY HEALTH COMMISSION AND CAROLINE KLEFISCH
Nursing aide; nursing home; instructions; wardsmen; insufficient use of lifting equipment; supervision

The case involved a nursing aide who worked in a nursing home. On the day of the injury in 1977, she was assisting with the moving of a resident for showering or bathing, who weighed 18 stone, and whom she had previously lifted without any problem. The aide was working under the direction of a nurse in order to move the patient from the bed to a bedside chair. The bed was not height adjustable. The manual handling involved the two staff linking arms behind the patient's back and linking arms under the upper part of the patient's legs. In so doing, and then subsequently going behind the chair to lift the patient higher up into the chair by the armpits, the aide felt pain in her back, and she could not stand up straightaway after the incident.

The aide alleged negligence of the employer on various grounds, including a lack of instruction in lifting heavy patients, failure of supervision on the day in question, failure to supply assistance to her in the form of wardsmen, and failure to supply assistance in the form of lifting equipment.

Instructions and wardsmen. The court found that the aide (on her own evidence) knew how to lift in the commonly accepted manner, and that she had also told the matron on coming to work at the nursing home that she had experience of lifting geriatric patients. Thus, there was no negligent omission to provide instruction. On the question of the use of wardsmen in nursing homes, the court found that at the time of the accident in 1977, the lack of wardsmen did not constitute negligence.

Lifting equipment. As to lifting equipment, the court found that a failure to have more than one lifting device was not negligent, but that the device was not used as often as it should have been. Thus:

> The defendant should have encouraged greater use of the mechanical aid. The defendant should have also sought to ensure that employees like the plaintiff and [the nurse], required to lift a patient of extraordinary weight, should have been placed in a position to make an informed choice as to how to perform the lift. The duty of the defendant is not simply to provide a reasonably safe system of work, it includes the duty to establish, maintain and enforce such a reasonably safe system. It is not enough simply to provide a device which will assist in minimising the risk of injury unless those susceptible to injury are at least encouraged to make use of the device. The evidence in the case establishes that the nursing staff entertained the belief, either correctly or mistakenly, that the lifting device was not available for practical purposes.

Supervision. The court also found that the second part of the move, in which the nurse allowed the aide to go to the back of the chair and take most of the patient's weight by pulling him up by the armpits, was negligence on the part of the nurse, albeit a momentary lapse. This lapse was indicative of a general failure to maintain and enforce a reasonably safe system of work.

Contributory negligence. The employer alleged contributory negligence in that the aide admitted that she knew she should not have been lifting in that way; and she had already felt some pain during the first part of the move. The court would have said that this failure to take care of her own safety was roughly equal to the nurse's lapse, and thus would constitute 50 per cent contributory negligence. However, the negligence of the employer was not just in respect of the nurse's lapse, but the overall system of work 'in the total context of the lack of male wardsmen, the failure of the defendant to keep the nursing staff aware of the need to employ a lifting device where necessary, and the nature of the defendant's enterprise where it was necessary for nursing staff in the position of the [aide] simply to try to get on with the job'. Therefore, the lack of reasonable care of the aide was not insignificant, but was overshadowed by the employer's lack of reasonable care; contributory negligence would therefore be fixed at 20 per cent only ([1988] ATSC 34, Supreme Court of the Australian Capital Territory).

CHILDREN

Children and the welfare of their carer parents, just as well as adults, might be at the heart of manual handling issues, in respect of both employee safety and the meeting of the children's needs.

Guidance. Royal College of Nursing and National Back Pain Association (now BackCare) guidance states that units dealing with babies and children should not concern themselves with rules not to lift; they should avoid the complexity of setting weight limits for lifting and concentrate instead on avoiding injury – by, for instance, considering issues like cot design which have greater implications for injury than the weight of the baby (RCN/NBPA 1997, p.24). It also contains a whole chapter on babies and children, which emphasises at its outset that staff and parents 'should not put their own health and safety at risk in the belief that the continuing welfare and development of the child is more important' (p.198). Other guidance from the Health and Safety Commission states that even small children with disabilities can present handling problems because of stiffness, weakness and their wearing of splints or braces (HSC 1998, p.44).

Cases. Manual handling cases involving children include alleged injuries suffered by: *school* assistants or teachers when attempting to restrain children (*Beasley v Buckinghamshire County Council; McLeod v Aberdeen City Council; Daws v Croydon London Borough Council*); a *foster carer* handling a disabled child placed with her by the local authority (*Beasley v Buckinghamshire County Council*); a residential social worker when a girl fell on her (*Wiles v Bedfordshire County Council*) and a care assistant filling a sandpit (*Schiliro v Peppercorn Child Care Centres*). It has also been reported that teachers sometimes incur injury through handling wheelchairs (Cassidy 2001).

CHILDREN ACT 1989

Section 17 of the Children Act 1989 places a general *duty* on local authorities in England and Wales to safeguard and promote the welfare of children in need, including disabled children. The duty also extends to other members of the family.

In one sense this is a very wide-ranging duty, and thus potentially strong, since it could embrace many services including personal assistance, manual handling, equipment, home adaptations and even provision of accommodation. However, in another sense the duty is vitiated, because the courts continue to state that in terms of individual entitlement of children and their families, it is a potentially weak duty, and places very limited obligations on local authorities (*A v Lambeth London Borough Council*). In other words, the courts give it the attributes of what they call a 'target duty' towards children in need generally, rather than a 'specific duty' toward each individual child in particular. Thus for manual handling related services, equipment and adaptations, disabled children are likely to be better served by the stronger duty under s.2 of the

Chronically Sick and Disabled Persons Act 1970 (see *R v Bexley London Borough Council, ex p B* which made this very point).

For the equivalent duty in Scotland, see s.22 of the *Children (Scotland) Act 1995*.

CHILDREN (SCOTLAND) ACT 1995

The Children (Scotland) Act 1995 places a duty on local authorities to safeguard and promote the welfare of children in need who are in the local authority's area (s.22), and to assess on request the ability of some *carers*, i.e. those providing substantial and regular care of disabled children (s.24). For discussion of the nature and strength of this duty toward children in need, see the *Children Act 1989* immediately above, which contains a similar duty. For carers' assessments generally, see under *carers*.

CHRONICALLY SICK AND DISABLED PERSONS ACT 1970 (CSDPA 1970)

The *duty* placed on local authorities (in England, Scotland and Wales) under s.2 of the *CSDPA 1970*, to arrange services to meet people's disabled needs, is a strong one, being an individual-orientated *duty*, rather than a general or target duty toward persons in general. The Act applies to both adults and children and is directly relevant to manual handling related issues.

Need and resources. Once a local authority has decided, against its eligibility criteria, that (a) there is a need, and (b) it is necessary for the authority to meet it, then a lack of resources is ultimately no defence for not meeting the need – although of two options, the local authority may choose the cheaper, so long as it genuinely meets the identified need (*R v Gloucestershire County Council, ex p Barry*). Furthermore, services can only be reduced or withdrawn following an individual reassessment, and on the basis of either a diminution of need or a change in the council's eligibility criteria. The implications of this duty were illustrated in the case of *R v Birmingham City Council, ex p Killigrew*, when a local authority attempted unlawfully to reduce services to a woman with multiple sclerosis following a manual handling assessment indicating that more staff were needed in order to deliver assistance safely.

Services. The services that fall to be provided under this Act are extensive and self-evidently relate to manual handling in some circumstances. For example, 'practical assistance' in the home might include personal assistance including manual handling; arranging attendance at activities or educational facilities or facilitating a holiday might involve manual handling issues; home adaptations or 'additional facilities' (including equipment) for a person's greater safety, comfort or convenience might be required to allow safe manual handling, or conversely to avoid the need for manual handling attended by unacceptable risk.

CHRONICALLY SICK AND DISABLED PERSONS (SCOTLAND) ACT 1972

This Act applies ss.1 and 2 of the *Chronically Sick and Disabled Persons Act 1970* to Scotland.

CLARKE v ADAMS

Physiotherapist; electrical treatment; following what had been taught; expert evidence from chief examiner; nevertheless liability; negligence case

A case illustrating that the following of what has been taught (or, by extension, guidance) is no substitute for the exercise of professional judgement in the particular circumstances.

A patient suffered burns to his left heel during electrical treatment provided by a physiotherapist. He had to have part of his leg amputated. The physiotherapist had given the following warning: 'When I turn on the machine I want you to experience a comfortable warmth and nothing more; if you do, I want you to tell me.' The chief examiner gave evidence that this was an entirely proper warning to give; and it was indeed the very warning that the physiotherapist had been taught. Nevertheless, the court found liability since in its view the warning had not been 'couched in terms which made it abundantly clear that it was a warning of danger' ((1950) 94 SJ 552, High Court).

CLARKE v OXFORDSHIRE HEALTH AUTHORITY

Student nurse; two-person lift; personal care; vulnerability of student nurses to injury; responsibility of higher management; negligence case

The plaintiff at the time of the accident in 1981 was a student nurse aged 18, and halfway through her course. She was working in a team of three, of whom the other members were a third-year student and an auxiliary nurse, lifting a highly dependent 12-stone patient. The 'orthodox' lift was used three times – with the plaintiff and one nurse lifting the patient, and the third washing the patient's buttocks, then drying, then changing the sheet. The plaintiff felt pain during the last of these tasks when she straightened up.

Australian lift, hoist and patient needs. The court accepted that the Australian lift could rightly have been rejected because it would cause pain to the patient and perhaps interfere with the healing process. Likewise, had a hoist been considered, the judge held that it would have been rejected on the grounds that the pressure exerted by the sling would have been likely to cause the patient considerable and unnecessary pain.

Three-person lift. However, in considering a three-person lift, the judge found that proper thought had not been given to the reduction from three to two nurses for the care of this particular patient. This was on the basis that the ward sister had stated that the reduction had been a:

natural progression. As they had been managing with two, I see no reason to have more... I can't remember if I was consulted about [the patient]... I don't say I wait until an accident before I recommend extra help, but if the patient is being lifted all right with two, there's no reason to have more; not if the two were quite happy with things. I find it very difficult to answer the question of how many nurses should have lifted [the patient].

The judge found that it had not been routine to apply thought, care and decision to student nurses in this situation. This was a fault in the system and represented a want of proper care. Damages were set at £2,700.

Creep factor. The court also accepted evidence about the 'creep factor', which meant that although the spine might recover from one heavy lift, the chance of recovery was significantly reduced if heavy lifts were repeated close together. Thus the judge accepted that the plaintiff had suffered injury through a repeated lifting procedure.

Student nurses. The judge:

had to bear in mind that it is student nurses who apparently are the class at greatest risk in orthopaedic wards because of their lack of physical development and experience, and also because they are, generally speaking, inherently less likely to be assertive and questioning. Is the high incidence of back injuries in the case of first year student nurses something which the defendants and other authorities can properly regard simply as the rub of the green; an inherent risk that has got to be run. Or are such students a class of young women, as they mostly are, who need particular care and protection? No problem, as it seems to me, financial, logistical or otherwise, would arise in giving special care, once it became routine to do so.

Responsibility at senior level.

It would be quite wrong and quite unfair for anyone to suppose that the ward sister is in any real sense the person who should bear any responsibility that thought was not given in the way that I have outlined. It is not for her to devise or enforce a system which takes special care for student nurses. The consciousness for such care must...begin at the top, and so must the initiation of appropriate measures so that they become routine.

Damages were awarded of some £11,500 (1986, High Court, unreported).

COAD v CORNWALL AND ISLES OF SCILLY HEALTH AUTHORITY
State enrolled nurse; delay in bringing case; whether case precluded by Limitation Act; negligence case
A case illustrating the court's preparedness in some circumstances to waive the legal time limit for bringing a compensation claim in respect of manual handling injury.

A state enrolled nurse was injured lifting a quadriplegic patient in August 1983 when she was 27 years old. She did not issue a writ until nearly 10 years later. She had acquired the relevant knowledge for the purposes of s.14 of the *Limitation Act 1980* (which imposes a limit of three years on bringing a negligence action) on the date of the accident. But the court chose to exercise its discretion under s.33 to disapply the limitation period, because she did not know and did not realise that she could bring an action against the defendants (because she had been able to return to work following the accident).

The Court of Appeal held that s.33 should be interpreted subjectively rather than objectively when looking to 'all the circumstances of the case and in particular to the length of and reasons for the delay on the part of the plaintiff'. One factor supporting the exercise of this discretion was the availability of good documentation to support the case. Some of the evidence referred to the fact that there was no lifting equipment in that part of the hospital on the evening of the accident, and that there was never a hoist in the bathroom of the ward and slings were never seen in the hospital ([1997] 8 Med LR 154, Court of Appeal).

COLCLOUGH v STAFFORDSHIRE COUNTY COUNCIL
Social worker; elderly client; helping him back to bed; injury; warning/instructions; negligence case

A case illustrating the high cost to a local authority of not providing even basic information or warnings about manual handling.

In 1989, a social worker aged 30 visited a client at home who weighed 15 stone. She found him lying half out of bed, with a neighbour there (a nurse). The nurse guided the social worker in moving him. She felt something give in her lower back. She had received no training in lifting techniques. Judgment was given on liability in the County Court in June 1994 on the basis that it was reasonably foreseeable that the plaintiff might be confronted with emergency situations. Although the situation was unusual, she should have been warned not to lift in such circumstances; even if a long training course was not warranted, the risks of lifting should have been brought to her notice. There was no contributory negligence.

Subsequently, a separate High Court hearing dealt with damages. Very detailed evidence was given relating to the woman's prior medical history and events subsequent to this injury. She was eventually awarded over £200,000 in relation to claims for both past and future loss of earnings, the cost of past and future domestic and gardening assistance, loss of pension rights and some minor expenses. She had claimed the injury led to pain, suffering, disability, stress, anxiety, breakdown of marriage, and loss of employment.

The council accepted that an injury had occurred but argued that the discs in her back were already vulnerable to injury through degeneration; that the injury itself gave rise to short-term symptoms only; that longer-term effects were due to pre-existing degeneration and complicated by emotional and psychological problems, difficulty in coping with work and with her family situation. These contentions, designed to reduce substantially any damages, were on the whole rejected by the court; damages of over £200,000 were awarded ([1994] CL 94/2283, County Court, on liability; and (1997) High Court, unreported, on damages: see Zindani 1998, p.189).

COMMONS v QUEEN'S MEDICAL CENTRE NOTTINGHAM UNIVERSITY HOSPITAL NHS TRUST
Nurse; use of fixed height beds; defective wheelchair; cumulative strain; MHOR 1992; Provision and Use of Work Equipment Regulations 1992

A staff nurse's claim for personal injury was based on repeated heavy lifting which could have been avoided by the provision of adjustable height beds, hoists or other mechanical devices for lifting patients. It also included alleged failure to provide a wheelchair safe for its purpose and a wheelchair with properly inflated tyres.

Height adjustable beds. For three weeks in 1994, prior to the wheelchair incident, she claimed that her back had been sore, although there was no identifiable incident to account for it. She reported this to colleagues and they assisted her with manual handling; however, when they were not available, she had to continue to lift, turn and support patients by herself. In other words, she asked for help, but only sometimes received it. This lifting, turning and supporting in the high dependency unit was made more arduous because of a lack of height adjustable beds – despite the fact that repeated requests for such beds had been made but none provided (until 1995, after the accident).

Wheelchair with a soft tyre. The wheelchair incident concerned a 20-stone lady in reception, barely mobile with two walking crutches, who needed to be pushed some 175 yards to the ward to see her husband who had suffered a suspected heart attack. At the time there was a shortage of porters, and one would not be available for an hour. The nurse went to reception where another nurse identified a wheelchair; however, the claimant nurse noticed that one of the rear tyres was soft and pointed this out to the other nurse – but was told that this was the only one available. The claimant then suffered an acute and extreme pain to her lower back during the wheelchair journey.

Liability. The court found that the heavy lifting that the claimant had been required to undertake would have been significantly reduced had a patient hoist and adjustable height beds been provided (as they later were). It considered that the note written by one of the claimant's colleagues – to the effect that it was ironic that the new beds finally arrived only after a wheelchair-pushing incident – 'singularly prophetic and accurate in the circumstances'. The wheelchair incident had significantly damaged her back, given the pre-existing soreness and stiffness from the general lifting she was having to undertake.

Cumulative strain. The evidence given in the case seemed mainly to argue that the cumulative strain involved prior to the wheelchair tyre incident was due to the soreness in the immediately preceding three weeks. At one point, one of the claimant's experts stated that increased strain had been placed on her back during that three-week period and 'possibly before this'. However, in his conclusions the judge stated firmly that there was 'repeated minor trauma to the claimant's back during the heavy lifting that she carried out over many years' on the ward.

Contributory negligence? The court rejected the suggestion of contributory negligence since it had not been obvious to the nurse that the soft tyre represented a risk of injury; and the NHS Trust anyway accepted that an alternative wheelchair was not available and that the wheelchair in question was not in a reasonable condition. Damages of about £330,000 were awarded (2001, County Court, unreported).

COMMUNITY CARE DIRECT PAYMENTS

When local authority social services departments have assessed people's needs and decided that services are called for under community care legislation, they have the power to make direct payments of money to clients so that the latter can arrange their own services, rather than the local authority doing so. The client must consent to the direct payment and in the view of the local authority be able to manage the payment (with or without assistance).

This power exists in England and Wales under the *Community Care (Direct Payments) Act 1996* and associated regulations in respect of disabled adults (as defined in the *National Assistance Act 1948*), carers (in relation to the *Carers and Disabled Children 2000*) - and under the *Children Act 1989* (s.17A) in respect of disabled children aged 16 to 17 years old, and the parents of disabled children. During 2002, it is expected that the power will become a duty and that direct payments will be extended to the disabled parents of children (ss.57-58 of the Health and Social Care Act 2001).

In Scotland, the power exists under ss.12B-12C of the *Social Work (Scotland) Act 1968* and associated regulations in respect of disabled people, disabled children aged 16 to 17 years old and disabled parents of children. It is intended through further legislation that, amongst other things, the power to make payments will become a duty, and to extend payments to the parents of children, and also to all community care clients.

Contracting with an agency. One way in which the recipients of direct payments may choose to spend the money in order to meet their assessed needs is on personal assistance, which might include manual handling. They may contract with a care agency, in which case the recipients are not employers but merely have a contract with the agency; then the *MHOR 1992* would apply as between the employer (the agency) and the assistant (employee). Otherwise, if the assistant wished to sue the recipient of the payment in case of accident, he or she would need to use the law of negligence.

Employing assistants directly. Alternatively, the recipient of the payment might employ one or more assistants directly and ostensibly be in the position of employer. In case of accident, the assistant would still have to sue in negligence, since it appears that the application of the *MHOR 1992* would be excluded by s.51 of the *Health and Safety at Work Act 1974*, which states that nothing in Part 1 of the 1974 Act (including, therefore, regulations made under it) applies 'in relation to a person by reason only that he employs another, or is himself employed, as a domestic servant in a private household' (s.51).

Manual handling issues. In case of accident, some local authorities are concerned that an assistant employed by the recipient might choose to sue the local authority which had made the payment, either instead of or as well as the recipient. In order to avoid this happening, local authorities might well – as part of their monitoring of the direct payment (i.e. to make sure that the recipient is spending it so as to meet his or her assessed needs) – consider manual handling aspects, and intervene if they believe that unacceptable risks are being taken.

The difficulty that local authorities have in this respect is that on the one hand, they remain ultimately responsible for the situation insofar as payments are made on the basis of statutory assessments of need and decisions about services under the *NHS and Community Care Act 1990* and *Social Work (Scotland) Act 1968*. On the other hand, the idea behind community care direct payments is to give clients greater independence and choice in organising their lives; and over-intrusion by local authorities would run counter to this purpose. The answer would appear to be that local authorities should steer a middle course and that any interference on health and safety grounds should be proportionate to the degree of risk identified. Certainly, authorities have the legal power to intervene; under the legislation they have the power ultimately to stop payments if they feel that the payment is not being used to meet the person's needs in an acceptable way. Of some reassurance to local authorities is the fact that the courts will presumably bear in mind the statutory context and recognise the arms-length nature of direct payments before imposing liability in a negligence case.

Liability of local authorities? Nevertheless, the case of *Smith v South Lanarkshire Council* has given some local authorities pause for thought as an illustration of how they might ultimately be held liable if things go wrong. The case involved two people with learning disabilities who ostensibly had a contract with a personal assistant, who was paid with money – not a community care direct payment – from the Independent Living Fund (a grant-giving body) and from a social work department. The assistant was bringing a case against her employer, based on allegations of sex discrimination and breach of contract, and was unsure who her employer really was. An employment tribunal held that because the local authority retained overall control of the situation in a number of respects, and conversely the two people with learning disabilities appeared to take little responsibility, it was the local authority which was in reality the employer.

However, this decision of the tribunal should arguably not cause undue concern in respect of community care direct payments, since one of the conditions which must be met for a direct payment is that the recipient be able to manage the payment

– i.e. that he or she retain ultimate control. This clearly did not happen in the *Smith* case (although the potentially restrictive comments made by the employment appeal tribunal, in the same case, should be noted).

(If an assistant wished to sue in *negligence* for an accident, and include the local authority in the case, he or she would not need to show that the local authority was employer, but simply that it owed him or her a duty of care. However, if an employment relationship were to be shown, then he or she would have the option of bringing – for instance, in the manual handling context – a case against the local authority not just in *negligence*, but also under the *MHOR 1992*.)

COMMUNITY CARE (DIRECT PAYMENTS) ACT 1996: see *community care direct payments*

COMMUNITY CARE SERVICES
Community care legislation gives local authorities duties and powers to arrange services for meeting the needs of adults with community care needs. Some of these duties are relatively strong, as demonstrated by the significant number of community care cases in the courts which local authorities have lost. Thus, when formulating and implementing manual handling policies both generally and in respect of individual clients, local authorities must bear in mind not just their health and safety work duties toward staff under the *MHOR 1992* and their duties towards clients under s.3 of the *Health and Safety at Work Act 1974*, but crucially also their duties to meet clients' needs under legislation such as the *NHS and Community Care Act 1990, National Assistance Act 1948, Social Work (Scotland) Act 1968* and *Chronically Sick and Disabled Persons Act 1970*. In other words, the decision-making process needs properly to balance manual handling concerns with client need in the overall assessment.

CONTRACTING SERVICES OUT: see *care agencies; care homes*

CONTRACTS
Well resourced, drafted, placed, monitored and reviewed contracts, placed by local authorities and NHS Trusts with care agencies and care homes, are likely – in relation to manual handling issues – to promote patient and client welfare and safety, agency employee safety, clarity of responsibility, and discharge of local authority and NHS statutory duties. They are likely also even to save money, by making unnecessary the typically disorganised and ad hoc commitment of staff time required to solve the confusion arising from unclear contractual arrangements. The Health and Safety Commission makes this sort of point in its manual handling guidance (HSC 1998, pp.26,39–40). It should also be noted that terms and conditions in contracts can exceed the so-called minimum standards demanded of care agencies and homes under regulatory legislation (i.e. the *Care Standards Act 2000* and *Regulation of Care (Scotland) Act 2001*).

CONTRIBUTORY NEGLIGENCE: see *negligence*

COOPERATION AND COORDINATION IN A SHARED WORK-PLACE

This is a specific duty placed on employers under the *Management of Health and Safety at Work Regulations 1999*. Clearly it could apply in the manual handling context – for example, in a person's own home, if there were more than one agency involved such as the local authority social services department, the NHS and a private care agency.

CREEP FACTOR: see *cumulative strain*

CULLEN v NORTH LANARKSHIRE COUNCIL

Lifting and handling; scope of tasks covered by the MHOR 1992; negligence case

A council worker was injured in 1993 when unloading fencing from a truck; whilst holding a section of fencing above his head, he caught his heel on some of the other fencing material and fell backwards out of the truck, striking his shoulder on the ground. The Outer House gave judgment against the pursuer under both negligence and the *MHOR 1992*, stating that the general mischief addressed by the regulations was strain injury through the handling of loads. (It was agreed that the load he had been holding above his head was not of excessive weight, either of itself or when considered in the light of other ergonomic factors.)

Relevant risk under the MHOR 1992 – not limited to back injury or heavy loads. However, the Inner House now overturned this decision, finding that no such restriction was to be implied. It considered the wording in article 2 of the original *European directive* on which the *MHOR 1992* are based, and concluded that the relevant risk was not limited to the risk of back injury or strain injury, or to risks arising from excessively heavy loads. Thus the definition of injury was largely unrestricted. The directive defined the manual handling of loads as a number of activities with a load:

> 'which by reason of its characteristics or of unfavourable ergonomic conditions, involves a risk particularly of back injury to workers'. It appears to us to be natural to interpret the involvement of risk as referring to those activities rather than to the load itself. In any event the article does not appear to us to make the characteristics of the load an essential component in the creation of the relevant risk.

Liability was established by the pursuer, since it was not in dispute that – assuming the manual handling operation did come under the *MHOR 1992* – the employer was in breach of the duty to avoid the risk posed by it. Indeed, the *MHOR 1992* were triggered even if the risk of injury was only a foreseeable possibility, rather than a probability – in which case the employer had therefore to turn its mind either to avoiding the risk or reducing it. This it had not done. Damages had already been agreed at £36,553 ((1998) SC 451, Inner House, Second Division, Court of Session, Scotland).

CUMULATIVE STRAIN

Many manual handling cases involve consideration not just of the injury which has precipitated some disability or inability to work, but also of the extent to which the employee had a pre-existing back condition. It would appear that often such a condition is due to repeated strain caused by manual handling at work over time; this is sometimes referred to as cumulative 'micro-trauma'. However, far from assisting employees, this fact has generally assisted employers who point to the pre-existing condition either to deny liability or at least to reduce the damages payable, on the grounds that the actual injury in question has merely accelerated or exacerbated a condition which would soon have made the employee unfit for work.

The problem facing employees in arguing cumulative strain has turned not only on legal *time limits* for bringing actions (e.g. *Daws v Croydon London Borough Council*) – although these could be overcome by arguing a lack of awareness of the cumulating injury – but more particularly on the inability to lead evidence and to prove such cumulative injury (*Channon v East Sussex Area Health Authority*).

Certainly the courts have long recognised the 'creep factor' as being a form of cumulative stress caused by repeated heavy manual handling over a short period of time, such as within a working day (*Blair v Lancaster Health Authority; Clarke v Oxfordshire Health Authority; Edwards v Waltham Forest Health Authority*). This is quite different from accepting cumulative injury over a longer period. Yet this very issue has been argued, apparently with some success, in a few recent cases. In the first, most of the evidence appeared to focus on cumulative strain developed over three weeks, although the judge stated in his conclusions that it had in fact arisen over a number of years (*Commons v Queen's Medical Centre*). In the second case, involving repeated awkward lifting in a stationery store, the court accepted that the injury sustained was unlikely to have been caused by one specific incident, but by a history of incidents during a two-year employment period (*Stone v Commissioner of Police for the Metropolis*). In a third, cumulative strain over two weeks was accepted as the cause of injury, as opposed to one specific injury (*Wells v West Hertfordshire Health Authority*). The Court of Appeal in a fourth case accepted that a condition of gastro-oesophageal reflux had been exacerbated by heavy lifting over a number of years, resulting in permanent impairment of the claimant's ability to work (*Welsh v Matthew Clark Wholesale*). Injury from repetitive tasks over a number of years was also accepted as at least arguable by the Court of Session in *Black v Wrangler*.

CUSTOM AND PRACTICE

If an employer is aware of and tolerates unsafe manual handling as a matter of 'custom and practice' – when it has failed to address the risk at all, when there is a policy to the contrary but efforts are not made to enforce it, or even sometimes when employees themselves know that they should not be following such practice – then the courts might impose liability. This might be in respect of routine lifts of 15-stone patients (*Blair v Lancaster Health Authority*); factory work (*Brown v Allied Ironfounders*); a prevailing ethos arising from staff shortages which meant that even experienced staff believed it their duty to perform unsafe lifting (*Forder v Norfolk Area Health Authority*); or the non-correction of bad lifting habits amongst nurses (*Salvat v Basingstoke and North Hampshire Health Authority*).

D v UNITED KINGDOM

Human rights; inhuman treatment; deportation of terminally ill man

This case illustrates a breach of article 3 of the *European Convention on Human Rights*, in terms of inhuman treatment. There is speculation that in some (extreme) circumstances, in the manual handling context, article 3 might be engaged (see e.g. *Price v United Kingdom*).

The applicant was suffering from the advanced stages of AIDS and challenged his removal to St Kitts on the grounds that there were inadequate medical facilities there. The court found that although as a general rule those facing deportation had no right to remain to benefit from medical, social or other forms of assistance, nevertheless in the exceptional circumstances, removal would be inhuman treatment under article 3 since it would have dramatic consequences for the applicant, including the hastening of his death ([1997] 24 EHRR 423, European Court of Human Rights).

DAMAGES

Damages awarded in manual handling compensation claims can be very substantial; for instance, over £300,000 (*Commons v Queen's Medical Centre*), £184,000 (*McGowan v Harrow Health Authority*), £205,252 (*McIlgrew v Devon County Council*). They are awarded under two main headings known as general damages (covering pain, suffering and loss of amenity) and special damages (covering loss of earnings, effect on pension, prospects of alternative work, personal assistance, equipment or home adaptations required, and so on).

DAWS v CROYDON LONDON BOROUGH COUNCIL

Teacher; restraining violent pupils in special school; back injury; modifying environment; cumulative nature of injury rejected; training; negligence case

A case involving injury sustained by a teacher, brought in *negligence*, but not for some reason under the *MHOR 1992* – although liability was anyway established. The teacher at a special school for emotionally and behaviourally disturbed children won compensation after suffering a back injury in 1996 when she was 53 years old; she had restrained a pupil who was swinging along a bar running across the ceiling of the classroom.

Regime for control of children's behaviour. The judge's decision hinged on a finding that, had there been a tighter regime for controlling the behaviour of children, there would have been significantly fewer incidents requiring staff to restrain pupils. The judge found that a pre-existing degenerative condition of her back was exacerbated by the incident, but would not entertain any argument relating to previous incidents which might have caused this condition, since in his view the *Limitation Act 1980* would preclude this. In addition, the judge found that the failure of the school to remove furniture giving access to the ceiling bars – despite the claimant having brought the problem to its attention some two years previously – also revealed a degree of inattention.

Training in restraint techniques. The judge did not find negligence in relation to the absence of training, on the basic ground that there was sparse evidence about specialist training and the extent to which other local authorities provided it, and because he was not convinced that such training would anyway have prevented the injury, given that it would substantially have been directed toward avoidance of injury to children rather than to staff. He also mentioned in this respect the fact that the education authority's resources were under substantial strain (2001, London County Court, unreported: but referred to in Hayes 2001).

DEGRADING TREATMENT

Degrading treatment, referred to in article 3 of the *European Convention on Human Rights*, is one ground on which human rights cases can be brought under the *Human Rights Act 1998*; there has been speculation about its application to manual handling situations. See *European Convention on Human Rights*.

DENTON v SOUTH WEST THAMES REGIONAL HEALTH AUTHORITY

Nurse auxiliary; faulty bed castor; no system for checking; negligence case

This case illustrates the importance of having a reasonable system of maintenance even under the law of *negligence* (the *Provision and Use of Work Equipment Regulations 1998* now impose stricter liability still in respect of such maintenance).

The plaintiff was a 46-year-old auxiliary nurse who was injured in 1977 when she was about to move, with another nurse, a heavy patient sitting up in bed from the bed to a chair. As they each went round to one side of the bed, the patient suddenly tipped toward the plaintiff, who found herself taking his weight in order to prevent him falling onto the locker on that side of the bed. She did not have the time to get into the proper position for handling him, and felt something 'pull away' in the middle of her back.

No system for checking safety of beds. Liability was established. The cause of the accident was a faulty castor assembly which had caused the bed to tip and partially collapse. The judge noted that a previous system for maintaining hospital furniture, beds and equipment had been abandoned because of cash limits and the pressure on hospital beds (this system had involved the wards being closed once a year, during which time the beds would be sent away for a general overhaul). The system now was that if something went wrong with furniture or equipment, the engineers would be called – but this would of course be on a reactive basis only. The district engineer was unhappy with this, foreseeing that if checks were not made periodically then patients could be seriously hurt, since he knew that wheels did come off beds about twice a year.

The judge found there was no system of checking beds for safety, but there should have been; the injury to the plaintiff was foreseeable, and the health authority's allegation of contributory negligence was rejected out of hand. Damages of £28,480 were awarded (1980, High Court, unreported).

DEWING v ST LUKE'S (ANGLICAN CHURCH IN AUSTRALIA) ASSOCIATION

Enrolled nurse; heavy patient; adjustable height beds; lifting straps; negligence case

A case illustrating the importance of using manual handling equipment. An enrolled nurse aged 38 was working in 1993 on a night shift in a nursing home, which had over seventy residents, most of whom were elderly, many of whom were bed-ridden or wholly or partially immobile, and many of whom suffered from dementia. She went with another nurse to rouse and to assist a 93-year-old resident to sit up. (Her duties were barely distinguishable in nature from those of this other nurse; but the latter was the sister-in-charge and night supervisor.) The resident had dementia and cardiac problems and sometimes stiffened his body to resist during manual handling. The plaintiff denied that she knew this; the court did not accept this assertion, although it did accept that she was not familiar with his care plan.

When he was being sat up by the two nurses using the 'cradle lift', the resident resisted and stiffened; the plaintiff was pulled sideways and twisted round; she suffered a back injury. The plaintiff claimed that the negligence lay in either the failure of the other nurse to use lifting straps or other equipment, or in an unsafe *system of work* insofar as the bed – which was not height adjustable – was unsuitable for its purpose.

Adjustable height beds. On the question of beds the court found no negligence. In 1993, when the accident occurred, some patients at the nursing home had height adjustable beds, their allocation being based on relative priorities. Given that the nursing home was a charitable operation, heavily dependent upon government funding, it 'would obviously be a very heavy expense to replace seventy-six standard, non-adjustable beds with the adjustable kind all at one time'. This would have been an unreasonable expectation; furthermore, the court was of the view that even an adjustable height bed would not necessarily have avoided the need for a similar type lift as was actually performed.

Lifting straps. The resident's care plan provided that lifts should be accomplished using blue lifting straps. The failure of the other nurse to use the straps, which were close at hand, or to direct the plaintiff to use them, was an act of casual negligence for which the employer was liable. The other nurse should have realised that 'there was a real risk of injury, both to herself and the plaintiff in adopting the procedure which she followed. That risk could have been avoided or minimised by the use of blue lifting straps'.

Contributory negligence. However, the court also found a high degree of contributory negligence, measured at 35 per cent, since the plaintiff – an experienced employee, as opposed to a more junior member of staff – would have been aware of the importance of using straps ([1999] TASSC 39, Supreme Court of Tasmania, Australia).

DICKSON v LOTHIAN HEALTH BOARD
Nursing assistant; ineffective training and tuition; underarm technique for lifting patients from the floor; custom and practice; negligence case

A case in which the court identified ineffective training and its consequences for manual handling on the wards, which meant that senior staff never interfered with unsafe lifts.

Lifting patient from floor. A 38-year-old nursing assistant had been one of two nursing staff who were lifting a patient from the floor of the hospital ward in 1986. The ward provided care for elderly, confused, male patients, some of whom were uncooperative, obstructive and occasionally aggressive. The patient in question frequently lay on the floor and refused to move. The pursuer and a colleague lifted him by each putting one hand under his armpit and beneath his shoulder, and then proceeded to lever him up from the waist to a sitting position without moving his bottom along the floor. As they repositioned their feet and hands, ready to stand the patient up, the pursuer experienced sharp back pain.

Differing views of experts and practising nurses. The expert evidence called roundly condemned this method of lifting; yet the practising nurses who appeared as witnesses approved of it. The judge commented on the lack of understanding – of the basic mechanics of lifting and of the risks to which they were exposed – of the practising nurses. Nevertheless, it was clear that neither the pursuer's colleagues, nor her superiors, criticised the lift she had used.

Ineffective tutorials. One of the witnesses (who referred to the Royal College of Nursing and Back Pain Association 1981 guidance, 'The handling of patients') was the health board's training officer who gave evidence that she had taught and trained nurses to the effect that this underarm technique was proscribed. However, the judge did not accept that any such proscription had been conveyed effectively, given that (a) in general the practising nurses denied that it had been, denied receiving instructions that three nurses should always be involved in lifting a patient from the floor, and denied that they had ever seen the relevant booklet or video; and (b) the tutorials had been held in the middle of the night in a relatively light-hearted atmosphere. Although the judge accepted that this was not an unreasonable method for the training officer to adopt given the shortage of time made available to her, nevertheless, 'the combination of the hour, the temporary release of nurses from ward duties, and the need to communicate a large amount of information provided a context in which it was all too likely that there would be less than full appreciation of the scope of the teaching'.

Inadequate system of work, toleration by senior staff of unsafe lifts. In any case, whatever went on in the tutorials, the court

> was clear beyond doubt that following the tutorials there was no effective system of any kind in operation within the hospital to ensure that any prohibition that was communicated to the nurses was enforced. The medium of enforcement of such a prohibition relied on was the control of operations by the senior nurses in charge of the wards…none of them ever in fact did interfere with an operation involving' the underarm technique. The health board should have taken effective steps to monitor the lifting techniques used in wards. Further, no question of contributory negligence arose since, as a nursing assistant, the pursuer was entitled to rely on the supervision available to her: she could 'hardly be blamed for continuing to use a technique which was not only tolerated but apparently approved of by her superiors on whom she was entitled to rely.

Damages were awarded of £31,000 ((1994) SLT 525, Outer House, Court of Session, Scotland).

DISABILITY DISCRIMINATION ACT 1995

The Disability Discrimination Act 1995 has a number of different parts; one concerns employment, another the provision of goods and services to the public.

Employees. As far as employees go, it has been suggested that, for example, the NHS will have to think seriously about finding alternative work for employees who have become disabled through manual handling injury, by making reasonable adjustments to working arrangements (RCN/NBPA 1997, p.12).

Goods and services. As far as discrimination in the provision of goods and services to the public goes – and the perceived adverse effects which NHS and social services manual handling policies and decisions sometimes have on patients and clients – the scarcity of case law under the relevant part of the Act makes it difficult to say quite how manual handling decisions might be challenged.

Education. It should be noted that with manual handling issues in mind, an amendment (contained in the *Special Educational Needs and Disability Act 2001*) to the 1995 Act extends it – in respect of provision of goods and services – to education. However, it should be noted that it expressly states that the duty to avoid discrimination by substantially disadvantaging disabled pupils does not require the provision of auxiliary aids (i.e. equipment) or services or alterations to premises (s.28C of the

1995 Act, expected to be in force from September 2002). This is potentially a significant limitation, since so often the meeting of manual handling related needs will involve equipment, human support or appropriate physical access to parts of the school. The government's explanation, that such needs will be covered by statements of special educational needs (in England and Wales) or records of need (in Scotland), would appear to be unsatisfactory, given that (a) such statements or records are for various reasons not always effective in regard to such matters; and also (b) that not all children with special educational needs will necessarily have a statement or record of needs anyway (SO 2001).

DISABLED PERSONS (SERVICES, CONSULTATION AND REPRESENTATION) ACT 1986

Under s.8 of this Act, a local authority has a duty to take account of a carer's ability to care for a disabled person when deciding what services to provide for the disabled person. The carer must be providing a substantial amount of care on a regular basis; but the duty does not depend on a request by the carer, nor does it appear to exclude carers from private or voluntary organisations, or simply those directly hired by the disabled person. See also *carers; Carers (Recognition and Services) Act 1995, Carers and Disabled Children Act 2000, Social Work (Scotland) Act 1968, Children (Scotland) Act 1995.*

DIVIT v BRITISH TELECOMMUNICATIONS
Telephone engineer; cutting hand on telephone box hinged flap; whether coming under MHOR 1992

This case demonstrates the potential scope of the *MHOR 1992*, in terms of the type of activity and load covered.

The pursuer was a British Telecom engineer. He was repairing a telephone kiosk, and standing on small folding steps. On completing the work, he closed the flap in the roof, cutting his hand on it. The matter in issue at the present hearing was whether the case could come under r.4(1)(a) of the *MHOR 1992* at all. The pursuer argued that the flap was difficult to manipulate and had a razor-sharp edge. The defenders argued that under the regulations, a load could only be something that was free to move about without connection or attachment to some other thing, and that injury must have arisen directly in relation to the strain or force involved in handling the load.

The court rejected the defender's argument, stating that a load could be hinged to something else and could be pushed, pulled or moved by hand or bodily force from one position to another around the hinge – which movement could constitute transporting or supporting as defined in regulation 2(1). Injury was not limited to strain injury and could include a cutting injury or burn (from the temperature of a load) received in the course of manual or bodily handling of the load – even though neither of these types of injury related to the weight of, or degree of force being applied to, the load (summarised in: (1997) SLG, 65(3), 130–131, Outer House, Court of Session, Scotland).

DOCUMENTATION

Legally, adequate documentation in relation to manual handling related policies and individual decisions is often essential as *evidence* that employers as a whole adhered to their duties – for instance, in maintaining hoists (*Eaton v West Lothian NHS Trust*). Indeed, under r.5 of the *Provision and Use of Work Equipment Regulations 1998*, under which the *Eaton* case was brought, there is a duty to keep maintenance logs up to date for work equipment. Likewise, under the *Lifting Operations and Lifting Equipment Regulations 1998*, there are duties of documentation in relation to the examination and inspection of lifting equipment used at work.

For any individual employees being accused of negligence or bringing compensation claims of their own, documentation might be crucial evidence. Adequate record-keeping is anyway demanded unconditionally of employees such as nurses and therapists by their professional bodies (e.g. CSP 2002, p.15; UKCC 1998, p.5; COT 2000, p.6).

Health and Safety Executive guidance nevertheless makes the point that while in general risk assessments should be recorded and kept accessible for as long as is relevant, this is not necessary if (a) the assessments can be easily repeated and explained because they are so obvious and simple; or (b) the manual handling tasks are quite straightforward, of low risk, will last only a short time, and it would be a disproportionate use of time to record them (HSE 1998, p.12).

DOHERTY v TUNBRIDGE WELLS HEALTH AUTHORITY
District nurse; stroke patient in own home; lifting; not credible evidence or nurse's own fault; discounting of changed care plan few weeks following accident; negligence case

The plaintiff was a nurse claiming for an injury sustained in 1983 when visiting a woman at home who had had a stroke and was chairbound during the day. Normally the visiting nurse would get her up, put her on the lavatory, sit her back on the bed and then put her into the wheelchair. This would be carried out with help from the husband who was still physically robust. When she required a bath, two nurses would visit. On the day in question, the plaintiff alleged injury when she placed her arms under the woman's armpits and raised her to her feet. She argued that she should not have been sent alone to provide such nursing.

However, three other nurses all gave evidence that they would lift the woman differently – under her armpit and legs, while the husband would lift her under her other armpit. The judge at first instance had held that this was a reasonable system, exposing the nurses to no unreasonable risk; that the plaintiff's account of her method of lifting was probably false; and that if she had indeed lifted in the way she described, then she was to blame for her own injury. He did not accept that the reason she would have carried out such a lift was because the husband did not help, since all the evidence suggested otherwise. Furthermore, the fact that by 30 November the woman's nursing notes disclosed efforts to use a hoist and the attendance of two nurses did not help the plaintiff, since the accident occurred on 5 November.

The Court of Appeal now upheld the judge's findings and dismissed the plaintiff's appeal (1988, Court of Appeal, unreported).

DUTIES

Duties in legislation impose obligations, as opposed to powers which can be exercised at the discretion of an organisation. However, duties themselves are not necessarily absolute or unconditional.

Duty to do what is reasonably practicable. In *health and safety at work legislation*, many duties are qualified by the term *reasonably practicable*, and can be contrasted, for example, with the apparently absolute duty on employers to maintain work equipment – including manual handling equipment – in r.5 of the *Provision and Use of Work Equipment Regulations 1998* (for its far-reaching effect see *Stark v Post Office*). Even so, if on the evidence risk is identified, then – unless the cost of doing something about it is grossly disproportionate to that risk – the courts will hold that it is reasonably practicable to do something about it (even if the cost is high), and so impose in effect an absolute duty in those circumstances (*Edwards v National Coal Board*). In principle, the same goes for the duty of care in *negligence*, involving reasonableness, owed by employers toward employees (e.g. *Fitzsimmons v Northumberland Health Authority*).

Individual welfare duties. In *welfare legislation*, there are at least two types of duty. The first type the courts treat as an individual duty imposed on public bodies, potentially enforceable by individuals in judicial review cases. These duties are relatively few, but include the provision in community care of residential and nursing home accommodation, and also of non-residential welfare services (including those related to manual handling) for disabled people under s.2 of the *Chronically Sick and Disabled Persons Act 1970*. However, even these duties are only triggered subject to clients' meeting of a local authority's eligibility criteria and so cannot be considered absolute. Likewise there is a duty to provide for the special educational needs of a child under s.324 of the *Education Act 1996*, and s.62 of the *Education (Scotland) Act 1980*, once those needs and the provision for them are enshrined in a statement, or a record, of needs.

General or target welfare duties. Alternatively, the courts identify in *welfare legislation* what they call general or target duties, which place a general duty on public bodies to provide services to the local population, but which are barely enforceable by individuals. Such duties include provision of services by the NHS under the *NHS Act 1977* and the *NHS (Scotland) Act 1978*; and by local authorities for children in need under s.17 of the *Children Act 1989* (and probably also therefore under s.22 of the *Children (Scotland) Act 1995*).

EASSON v DUNDEE TEACHING HOSPITALS NHS TRUST
Hospital laundry worker; question of adequate specificity in bringing case; MHOR 1992

A laundry worker alleged injury in 1995 when a 17–18kg bag slipped from her grasp whilst she was manually unloading bags from a barrow. The employer argued for dismissal of the case on grounds of lack of specificity. However, the court found adequate specification in relation to (a) the lifting of the bag being a manual handling operation under r.2 of the *MHOR 1992*; (b) the circumstances in which the injury had allegedly occurred; and (c) references to the bag's weight, awkwardness, lack of rigidity, fabric handles and position on the barrow. The case should therefore proceed ((2000) SLT 345, Outer House, Court of Session, Scotland).

EATON v WEST LOTHIAN NHS TRUST
Student nurse; hoist; jamming of handle; credibility of evidence; Provision and Use of Work Equipment Regulations 1992; negligence case

A student nurse claimed that she had been injured in 1995 when she was operating a hoist, the handle of which jammed and caused a jerk to her back. On the evidence, the hoist was not defective (in terms of a stiff handle) and the court accepted that she probably twisted her back when using a perfectly satisfactory hoist, because her back was vulnerable and susceptible. If the hoist had been defective, the case would have been made out under breach of statutory duty (i.e. *Provision and Use of Work Equipment Regulations 1992* – see now the 1998 regulations of the same name) but not in common law, because the jamming was unforeseeable in all the circumstances, and there was a satisfactory system for dealing with defective equipment – namely labelling it as faulty and withdrawing it from use. The pursuer had claimed that there was a sticker on the hoist indicating it was faulty, but that it was on the side of the hoist away from the handle and was only pointed out to her afterwards.

Maintenance of hoists. The court responded:

> The pursuer led no evidence to support her contention that there was a label there then present and no evidence that the particular hoist she used was faulty. Although two auxiliary nurses were present in the ward, no evidence was led from either of them as to events of the day. There was no acceptable evidence from which I could conclude that the hoist did in fact bear a label indicating it was faulty. If it had I fail to understand why the pursuer would not have seen it when installing the patient. No steps were taken, according to the records kept for the defenders about the maintenance of equipment, to deal with any alleged or reported defect in any hoist from the date of the incident until October 1995. Specifically, there was no evidence that the hoist was in any way faulty at the time of the incident. It had been maintained along with the other hoist by way of a complete overhaul when the new engineers charged with that duty took over the contract for maintenance in March 1995. On 17 July one hoist was reported as stiff and that report was

attended to on a brief visit by an engineer. No other complaint or attendance by maintenance staff was noted and in particular the pursuer did not convey to any of the senior staff to whom she reported the accident any information which indicated a faulty hoist. Nothing was done by either of the senior staff to check the hoist or have it checked. Had it caused an accident it would have been checked. Both senior staff reported many defects in equipment as both their evidence and the Maintenance Record Book...confirmed ([1999] GWD 23–1114, Outer House, Court of Session, Scotland).

EDUCATION

Not always apparently appreciated by those working in the education field, is the extent to which *health and safety at work legislation* concerning *employee* safety applies to *schools* and education authorities (as employers) (a) in respect of manual handling of disabled children or *restraint* of children with behavioural problems; and (b) in respect of duties to provide and maintain *equipment*. See also *children; Education Act 1996; Education (Scotland)Act 1980; restraint; schools.*

EDUCATION ACT 1996

In respect of children with statements of special educational needs in England and Wales, s.324 of the *Education Act 1996* states that education authorities must arrange provision deemed in the statement to be 'educational' provision; whereas there is no duty, but only a power, to arrange provision deemed 'non-educational'. This distinction underpins sometimes protracted disputes as to who, if anybody, will arrange services and equipment for disabled children – including manual handling related services and equipment, therapy and rehabilitation – and consequent delay in the meeting of a child's needs.

Educational provision. The duty to make educational provision contained in a statement is a strong, specific one, enforceable in individual cases; it is not simply a target duty. Thus for a child with manual handling related needs, specific provision included in such a statement – in terms of equipment and human support or assistance – will be more surely provided if it is in the educational, rather than the non-educational, part. For instance, when occupational therapy, physiotherapy, speech and language therapy, and related equipment were deemed educational, then in the absence of the NHS deciding to provide them, the education authority was under a duty to do so (see e.g. *R v Harrow London Borough Council, ex p M*).

Non-educational provision. Conversely, if services are deemed non-educational then no duty arises; for instance, in one case the court stated that, as a matter of law, the need for a lift to access a classroom could not be educational, and so no duty on the education authority could be triggered (*R v Lambeth London Borough Council, ex p M*). Similarly, it has been held that nursing care at school cannot in law be deemed to be educational, and so would have to come into the non-educational part of a statement (*Bradford Metropolitan District Council v A*). Even where there is in principle a discretion as to whether any particular service or equipment is deemed educational or non-educational, it might well be that in practice education authorities will generally view manual handling issues as not primarily educational, even if school-related, and so relegate provision of assistance to non-educational status.

NHS provision. As to provision by the NHS for children's manual handling and related needs in the school context, whether deemed educational or non-educational, there is considerable difficulty in enforcement. Under s.322, the 1996 Act imposes a significantly qualified duty on the NHS, if assistance is requested by an education authority. The health authority does not have a duty to comply with the request if it considers that such compliance would not be reasonable, having regard to the resources available to it (see e.g. *R v Brent and Harrow Health Authority, ex p Harrow London Borough Council*).

Children without statements. For children with special educational needs but without statements or records of need, any duties on schools and education authorities that exist to meet their special educational needs are basically general or target duties, and therefore barely amenable to specific enforcement in individual cases.

Disability discrimination. See *Disability Discrimination Act 1995*.

Scotland. For Scotland, see *Education (Scotland) Act 1980*, where the position is in principle the same, but differs in detail.

EDUCATION (SCOTLAND) ACT 1980
In respect of children with a record of need in Scotland, s.62 of the *Education (Scotland) Act 1980* states that education authorities must arrange provision of special educational needs in the record if they are not otherwise being suitably arranged. Such needs might be manual handling related.

Record of need. Unlike corresponding English and Welsh legislation in respect of statements of special educational needs, there is in Scotland no explicit statutory distinction between educational and non-educational provision made in a record of need. In Scotland, it appears that the record of need is to contain details only of special educational needs, but not what in England and Wales would be called 'non-educational' needs.

Extent of special educational needs and provision specified in a record of need. Thus by default, if needs and provision are contained within a record of need, it follows (a) that they have been deemed to be special educational needs; and (b) that ultimately, the education authority has a duty to see that they are met (if, for example, the NHS declined to provide any of them). This is the clear duty in s.62 of the 1980 Act, reiterated in Scottish guidance (see Scottish Office 1996, p.36). However, this guidance appears to suggest that this could apply, for instance, even to the provision of a prosthesis (p.35). Yet, in the light of English case law stating that neither nursing nor a lift could be deemed to be special educational provision, there may be a question of whether the Scottish courts would rule that such an item such as a prosthesis could not in law possibly be a special educational provision, and so should not come within the record of need at all. Obviously from the point of view of the child, especially given the difficulty of enforcing NHS provision, the more provision specified in the record of need, the better.

For further discussion as to the distinction between educational and non-educational needs, see *Education Act 1996.*

Children without a record of need. For children with special educational needs but without records of need, any duties that exist to meet their special educational needs are basically general or target duties, and therefore barely amenable to specific enforcement in individual cases. Therefore, given the shortage of resources which chronically afflicts local authorities, the statement in Scottish guidance – that a record of needs should not necessarily trigger the commitment of resources any more than the needs of a child without a record – is perhaps somewhat over-optimistic (SO 1996, p.8).

Disability discrimination. See *Disability Discrimination Act 1995.*

England and Wales. See *Education Act 1996.*

EDWARDS v NATIONAL COAL BOARD
Meaning of 'reasonably practicable' in health and safety at work legislation

A case in which the courts stated that the term 'reasonably practicable' did not mean 'physically possible'. Instead it meant that a:

> computation must be made by the owner in which the quantum of risk is placed on one scale and the sacrifice involved in the measures necessary for averting the risk (whether in money, time or trouble) is placed in the other, and that, if it be shown that there is a gross disproportion between them – the risk being insignificant in relation to the sacrifice – the defendants discharge the onus on them.

In other words, it would in those latter circumstances not be reasonably practicable for the employer to do something about the risk ([1949] 1 All ER 734, Court of Appeal).

EDWARDS v WALTHAM FOREST HEALTH AUTHORITY
State enrolled nurse; bathing a patient; application of guidance; responsibility of employer for non-provision of equipment; negligence case

An accident occurred in April 1982 to the plaintiff, a state enrolled nurse aged 29. She was being assisted by a newly qualified nurse and a student nurse to bath a hemiplegic patient in his late fifties and weighing 16 stone. They had already bathed four patients successfully. The bathing was necessary regularly because all the patients were incontinent. The plaintiff had suffered an annular tear to a disc in her back in a previous incident; this now protruded as a result of the incident in question. She gave up nursing and trained as a teacher.

Creep factor. The court accepted evidence about the effect of the 'creep factor', involving a series of heavy compressions of the spine in a short space of time, water being squeezed out of the spinal disc each time, and the disc not restoring itself quickly enough each time and so losing its resilience.

Hoists: unsafe system of work. The judge concluded that the employer 'ignored an obvious danger to their nurses by requiring their nurses to lift patients from the bath... It was a danger of injury to the back...well known to the nursing profession as a perusal of the 'Handling of patients', which was in circulation at the material time, clearly shows. In my view it was not reasonable to expect [the plaintiff] to take the initiative to avoid the danger of injury to her back'. The employer had done nothing to bring to the attention of the plaintiff the availability of a hoist; yet 'it was the duty of the defendants to consider the situation that arose when patients had to be bathed, to devise a suitable system, and to instruct [the plaintiff] what she must do, and to supply an ambulift that was, as I am satisfied, required'. Damages of £33,300 were awarded (1989 High Court, unreported).

EMERGENCY SITUATIONS
To the extent that they are foreseeable and constitute a risk of manual handling injury, emergency situations clearly come under the *MHOR 1992*, in terms of risk assessment and avoiding or reducing risk. One Scottish case suggested that emergency situations would not be so covered (*Fraser v Greater Glasgow Health Board*); but this decision has not been followed in England (*Purvis v Buckinghamshire County Council*) and its correctness has been doubted in Scotland (*Fleming v Stirling Council*).

EMPLOYEES
Employees have various duties toward themselves, which are spelt out under *health and safety at work legislation*, including the *MHOR 1992* (see also Overview).

In manual handling cases, the courts look to see whether employees have reasonably discharged their responsibilities, are solely to blame for the accident they have suffered, or are at least contributorily negligent.

Employees asking for assistance. For instance, the courts might take into account the futility of asking for assistance if it was not anyway available (*Bearman v Australian Capital Territory Community and Health Service; O'Neill v Boorowa District Hospital; Swain v Denso Martin*); not expect auxiliary, as opposed to trained nurses, to decide whether to ask for assistance (*Moore v Norfolk Area Health Authority*); and not necessarily expect even experienced employees to make decisions in certain types of situation (*Bunter v Liftwise*).

Employees making decisions and experience. Equally, the courts sometimes find that employees – particularly, but not always, experienced employees – should have made their own decisions, whether they are nurses (*Woolgar v West Surrey and North East Hampshire Health Authority*) or bakery manageresses (*Black v Carricks*). A nursing auxiliary competent to carry out the accepted lift she was using, but who was injured through failing to apply common sense to the situation, was to blame for her own injury (*Bohitige v Barnet Healthcare NHS Trust*). A risk might have been so obvious that some responsibility for the accident must be borne by the employee (*Blanchflower v Chamberlain*). Experience on the part of an employee may tempt the court to find some degree of contributory negligence (*Dewing v St Luke's; McCaffery v Datta*) or simply no employer liability at all (*Koonjul v Thameslink Healthcare NHS Trust*).

In an older case (which perhaps would be decided differently today), when an employee simply failed to follow clear instructions, then even though she was only a 17-year-old student nurse, the court found that she was to blame and the employer not liable at all (*Gower v Berks*). More recently, when an employee did not follow a system of work which avoided manual handling with risk – a specific duty he has under the *MHOR 1992* – there was no liability (*Gordon v British Airways*).

Judicial protection of employees. Nevertheless, it is clear that the courts also extend a certain amount of protection to employees, by taking into account matters such as the altruism and enthusiasm of care professionals in assisting patients or clients (*Moore v Norfolk Area Health Authority*); the pressure employees are sometimes under (*Bearman v Australian Capital Territory Community and Health Service*); inexperience such as that of student nurses (*Clarke v Oxfordshire Health Authority; Shirley v Wirral Health Authority*); the particular exposure to risk of district nurses in the community (*Hammond v Cornwall and Isles of Scilly Health Authority*); lack of *training* even after ten years on the job (*Skinner v Aberdeen City Council*); natural reliance on senior staff (*Dickson v Lothian Health Board; Gower v Berks; Shirley v Wirral Health Authority*) or on the *system of work* in place even though it was unsafe (*Williams v Gwent Health Authority*); even experienced staff believing it their duty to perform unsafe lifting because of staff shortages and the prevailing ethos in the hospital (*Forder v Norfolk Area Health Authority*); misjudgements in the heat of the moment if the employer has otherwise not provided an adequate system of work (*Fitzsimmons v Northumberland Health Authority*); or lapse of concentration when tedious tasks are involved (*King v RCO*). Even where there is some contributory negligence on the part of an employee (e.g. a nurse lifting in a way she knew she should not), the courts might downplay its extent if it is 'overshadowed' by a failure in the overall system of work (*Charnock v Capital Territory Health Commission*).

EMPLOYERS

Employers have extensive duties in *health and safety at work legislation* and in the common law of *negligence* toward *employees*, and also toward non-employees. In the particular context of this book, employers include NHS Trusts, local social services authorities, local education authorities, care homes and domiciliary care agencies.

In manual handling cases, the courts often ask questions such as whether there is any *evidence* that the employer applied its mind to the risk involved, or whether a 'senior mind' in the organisation did so. An answer in the negative has often resulted in liability being imposed (*Blair v Lancaster Health Authority; Hall v Edinburgh City Council; Logan v Strathclyde Fire Board; McGowan v Harrow Health Authority; Stuthridge v Merseyside Metropolitan Ambulance Service*). A ward sister might not be a senior mind, if the court believes responsibility should start 'at the top' (*Clarke v Oxfordshire Health Authority*). This is part of considering whether the employer had been operating a safe *system of work* in its various manifestations, including *supervision, instructions and information*, protection of *employees*, adequate *risk assessment*, balancing *patient and client need* with staff safety, putting a stop to unsafe *custom and practice, training*, ensuring provision and use of *equipment*, paying attention to national manual handling *guidance*, and so on. See the entries for these italicised terms, and also under *employees*.

EPSOM AND ST HELIER NHS TRUST
Health service ombudsman; wheelchair provision; fettering of discretion; maladministration

A health service ombudsman investigation illustrating that, just like the courts, the ombudsman might find a *fettering of discretion* when a policy is applied too restrictively; this case involved electric wheelchairs (but the principle applies to all services and equipment provision, including those which are related to manual handling issues; of course wheelchair provision might anyway have direct manual handling implications for assistants or carers).

The ombudsman found that the NHS Trust had failed to consider adequately the parents' request that their disabled son be provided with an electric indoor/outdoor wheelchair. The Trust had applied both local and national guidance too restrictively; had not taken into consideration the son's previous experience of using such wheelchairs; and had not considered adequately whether the son had exceptional needs which were not covered directly by the guidance (Investigation E559/99–00; contained in HSO 2001).

EQUIPMENT
The appropriate use of equipment in manual handling is a crucial part of the ability of health and social care providers to reduce the risk to their staff entailed in the manual handling of clients and patients – and also, by its appropriate provision, to meet the needs of patients and clients. It is beyond the scope of this book to set out in detail the law, policy and practice applying to equipment provision by the NHS and social services, care homes and domiciliary care agencies, but the following points should be borne in mind.

Equipment: health and safety at work legislation. Under health and safety at work legislation, equipment (including manual handling equipment) used at work by employees is covered explicitly, for instance by the *Health and Safety at Work Act*

1974, ss.2 and 6, by the *Provision and Use of Work Equipment Regulations 1998 (PUWER 1998)* and by the *Lifting Operations and Lifting Equipment Regulations 1998*. In particular, the duty under *PUWER 1998* to maintain equipment in good repair and efficient working order should be noted; it imposes strict liability, something that was perhaps not clear until the major case in 2000 of *Stark v Post Office*. Employees might also sue in negligence for injury from defective equipment. Along with this legislation goes, for instance, an approved code of practice and guidance on work equipment (HSC 1998a) and on lifting equipment (HSC 1998b).

In respect of the risk of, or actual, harm to non-employees arising from equipment provision, the general duty under s.3 of the 1974 Act – together with r.3 of the *Management of Health and Safety at Work Regulations 1999* – is relevant to potential Health and Safety Executive improvement notices and criminal prosecution.

Equipment: cost of not providing or maintaining appropriately. The importance of equipment to manual handling is signified in the separate chapter accorded it in the Health and Safety Commission's guidance on *Manual handling in the health services*. The guidance also gives an example of an NHS Trust which was so concerned about manual handling injury to its staff and lost work time, that it spent the best part of £100,000 the next year on patient handling equipment and also set up a comprehensive training programme. Subsequently an 84 per cent reduction in lost work hours from manual handling injury was demonstrated with estimated savings of £400,000 (HSC 1998, p.7). Another Trust was reported to have made available, following the introduction of the *MHOR 1992*, £250,000 for equipment that would avoid the need for manual handling (Snell 1995).

Indeed, the cost of not providing appropriate equipment – and of failing to maintain equipment adequately – might be very high indeed in particular cases. For instance, when a nurse was injured because of the lifting she had to undertake in the absence of height adjustable beds and because of pushing a heavy patient in a wheelchair with a flat tyre, the court awarded over £300,000 (*Commons v Queen's Medical Centre*); and a physiotherapist who was injured when operating a defective height adjustable bed settled the case in court at £117,000 (HSC 1998, p.6).

Equipment: examples of occurrence in legal cases. Reference to equipment occurs in many manual handling cases in a number of different circumstances. Hoists might be: simply not considered by the employer when they should have been (*McGowan v Harrow Health Authority*), or unavailable (*Edwards v Waltham Forest Health Authority*); available but deemed a danger to patients (*Bearman v Australian Capital Territory Community and Health Service*); available but not used because of lack of employer encouragement (*Charnock v Capital Territory Health Commission*), or only used for some tasks (*Salvat v Basingstoke and North Hampshire Health Authority*); allegedly not available in the right place and anyway lacking slings (*Coad v Cornwall and Isles of Scilly Health Authority*); having faulty wheels that lock and cause injury (*Moran Health Care Services v Woods*); or subject to a sound maintenance system backed up with appropriate documentation (*Eaton v West Lothian NHS Trust*).

Otherwise, manual handling legal cases have considered: failure to use lifting straps (*Dewing v St Luke's*); inappropriate patient armchairs (*Bearman v Australian Capital Territory Community and Health Service*); fixed height beds (*Commons v Queen's Medical Centre*); faulty bed castors and the effect of abandoning proper systems of bed maintenance (*Denton v South West Thames Regional Health Authority*); injury caused by an inappropriate type of bed rail (*Bearman v Australian Capital Territory Community and Health Service*) or by misuse of a bed rail (*Kempsey District Hospital v Thackham*); flat wheelchair tyres (*Commons v Queen's Medical Centre*); equipment for foster carers (*Beasley v Buckinghamshire County Council*); hospital food trolleys (*McMenamin v Lambeth, Southwark and Lewisham Health Authority*); wheeled ambulance trolleys on icy ramps (*Lang v Fife Health Board*); and sound maintenance systems for beds (*Pearson v Eastbourne Area Health Authority*). Even with the existence of an apparently sound maintenance system, there needs to be some evidence that it was operated in respect of the particular equipment (traction couch) and defect in issue (*McMenamin v Lambeth, Southwark and Lewisham Health Authority*).

Equipment: Medical Devices Agency (MDA) guidance and advice. The Medical Devices Agency issues various *guidance* and advice, some of which applies to all equipment (including manual handling equipment) and some to manual handling equipment alone. General guidance includes a comprehensive publication on the management of equipment (MDA DB9801); a supplement to this on checking and testing new equipment (MDA DB9801 supplement 1); and a further publication on repair and maintenance (MDA DB(2000)2).

Advice on manual handling equipment has been issued by the MDA (or its predecessor) over the years, some relating to specific products, some of wider application. For instance, on specific product failure or misuse, it has covered detachment of a hoist spreader bar (SIB8403); dropping of the jib arm of a hoist (MDA SN9627); faulty installation of a bath lifter (MDA SN9705); hoist mast failures (MDA SN9817 and SN9838); collapse of an unmodified hoist because neither the manufacturer nor the NHS Trust involved knew the whereabouts of the hoist to modify it (MDA SN9828); cracked and fractured plastic attachment clips on slings (MDA SN9829); wrongly set springs on manual self-lift chairs (MDA SN9832); cross straps incorrectly assembled on stretchers (MDA SN9938); collapse of a variable height examination couch through misuse as transportation equipment (MDA HN2000(11)); and failure of pivot pins of a folding wheelchair/carry chair (MDA SN2001(21)).

Other MDA advice, not product specific, has dealt with the regular inspection of hoist slings, harnesses, straps, and attachment clips – normally every six months (MDA SAB8914 and SN9929) – general use of transfer and lifting equipment (MDA SN9637), and careful assessment of whether a two-piece band sling is appropriate (MDD HN9418).

Equipment provision under welfare legislation. Of course, logically prior to health and safety issues in respect of equipment use by employees and patients or clients, is the question of whether any particular patient or client is eligible, either at all or how urgently, for NHS or social services provision. This is determined ultimately under the *NHS Act 1977* and *NHS (Scotland) Act 1978* – and under community care legislation such as the *NHS and Community Care Act 1990, Chronically Sick and Disabled Persons Act 1970* and *Social Work (Scotland) Act 1968* – by setting professional assessment against priorities, eligibility criteria and waiting times. See also *patient and client need.*

Equipment services in the NHS and social services have for many years been regarded as substandard, and have been reported as such by many different bodies over three decades (see e.g. Mandelstam 1997, p.78). Following yet one more report to this effect by the Audit Commission (2000) and a good practice guide produced by the Disabled Living Centres Council (Winchcombe 1998), the Department of Health has issued *guidance* covering England and instructing the NHS and local authorities to improve services significantly by 2004 (HSC 2001/008). Likewise guidance has been issued by the Scottish Executive (SE 2000, pp.28–30).

Equipment: practical problems in using manual handling equipment. Clients and patients might wish not to use, or find difficulties in using, manual handling equipment. Reasons commonly cited for this in the past have included lack of confidence on the part of staff using the equipment, discomfort, concerns about safety, the look of the equipment in the home, or lack of space in the home allowing the equipment properly to be used – although it is not clear how widespread such feelings actually are (McGuire *et al.* 1996). Another study identified a range of issues affecting people's acceptance of equipment, including comfort and security in a sling, compatibility of equipment with the physical and social environment, the psychological effect of hoists which might emphasise a person's loss of ability – and the need for professionally competent staff to assess what equipment is appropriate and to take a consultative approach with patients and clients, so as to avoid further feelings of loss of control (Conneeley 1998). For instance, it might take parents months or even years to accept that their child needs a hoist (Oliveck 1998).

Equipment: examples of manual handling items. Manual handling equipment, and also equipment relevant to manual handling situations, includes hoists and slings of many types, bath lifts, handling belts, transfer boards, sliding sheets, turning discs, adjustable height beds and chairs, trolleys, chairs and beds of suitable height, riser-recliner chairs, non-slip sheets and mats, ambulatory rehabilitation aids, and so on.

EUROPEAN CONVENTION ON HUMAN RIGHTS
The European Convention on Human Rights has since October 2000 been incorporated into United Kingdom law by means of the *Human Rights Act 1998*. It sets out a number of wide-ranging rights; two of the most obvious with potential application to manual handling are article 8, concerning the right to respect for privacy, home and family life; and also article 3 concerning the right not to be subjected to degrading and inhuman treatment. For an outline of the potential implications of these arti-

cles, see further below. Immediately below, however, is a brief explanation of how the courts approach human rights issues.

Incompatibility of local policies, of individual decisions or of legislation itself. The *Human Rights Act 1998* is primarily about ensuring that public bodies (such as local authorities, NHS Trusts, health authorities and even the law courts themselves) do not breach the rights set out in the Convention. It was expected that perhaps under s.6 of the 1998 Act, residential and nursing homes – and perhaps domiciliary care agencies – might be considered to be public bodies, insofar as they were carrying out public-type functions by providing services on behalf of the NHS and local authorities. However, at the time of writing at least, the case of *R (Heather, Ward and Callin) v Leonard Cheshire Foundation* appears to have dispelled this expectation.

The courts ultimately might have to consider whether such a breach by a public body is due to a piece of legislation (e.g. the *MHOR 1992*) itself, under which the public body (e.g. NHS Trust) had a duty to act in the way in which it did (so being unable to avoid the breach). In the case of so-called secondary legislation, such as regulations, the courts have the power in some circumstances to strike it down; otherwise, in the case of primary legislation – i.e. Acts of Parliament – the courts may only go so far as to make a declaration of incompatibility. Such a declaration does not immediately invalidate the legislation which, technically now unlawful, would continue paradoxically to remain law until such time as central government passes a remedial order.

However, before considering such a drastic step as a declaration of incompatibility, the courts will consider whether any breach of human rights is due instead to the public body (e.g. local authority) having adopted an overly restrictive local policy. Indeed, a striking down or declaration of incompatibility in respect of the *MHOR 1992* is highly unlikely; if any manual handling decisions do fall foul of the *Human Rights Act 1998*, it is much more likely to be in respect of a local decision and policy. This is because the courts have a far-reaching duty under the 1998 Act to, if possible, read and give effect to legislation such that it is interpreted compatibly with Convention rights.

Human rights: degrading or inhuman treatment. Article 3 states simply: 'No one shall be subjected to torture or to inhuman or degrading treatment or punishment.' It places a duty on public bodies to ensure that people are not subjected to these things.

In the context of manual handling, it has been suggested that for the NHS or local authority effectively to force a disabled person to use a hoist in their own home (i.e. by refusing to offer manual handling assistance) – where there are implications for dignity, privacy or safety – might in some circumstances breach article 3. However, case law directly relating to this sort of situation and supporting this view is lacking; and in general, on the evidence of past case law involving article 3, fairly extreme circumstances have to be identified before a breach is found by the court.

Examples of a breach of article 3 found by the European Court of Human Rights against the United Kingdom include a decision to deport a man in an advanced stage of terminal illness back to a country where there were inadequate facilities and where his death would be hastened (*D v United Kingdom*); the failure of a local authority over a number of years to take effective child protection measures in the case of four children subject to severe parental neglect and abuse (*Z v United Kingdom*); and the failure of the police and prison authorities to provide for a disabled woman – who had been imprisoned – adequate facilities relating to her personal care and manual handling needs (*Price v United Kingdom*). Reading this last case across into the health and social care context might be tempting, but it should be borne in mind that the courts might be more ready to intervene in the case of prisoners, given the compulsory and punitive nature of the situation, than in the case of hard-pressed health and social care agencies struggling to meet people's needs.

Even so, one imagines that the sort of circumstances identified by one particular investigation of the Commission for Health Improvement – if put before a court – might well represent a breach of article 3. The Commission discovered that in one NHS Trust, patients with mental health problems were tied to commodes, fed on them, and denied food, clothing and blankets, and so were subjected to abuse – owing to a working culture that allowed unprofessional, counter-therapeutic, degrading and even cruel practices. One matter, about which the Commission was unable to reach a conclusion, concerned allegations that a wooden board and harness used for restraint on one of the wards had been made in the occupational therapy department (CHI 2000).

Human rights: privacy, home and family life. Article 8 sets out both a right and an explicit qualification to that right:

> 1. Everyone has the right to respect for his private and family life, his home and correspondence.
>
> 2. There shall be no interference by a public authority with the exercise of this right except such as in accordance with the law and is necessary in a democratic society in the interests of national security, public safety or the economic well-being of the country, for the prevention of disorder or crime, for the protection of health or morals, or for the protection of the rights and freedoms of others.

The first part of this article, 8.1, requires respect for a person's home, private and family life, and correspondence. In principle, this article sets a lower threshold than article 3 for a breach to be established. Clearly its content would appear potentially relevant to manual handling decisions, since in some situations they can profoundly affect a person's home, private and family life. However, it should be noted that article 8.2 allows interference by a public body with this right to respect, if that interference is in accordance with the law, is necessary in a democratic society and is, amongst other things, in the interests of the economic well-being of the country, for the protection of health or for the protection of the rights and freedoms of others. In other words, unlike article 3, the right in article 8 is qualified and not absolute.

(a) **Importance of existing law**. Assuming a court were to accept that a particular manual handling decision taken by the NHS or a local authority did breach article 8.1, then the decision would have to be defended under article 8.2, first of all, on the grounds that it was 'in accordance with the law' – that is, the relevant *welfare legislation, health and safety at work legislation* and associated *guidance*. So, when a local authority could show that its decision to offer residential care but not full home care support was supported by a full and balanced assessment under community care legislation and guidance, the court on that basis accepted that the local authority had complied also with article 8 of the Convention (*R (Khana) v Southwark London Borough Council*).

In another case, involving the proposed closure of a residential home, the court ruled that the local authority had not *taken account of all relevant factors* (such as the reference in the home's handbook to a 'home for life'), and that therefore the local authority should reconsider its decision. In so holding, the court was deploying a well-used common law principle, employed frequently in judicial review cases and not dependent on the *Human Rights Act 1998*. As the judge put it: 'it is unnecessary to visit the Human Rights Act... As is so often the position, the common law by its adaptability has demonstrated that it is capable of meeting human rights standards unaided' (*R(Bodimeade) v Camden London Borough Council*).

It seems clear therefore, that for practitioners and managers in the NHS and in local authorities to concern themselves with the *Human Rights Act 1998* – without first understanding the implications of existing legislation and the common law principles applied in judicial review – represents not only a failure to understand how the 1998 Act works, but also does a disservice to their clients and patients.

(b) **Proportionate decisions**. A decision under article 8 has also to be a proportionate and balanced one. This principle derives from the phrase 'necessary in a democratic society' in article 8.2.

For instance, when a local authority sought a care order for a child, the Court of Appeal found that this would have been disproportionate in all the circumstances, and that a less drastic supervision order would be more appropriate (*Re O*). Thus, if a decision that no manual handling could be provided was based on the application of a blanket policy – irrespective of the actual risk to staff in an individual situation, or of the needs and welfare of the patient or client – this might begin to look like an unbalanced decision. It might anyway indicate a breach of the duty under existing legislation (such as community care legislation) to assess individual need, and also offend against the principle that public bodies should not *fetter their discretion* – and so in either case not be 'in accordance with the law'.

(c) **Health and safety under article 8**. If a decision not to provide the manual handling wanted by a client could be justified on genuine grounds of a serious and real risk to staff and perhaps to the client or patient, then clearly reference in article 8 to health and to the protection of the rights of others is relevant. Thus, there is nothing in article 8 which simply sweeps aside genuine health and safety at work concerns in the face of untrammelled client and patient wish or choice.

(d) **Economic well-being of the country**. If a local authority could justify before the court, on the basis of a thorough assessment, that a person's needs could be met either by manual handling or by equipment – but that the latter option was chosen because it was cheaper or more cost-effective – then the reference in article 8.2 to the economic well-being might be relevant. Obviously, decisions about cost-effectiveness relate to health and social care rationing and the inevitable limits to available resources. Indeed in one community care case, in which the local authority argued that to keep a particular residential home open would cost £3,000 per week per resident, the judge stated – when denying permission for a judicial review – that the economic well-being of the council and of all those people in need of its services would surely justify the proposed closure of the home (*R (Rowe) v Walsall Metropolitan Borough Council*). The court concluded likewise, though less explicitly, in *R (Khana) v Southwark London Borough Council*, in which it concluded that cost-effectiveness was a legitimate factor to take into account under both community care legislation and, by extension, under article 8.

Even so, in a case when the closure of a specialist NHS residential unit – without an overriding reason of public interest – involved the breaking of a specific promise made to a group of disabled people that they had had a 'home for life', the Court of Appeal found a breach of article 8, because of the explicit nature of the promise and the absence of an overriding reason why the unit should be closed. This outweighed any argument by the health authority that closure represented best use of its resources (*R v North and East Devon Health Authority, ex p Coughlan*).

(e) **Health and social care policy**. It should be borne in mind that the courts in the United Kingdom have traditionally given a wide, though by no means unlimited, discretion to central and local government when it comes to rationing policies in health, social care and housing. Even the European Court of Human Rights has, broadly, done the same. Therefore, it should not be expected, even in the light of article 8, that the courts will make sweeping decisions affecting health and social care policy, practice and expenditure, whether in respect of manual handling or any other issues. More likely is that some decisions in health and social care will be subjected to greater scrutiny than previously, and may in some individual and limited circumstances enable clients or patients to win cases they would previously not have won.

EUROPEAN DIRECTIVE ON MANUAL HANDLING
The *MHOR 1992* transpose a European directive (see below), a number of extracts of which follow immediately below. The directive in turn comes under the umbrella of

a general health and safety at work 'framework directive' ('89/391/EEC on the introduction of measures to encourage improvements in the health and safety of workers at work' – not set out in this book), which is transposed into United Kingdom law through the *Management of Health and Safety at Work Regulations 1999*.

Referring to the original directive. The wording in the *MHOR 1992* differs from that of the original directive; were a court to find a difference in meaning between the two, the terms of the directive would prevail. Indeed in a recent case concerning product liability under Part 1 of the Consumer Protection Act 1987 – likewise derived from a European directive and departing from the wording of the original directive – the High Court concentrated on the wording of the directive rather than the Act, thus going 'straight to the fount' (*A v National Blood Authority*). More specifically, in the manual handling case of *Cullen v North Lanarkshire Council*, the court went beyond the *MHOR 1992* back to the original directive, in order to ascertain the scope of definition to be applied to different types of loads and attendant risks.

Reasonable practicability and foreseeability of risk. Some commentators have suggested that the term *reasonably practicable* – which appears in the *MHOR 1992* but not in the directive – might have the effect of reducing the intended strength of both the manual handling directive and the framework directive, if the term is given its traditional meaning in United Kingdom law (e.g. RCN/NBPA 1997, p.15; Zindani 1998, p.44). Nevertheless, to date, the courts have not adopted this view (e.g. *Hawkes v Southwark London Borough Council*). Likewise it has been argued that the risk referred to in the *MHOR 1992* not only need not be reasonably foreseeable, but also need not be even foreseeable, in order for a duty to arise. This would amount to potentially strict liability; and when a question about it was posed, the Court of Appeal did not answer (*King v RCO*). It is beyond the scope of this book to speculate in detail on this question. Ultimately a reference could be made to the European Commission and European Court of Justice as to whether the regulations do indeed correctly transpose the directive.

Selected provisions of the European directive (90/269/EEC, 'Council directive on the minimum health and safety requirements for the manual handling of loads where there is a risk particularly of back injury to workers') are as follows:

1. **Directive: minimum requirements**. 'This Directive, which is the fourth individual Directive within the meaning of article 16(1) of Directive 89//391/ EEC, lays down minimum health and safety requirements for the manual handling of loads where there is a risk particularly of back injury to workers' (a.1).

2. **Directive: definition**. 'The "manual handling of loads" means any transporting or supporting of a load, by one or more workers, including lifting, putting down, pushing, pulling, carrying or moving of a load, which, by reason of its characteristics or of unfavourable ergonomic conditions, involves a risk particularly of back injury to workers' (a.2).

3. **Directive: avoiding manual handling.** 'The employer shall take appropriate organisational measures, or shall use the appropriate means, in particular mechanical equipment, in order to avoid the need for the manual handling of loads by workers' (a.3).

4. **Directive: reducing the risk**. 'Where the need for the manual handling of loads by workers cannot be avoided, the employer shall take the appropriate organisational measures, use the appropriate means or provide workers with such means in order to reduce the risk involved in the manual handling of such loads, having regard to Annex 1' (a.3).

5. **Directive: organisation of workstations**. 'Wherever the need for manual handling of loads by workers cannot be avoided, the employer shall organise workstations in such a way as to make such handling as safe and healthy as possible and:

    (a) assess, in advance if possible, the health and safety conditions of the type of work involved, and in particular examine the characteristics of loads, taking account of Annex 1;

    (b) take care to avoid or reduce the risk particularly of back injury to workers, by taking appropriate measures, considering in particular the characteristics of the working environment and the requirements of the activity, taking account of Annex 1'.

6. **Directive: information and training**. 'Employers must ensure that workers and/or their representatives receive general indications and, where possible, precise information on:

    – the weight of a load,

    – the centre of gravity of the heaviest side when a package is eccentrically loaded...

    ...employers must ensure that workers receive in addition proper training and information on how to handle loads correctly and the risk they might be open to particularly if these tasks are not performed correctly, having regard to annexes I and II'.

7. **Directive: annexes I and II**. These are along the lines of schedule 1 of the *MHOR 1992* – although they are not set out or phrased in the same way – and deal with reference factors to be paid regard to in respect of the characteristics of the load, the physical effort required, the characteristics of the working environment, the requirements of the activity, and risk factors for individual workers. They are not set out in detail here.

EVERYDAY TASKS

It is possible to detect a theme in manual handling cases, in which the courts more or less deem the manual handling in question to be an everyday, perhaps straightforward 'commonsense' task – such as bedmaking, light furniture removal, routine labouring – and shy away from imposing liability. However, the definition of everyday tasks is not hard and fast, and the courts might anyway impose liability in some circumstances.

The courts did not impose liability for injury incurred when a nursing home employee reached and fell into a deep freezer chest (*Cantillon v London Nursing Homes*); care assistants were making beds (*Koonjul v Thameslink Healthcare NHS Trust; Miletic v Capital Territory Health Commission*); an ambulance worker was walking backwards up steps with a stretcher (*Parkes v Smethwick Corporation*); a scrap metal yard worker slewed round a piece of lead (*Chalk v Devizes*); a road worker lifted a box into a truck (*Forsyth v Lothian Regional Council*); another road worker lifted a heavy load of stone (*Gilchrist v Strathclyde Regional Council*); a packer of crisp boxes suffered injury (*Gissing v Walkers Crisps*); a post office worker lifted a 10kg box (*Rozario v Post Office*); a child care assistant put sand into a sandpit (*Schiliro v Peppercorn Child Care Centres*); or an employee moved a cupboard up stairs in school (*Taylor v Glasgow City Council*).

On the other hand, liability was established in relation to unloading relatively light fencing out of a truck (*Cullen v North Lanarkshire Council*); carrying a sheet of glass (*Fotheringham v Dunfermline District Council*); lifting and laying pavement slabs (*Skinner v Aberdeen City Council*); lifting a bucket of water out of a deep sink (*Warren v Harlow District Council*); moving furniture in a crowded social work office (*Watkins v Strathclyde Regional Council*); and lifting gravel into a compactor (*Wilson v British Railways Board*).

EVIDENCE

Obviously, court cases can only be decided on the court's view of the evidence which has been presented. Thus, the reliability and credibility of the evidence presented by the employee (e.g. *Aitken v Board of Management of Aberdeen College; Callaghan v Southern General Hospital NHS Trust; Doherty v Tunbridge Wells Health Authority; Hillhouse v South Ayrshire Council; Wild v United Parcel Services; Wilson v British Railways Board; Young v Salford Health Authority*) – or by the employer (e.g. *Williams v Gwent Health Authority*) – may be crucial to the outcome of the case. Specificity of evidence might also be an issue (*Boyd v Lanarkshire Health Board; Channon v East Sussex Area Health Authority*).

It is also notable that employers breach their duty in a substantial number of cases, because they are unable to convince the court that they put their mind to the situation in question – for instance, by considering whether it was reasonably practicable either to avoid or reduce risk under the *MHOR 1992*. They simply fail to lead evidence on these matters (e.g. *Anderson v Lothian Health Board; Boyd v Lanarkshire Health Board; Hall v Edinburgh City Council; King v RCO; Logan v Strathclyde Fire Board*). Adequate *documentation*, albeit backed up by other corroborative evidence, might be of great assistance to employers in demonstrating that they did not breach their duties – for example, in maintaining hoists (*Eaton v West Lothian NHS Trust*). Even then, a court might require evidence that such a system of maintenance actually covered the equipment and particular defect in question (*McMenamin v Lambeth, Southwark and Lewisham Health Authority*).

In any case, a court is unlikely to be impressed by evidence that a man known as 'Harry' did a risk assessment, that his surname could not be recalled, and that in any case no supporting documentation could be found or produced (*Wells v West Hertfordshire Health Authority*). And sometimes the court will simply be faced with two sets of inadequate evidence – for instance, about the training a nursing auxiliary received – and have to choose the most credible (*Sommerville v Lothian Health Board*).

FACTORIES ACT 1961
Now rendered obsolete by the *MHOR 1992*, s.72(1) of this 1961 Act stated: 'A person shall not be employed to lift, carry or move any load so heavy as to be likely to cause injury to him.' A few cases heard under this Act are included in this book.

FETTERING DISCRETION
Fettering of discretion is a ground on which the decision-making of public bodies such as the NHS and local authorities are challenged in *judicial review* cases by clients and patients. Courts will strike decisions down if they represent the application of a blanket policy which gives no room for exceptions (e.g. *R v North West Lancashire Health Authority, ex p G, A and D*). The ombudsmen too apply the principle (see e.g. *Bristol City Council*, a local government ombudsman case which had manual handling implications for the parents of a disabled child; and the health service ombudsman's finding that eligibility criteria for NHS wheelchair provision had been applied too rigidly (*Epsom and St Helier NHS Trust*)). In principle therefore, an over-rigid manual handling policy might in some circumstances be challengeable – for instance, were it applied irrespective of the actual risk to staff involved and of the individual client or patient's need.

FITZSIMMONS v NORTHUMBERLAND HEALTH AUTHORITY
Auxiliary nurse; whether hoist appropriate; liability for unsafe system of work; three nurses required; approach of experienced nurse who was sceptical about teaching safe lifts; principle of reasonableness; negligence case

The plaintiff was an auxiliary nurse aged 22 who in 1981, together with a student nurse of less than one year's experience, was lifting a man with multiple sclerosis, weighing nine stone and six feet tall, from bed to wheelchair. He had no control over his limbs and had frequent uncontrollable spasms. When he was standing, his legs started wobbling. The student nurse relaxed her support, but the plaintiff kept hold of him and went down with him to a half-kneeling position. When she stood up she felt she had been stabbed with something hot at the base of her spine.

The plaintiff claimed that (a) a hoist should have been used; (b) three nurses were needed; and (c) she should have been trained not to try to catch patients. The health authority argued that the whole incident was not foreseeable since it was not foreseeable that the student nurse would withdraw support. It also maintained that using a hoist would have been difficult and carried the risk of further damaging (through the shearing action of the sling) the patient's buttocks which were already sore. However, the defendant's expert accepted that with hindsight three nurses should have been used.

Hoist or third nurse? The court was not satisfied that a hoist was appropriate, given the patient's soreness, the risk of a sling's shearing action on his buttocks and his probable lack of confidence in being hoisted by young unknown nurses. However, the court took note of the fact that the defendant's lifting expert 'readily accepted that a third nurse could have been made available for lifting this patient and that the third nurse, therefore, without undue disturbance to the nursing system in the ward could have been made available, and if the third nurse had been made available the plaintiff's accident would not have occurred'. So:

> this was a risk which could reasonably be foreseen by a reasonably prudent employer. If a patient behaved in the way that this 28-year-old patient with multiple sclerosis did behave, then it was reasonably foreseeable, in my judgement, that a student nurse of less than two years' experience could behave in the way that [the student nurse] did behave in the emergency of the moment. If that is right, and I am satisfied having thought about it carefully that this was a risk which the employers should have reasonably foreseen, then the system of work which they adopted was not, in my judgement, a reasonably safe system.

Contributory negligence? The court dismissed the heath authority's argument that there was contributory negligence since the overall duty was to protect the employee from reasonably foreseeable risk and nothing turned 'on the point that the plaintiff, who no doubt had had training in theory as to how to cope with an emergency, failed to behave in the split seconds in which this incident occurred in such a way that she protected her spine'. Damages of £157,000 were awarded.

Approach of experienced nurse. One of the witnesses, a very experienced nurse and a clinical teacher of nurse students, was sceptical about expert evidence as to what would have been a safer lift. Her method of teaching was:

> to tell the nurses that, if they needed help, they should ask for it and get it and she stressed the importance of teaching the principles of nursing rather than teaching the details of a number of different alternative lifting techniques without a very firm grounding in principle…she was aware that the risk of back injury was a serious problem… She considered most back injuries were avoidable… She considered that most of the responsibility lay on the girls to

look after their patients and to look after themselves when they undertook lifting.

Appeal: reasonable precautions to be taken and resource implications. The Court of Appeal upheld the judge's decision, and in doing so considered the test in negligence cases as to what reasonable precautions should be taken in the light of the magnitude of risk identified:

> It is common ground that that which is required of a reasonable employer is to deal with a known risk by such precaution as, having regard to the severity of any possible injury, the likelihood of the injury being suffered if the event happened, and the difficult and expense of any precaution against the risk, it is reasonable should be taken... It was argued that it was not foreseeable that [the student nurse] would lose her grip. But...the judge viewed the case on the basis that if the defendants should have foreseen that the state of the patient was such that one of a two-nurse team of lifters might lose her grip in the course of a lift, then the magnitude of risk, having regard to the possible severity of potential injury resulting from such an incident, was such as to justify the requirement of the proportion proposed, that is the employment of a third nurse. I consider that the judge's conclusion cannot be faulted...

> It seemed that it might be regarded as a decision to the effect that two nurses of sufficient strength and adequate training to lift a disabled patient could not be properly allowed to lift him from bed to chair without a third nurse taking part. Such a decision would naturally cause grave concern to health authorities.

However, the court accepted that the judge's decision did not have this general effect but was directed towards the particular patient who was prone to spasm and likely to panic in the process of lifting because of lack of confidence in those lifting him ((1989) 5 BMLR 48, High Court; and 1990, Court of Appeal, unreported).

FLEMING v STIRLING COUNCIL
Care assistant; residential home; emergency situations; MHOR 1992; negligence case

A care assistant working in a residential home claimed that in 1994, on duty alone in a unit for elderly people with dementia, she had suffered injury when she had tried to prevent a resident from falling. She claimed that she had accompanied a nine-stone woman to the lavatory. Whilst she was there, another patient needed helping back to the ward, and the first woman asked to remain seated until the assistant returned. On the latter's return, the patient tried to stand up and fell sideways, and the assistant tried to prevent this but took her full weight.

The council sought to have the case dismissed on the grounds that (a) the complaint was about the single act of catching rather than the whole procedure of getting the resident to and from the bathroom – and that it was not clear that such a single act would come under the *MHOR 1992*; (b) the assistant was merely coping with an emergency situation, and that such a situation did not come under the *MHOR 1992*; and (c) the negligence case, as far as training and adequacy of staffing went, lacked specification.

The judge found that the case should proceed, (a) not being impressed with the attempt to break up the whole operation of toileting into discrete acts and then attempting to exclude one of them; (b) doubting the view in *Fraser v Greater Glasgow Health Board* that the *MHOR 1992* did not apply to emergency situations; and (c) finding that the claims about training and adequacy of staff should be heard in respect of the negligence claim and decided on the evidence – i.e. as part of the general issue as to whether there was a foreseeable risk of injury which had been inadequately guarded against ([2000] GWD 13–499, Outer House, Court of Session, Scotland).

FORDER v NORFOLK AREA HEALTH AUTHORITY
Nurse; moving a patient up a bed; parameters of what should be expected of employees; unsafe custom and practice; staff shortages; negligence case

In 1975, a 29-year-old nurse was moving a 15-stone patient up in bed assisted by an auxiliary nurse, using a 'drag' lift. Liability was established.

The court stated that it should have been made clear to nurses working on the orthopaedic ward that patients of that weight should not have been handled by two nurses alone, if the 'shoulder' or 'Australian' lift could not be used. It accepted that there 'is a large area of discretion which has to be entrusted to the individual nurse in charge', but this would be within certain 'parameters'; however, the present case went beyond such parameters. Instead the health authority had allowed an atmosphere to prevail where, because of staff shortages, nurses were encouraged to move patients without sufficient assistance. Thus, although there were four nurses working on the ward at the time of the accident and the plaintiff was an experienced nurse, the court did not blame her for this – because of the prevailing ethos in the hospital which meant that nurses thought it their duty to perform such lifting with only limited assistance. Damages of £5,600 were awarded (1982, High Court, unreported).

FORSYTH v LOTHIAN REGIONAL COUNCIL
Roadman; lifting box; routine heavy work; system of work not required; negligence case

The pursuer was a roadman who suffered an injury in 1990 when assisting the foreman of the roadworking team to lift a tamper box (for heating tools to stop asphalt sticking to them) weighing 62kg onto a lorry.

At first instance, the Outer House of the Court of Session concluded that there was no foreseeable risk to workmen through the lifting of the tamper box; that the handling of the box had been performed for many years, as one of many manual jobs carried out by men accustomed to heavy work; and that there was no requirement for a system of work to be laid down in relation to the handling of the box. Reference was made to 1982 proposals by the Health and Safety Commission, under the title 'Health and Safety (Manual Handling of Loads) Regulations and Guidance', which stated that the handling of weights above 34–55kg required either mechanical handling, or supervised, selected and trained individuals.

The Inner House now upheld this decision, even taking account of the Health and Safety Commission's consultative document. As to any special duty towards him, there was likewise no obligation. He had undertaken heavy work for the council from 1981 until 1990, and even after suffering a hernia in 1986, he had carried on heavy work for four more years. Thus, there was no duty to set up a special system for this employee, effectively for one day (since the pursuer had volunteered for Sunday work, and so another labourer, who usually undertook heavy lifting for the pursuer, was not present) (1994, Inner House, Court of Session, Scotland, unreported).

FOSTER CARERS

Foster carers sometimes look after children on behalf of local authorities, whose care involves manual handling. Under foster care arrangements, which are governed by the *Children Act 1989* and *Children (Scotland) Act 1995* and derivative regulations, there is neither a contract of employment nor even an enforceable contract for services (*W v Essex County Council*); but even so, this would not stop a local authority owing obligations to a foster carer. First, under this children's legislation itself agreements with foster carers should cover matters such as support and training. Second, in respect of safety, even if the Health and Safety Executive and courts choose not to apply the *MHOR 1992* covering duties towards employees, nevertheless s.3 of the *Health and Safety at Work Act 1974* (duty toward non-employees) would still apply; and local authorities anyway potentially owe a duty of care in *negligence* toward foster carers (see e.g. *Beasley v Buckinghamshire County Council*).

FOTHERINGHAM v DUNFERMLINE DISTRICT COUNCIL
Factory; moving sheet of glass; Factories Act 1961; negligence case

The case was brought in *negligence* under s.72 of the *Factories Act 1961* (now obsolete).

The employee was in 1985 manoeuvring a sheet of glass weighing 29.1kg in the glass shop of the employer's Cowdenbeath depot. The common law case was made out on the basis that the evidence was that such an awkward load was likely to injure the average untrained employee. (The Health and Safety Commission's consultative document of 1985, 'Manual handling of loads', was cited in relation to loads up to 75lb being safe to lift, but that that figure dropped in case of awkwardness, difficulty of grip or centre of gravity being at a distance from the handler.) The statutory case, under s.72, was also made out (more easily) since the test of foreseeability was unnecessary. Damages were agreed at £96,500 ((1991) SLT 610, Outer House, Court of Session, Scotland).

FRASER v GREATER GLASGOW HEALTH BOARD
Nursing auxiliary; moving patient up bed; emergency situation; training; negligence liability but no breach of MHOR 1992

A nursing auxiliary aged 40 sustained a back injury in 1993 when she was assisting another nurse in moving an elderly patient up the bed. The accident arose from an emergency situation, when the patient collapsed onto her bed and had to be returned to an upright position as soon as possible (in case she drowned in her own chest fluid). The nurse in charge had asked the pursuer to help her lift the patient (weighing 14 stone) back up, by employing the 'Australian lift'; the pursuer injured her back when using this lift.

Negligence liability for lack of training. The court held that the employer owed a duty of care to provide adequate and proper training for nurses, in the safe lifting and moving of patients. This duty had not been performed satisfactorily; the evidence established that the instructions given 'were so inadequate and insufficiently clear' that nurses such as the pursuer 'reasonably formed the view' that their free hand should be placed round the back or at the base of the scapula, instead of used like a strut on the bed or bed head. The court also found that the nurse in charge had failed to check where the pursuer's free hand was. Liability in negligence was thus established; damages were awarded at £4,515.

No liability under MHOR 1992: emergencies not covered. The court also considered the *MHOR 1992*. It concluded that, first, the nature of the emergency situation meant that the operation, though involving a risk of injury, could not reasonably practicably have been avoided (r.4(1)(a)). Second, it was difficult to see how r.4(1)(b) – which imposed a duty to carry out a risk assessment and to take appropriate steps to reduce the risk of injury to the lowest level reasonably practicable – applied in the circumstances. This was because the regulation was:

> applicable to manual handling operations regulations which are regularly undertaken as a matter of course in the furtherance of the employer's business, and that it does not apply where a manual handling operation is undertaken as an emergency on the initiative of an employee. Besides, the defenders supplied mechanical assistance to avoid the need for a manual handling operation. It just was not sufficiently to hand to be used on the particular occasion.

In addition, if there was a breach of either or both subparagraphs of r.4, the court could not 'understand how such breach caused the accident' ((1996) Rep LR 58, Outer House, Court of Session, Scotland).

Note. The reader should note that the exclusion of emergency situations under the *MHOR 1992* has been since doubted in Scotland in *Fleming v Stirling Council*, and anyway not followed in England in *Purvis v Buckinghamshire County Council*.

GENERAL CLEANING CONTRACTORS v CHRISTMAS
Custom and practice; burden on employer; system of work; instructions; negligence case

An influential older negligence case, concerning the burden on the employer to ensure a safe *system of work* in operation.

    The case involved a man cleaning the windows of a library, who fell when a sash window came down on his fingers. In finding liability, the House of Lords made the point that where:

> a practice of ignoring an obvious danger has grown up I do not think that it is reasonable to expect an individual workman to take the initiative in devising and using precautions. It is the duty of the employer to consider the situation, to devise a suitable system, to instruct his men what they must do and to supply any implements that may be required. ([1953] AC 180, House of Lords)

GILCHRIST v STRATHCLYDE REGIONAL COUNCIL
Roadworker; rebuilding wall; whether mechanical assistance required; routine heavy work; negligence case

This negligence case, brought on the basis that a 38-year-old road worker should have been provided in 1991 with a small crane or lifting appliance for rebuilding a retaining wall, failed.

    The court referred to three Health and Safety Commission sets of proposals on manual handling published in 1982 ('Proposals for Health and Safety (Manual Handling of Loads) Regulations and Guidance'), 1988 ('Handling loads at work: proposals for regulations and guidance') and 1991 ('Manual handling of loads: proposals for regulations and guidance') and accepted that, though these were proposals not enacted in legislation, nevertheless local authorities and industry would have been aware of the recommendations on the weight of loads. However, the court concluded that the 84lb weight of the stone involved was not excessive; and that the pursuer, having received training as a labourer, should have been able to gauge what was safe for him to lift (1994, Outer House, Court of Session, unreported).

GISSING v WALKERS SMITH SNACK FOODS LTD
Packing crisps; wrist injury; MHOR 1992; negligence case

The plaintiff worked 12-hour shifts packing up bags of crisps in boxes of 48. He suffered wrist pain. Medical evidence suggested either tenosynovitis or per-tendinitis crepitans. The court concluded that the work was rapid but not forceful, it was not reasonably practicable to do it any other way, and the plaintiff was fully trained and had undergone a satisfactory probation period. He had also been warned about the risks and signed a health and safety form on commencement of employment. He was exposed to risk only at the lower end of the scale. The employer had not acted negligently; and the *MHOR 1992* did in any case not apply to this type of work. Even if they did, they had not been breached ([1999] CL 99/Nov, County Court).

GORDON v BRITISH AIRWAYS PLC

Airport worker; hydraulic pump; MHOR 1992; Provision and Use of Work Equipment Regulations 1992; adequate system of work; negligence case

A case in which the court found an adequate system of work and an accident caused by the employee's not following that system. In 1995, the plaintiff was operating a towbar with hydraulic pump. The pump had not jacked up the towbar quite enough; the plaintiff manually raised it another 1.5 inches and suffered a searing pain in his back.

Negligence. As to breach of duty of care in negligence, the court found that there was a system for repairing and maintaining equipment such as the towbar; that the system was that employees would report the defect; and that it was not the case that employees were in the habit of lifting the towbar themselves (so there was no need to issue instructions not to do so).

Work equipment. Under r.6 of the *Provision and Use of Work Equipment Regulations 1992* (since superseded by the 1998 regulations of the same name) concerning maintenance of equipment in an efficient state of repair, there was no proof that the hydraulic pump had not been working properly; and even were there a breach of the 1992 regulations, it was not the cause of injury. The cause was the fact that the claimant moved the towbar.

MHOR 1992: avoidance of risk. As for the *MHOR 1992*, no breach was shown, since the tractor/towbar operation did not require any manual handling: if 'the hydraulics failed, it was not then the defenders' system that the towbar be connected manually. They had avoided the need for manual handling of this operation by providing a hydraulically operated system and a system for reporting and repair in the event of a defect'. The court added also that even if liability had been shown, the pursuer would have been held contributorily negligent and substantially at fault (1998: Outer House, Court of Session, Scotland, unreported).

GOWER v BERKS

Student nurse; blocking a bed; example of senior staff; pressure on junior staff; training; reliability of evidence; effect of injury; negligence case

In 1977, a 17-year-old student nurse 'blocked' a bed by herself; her argument that she had been set a bad example by a senior nurse failed on the grounds that, on the evidence, there was in fact no systematic bad example set by senior staff. It is possible that this case might be decided otherwise today.

Blocking a bed. The plaintiff had enrolled as a student nurse at the age of seventeen and began work on the orthopaedic wards of a hospital. A year later, in 1977, on an afternoon shift, she was allegedly asked by a nurse to 'block' a bed – that is, to lift the foot of it and put two large wooden blocks under the frame, in order to tilt the bed so that the patient could be given traction. She claimed that there were no other nurses to ask assistance of on the ward, other than the nurse who had issued the instruction, and she did not ask her because she knew that this nurse suffered from a bad back. She also claimed that she had seen a senior member of the nursing staff regularly performing this task alone. The patient, weighing over 13 stone, realised the plaintiff would be at risk and advised her not to attempt to block the bed alone. She disregarded the advice, suffered severe pain in her back, and found she could not straighten her body.

Instruction and example of senior staff. The plaintiff, eventually on her own admission, had received instruction which would have advised against carrying out such a task alone, so the chief question centred on whether senior staff had set a bad example to junior staff – in which case it could only be 'expected that pupils, perhaps in any other field as well but particularly in the nursing profession, would follow the example of those who were immediately superior to them; were trained, experienced and working with them on the ward'. The judge recognised the pressures on junior staff to do what they are told; however, 'it must be obvious that the mere fact that you are under pressure does not mean to say that you could act in a way which you had been taught is dangerous'.

However, on the evidence, the judge concluded that the senior member of the nursing staff involved did not block beds in that way; and that furthermore, the possible justification of urgency in the situation did not arise, even had there been no other nurses present. The judge found on the evidence that the plaintiff could reasonably have asked assistance from what was regarded as the 'senior nursing officers' sanctum' a mere few paces from the patient's bed. The judge also stated that the plaintiff had probably seen some other nurses blocking beds alone from time to time, but that could not amount to a systematic example set by senior staff. The judge sympathised with the plaintiff and wished she could have some redress, but the evidence did not allow it.

Effect of injury. Since the accident, the plaintiff had to wear a corset, take analgesics, sometimes lie down to relieve the pain, abandon sports and recreations (e.g. badminton, dancing, riding, squash). She found difficulty looking after the house, hanging up the washing or making the beds. She could not drive properly because she could not turn her head. She had to give up nursing, the career she had set her heart on. The pain was exacerbated by menstruation, sexual intercourse, driving and sneezing (which caused the pain to shoot up her back). A spinal injury expert stated that the pain had turned a happy, willing nurse into someone suffering from chronic pain and all its features of depression (1984, High Court, unreported).

GUIDANCE
Apart from legislation and case law, relevant national guidance must be taken account of by the NHS and local authorities.

Guidance as quasi-legislation. Such guidance occupies to some extent a 'no-man's-land' and is sometimes referred to as quasi-legislation. This is because whilst it is not by definition law, a failure to follow it may sometimes – but not always

– be taken by the courts to indicate breach of legal duty. For example, the 'Guide to the safer handling of patients' (current edition: RCN/NBPA 1997) and its predecessors have been frequently looked to for information about safe handling techniques (as in *Edwards v Waltham Forest Health Authority*, and many other cases) – but not always (e.g. *McLean v Plymouth Health Authority; Wright v Fife Health Board*).

Points to note about guidance. The following points can be made about guidance:

(a) **Usefulness.** First and foremost, guidance is very useful and normally an essential tool for employers, in order to achieve health and safety for employees and non-employees and comply with legal duties.

(b) **Currency.** It might become obviously out of date, in which case blind adherence to it could itself constitute incompetent practice.

(c) **Situations not envisaged by guidance.** Situations may arise not covered by guidance; in which case inappropriate application of the guidance might likewise constitute poor professional practice and even breach of legal duty.

(d) **Guidance only part of the picture.** In similar vein, ultimately, the courts are looking to see whether – in all the circumstances of the case – an employer has complied with legal duties. Compliance with guidance might or might not be relevant, or at least only part of the picture.

(e) **Alternative expert views.** As already stated above, even where aspects of guidance are relevant, the court may choose alternative expert evidence or adopt its own view (see also a case involving a physiotherapist who was found negligent despite doing what had been taught and expert supporting evidence given by the chief examiner of the Chartered Society of Physiotherapy: *Clarke v Adams*).

(f) **Different guidance and different professionals.** Depending on the context and the professionals involved, the following of one set of guidance might not appear totally consistent with another set of guidance. For instance, the guidelines for physiotherapists (CSP 2002, p.11) state that Royal College of Nursing guidance (RCN/NBPA 1997) is not necessarily appropriate for physiotherapists.

(g) **Erroneous interpretation of guidance.** Employers and employees might develop their own interpretations and beliefs about what national guidance states, with little reference to the guidance itself.

(h) **Assisting professional judgements.** Guidance is meant to assist and not to stultify the exercise of professional judgement (see generally Hurwitz 1998).

National guidance on manual handling. Relevant national guidance on manual handling specifically includes:

(a) 'Changing practice, improving health: an integrated back injury prevention programme for nursing and care homes' (RCN 2001)

(b) 'Guidance for safer handling during resuscitation in hospitals' (Resuscitation Council (UK) 2001)

(c) 'Guidance on manual handling for chartered physiotherapists' (CSP 2002)

(d) 'Guide to the handling of patients' (RCN and NBPA 1997, 4th edition)

(e) 'Handle with care: a midwife's guide to preventing back injury'(RCM 1999, 2nd edition)

(f) 'Manual handling assessments in hospitals and the community' (RCN 1996)

(g) 'Manual handling: Manual Handling Operations Regulations 1992, guidance on regulations' (HSE 1998)

(h) 'Manual handling in the health services' (HSC 1998)

(i) 'Paediatric manual handling: guidelines for paediatric physiotherapists' (APCP, undated)

(j) 'Safer handling of people in the community' (BackCare 1999).

Royal College of Nursing and National Back Pain Association (now BackCare) guidance. Of this guidance, the 'Guide to the handling of patients'(RCN/NBPA 1997) is certainly the most substantial and influential, and is commonly referred to in NHS manual handling cases in the courts. Overall it runs to some 260 pages and includes chapters on, for instance, legal and professional responsibilities, introducing a safer handling policy, management responsibility, risk assessments, equipment, special handling situations, babies and young children, emergencies and unsafe lifting practices.

Other national guidance. However, each of the above pieces of guidance comes at the subject from a different angle or involves different professions; therefore all of it should be taken account of generally in the health and social care context. A joint statement about manual handling by the Chartered Society of Physiotherapy, the College of Occupational Therapists and the Royal College of Nursing recognises that different approaches and even disagreement might exist between professions in respect of individuals or groups of patients, and that efforts are required to solve these (CSP, COT and RCN 1997). Thus, while the Royal College of Nursing guidance (RCN/NBPA 1997) refers to the 'heated debate' about manual handling and rehabilitation (p.4), guidance for physiotherapists states that therapists are in danger of being subjected inappropriately to the Royal College of Nursing guidance – which has adopted a 'different philosophical response' to manual handling (CSP 2002, p.11).

GYSEN v ST LUKE'S (ANGLICAN CHURCH IN AUSTRALIA) ASSOCIATION

Care assistant; nursing home; move from bed to commode; in accordance with care plan; time limits for bringing case; whether arguable case; breach of statutory duty (Australian legislation); negligence case

The applicant, a care assistant, was allegedly injured in 1993 while she was assisting in moving an elderly resident from her bed to a commode. The commode was at the bottom of the bed in the resident's room; as they began to walk her, the applicant alleged that instead of taking her weight by using her legs, the resident simply raised her feet off the ground, thus causing the applicant injury. The case was now being brought out of legal time limits, and as part of deciding whether to allow it to proceed, the court considered whether the case was arguable.

First, the applicant's terms of employment included those which under Tasmanian law were implied into all contracts of nursing home staff. These terms stipulated what staff were and were not allowed to do in terms of manual handling. Because the resident's care plan showed that the resident could herself provide reasonable assistance when she was moving over short distances, and there were also two staff, these terms were not breached. Second, the manual handling causing the alleged injury was consistent with the care plan – i.e. that the resident could weight-bear for short distances, that equipment was not required and that two staff should assist her in such circumstances. Furthermore, the applicant had been trained in such manual handling; and the distance was in fact about one metre. Thus the applicant's case in negligence was weak; and the court went on to rule that the time limits should not be extended for the applicant to pursue her case (1997, Supreme Court of Tasmania, Australia, transcript).

HADFIELD v MANCHESTER HEALTH AUTHORITY

Nursing auxiliary; walking elderly patient; legs buckling; lack of instruction; training; negligence case

An accident occurred in 1976 to a 38-year-old nursing auxiliary who had just completed her training. She was on an unaccompanied home visit to an 89-year-old, eight-stone patient who was slightly taller and heavier than her. The patient was frail, lived alone, could not stand or walk without assistance; her movements became increasingly limited after periods of immobility. Most of the time she was alert and lucid, but she was also doubly incontinent. She had suffered three falls over the previous twelve months. On the day in question, the plaintiff had begun to walk with the patient when the latter's legs buckled; the plaintiff stood up as straight as possible to prevent the patient falling and felt a sharp pain in her lower back. Liability was established.

Lack of instruction or training. The court found that the plaintiff should have been instructed to deal with such a situation – by giving at the knees and going down with the patient – since it was reasonably foreseeable that this patient might slump or collapse. However, on the evidence, it accepted that she had received no such training. It took the view that had she received it, she might of course 'on the spur of the moment' have ignored or forgotten such instruction – but that, given that the court believed she was 'careful, conscientious and intelligent', it was likely that in an emergency she would have followed any such training instruction.

(However, the court thought that it was reasonable for the plaintiff's immediate supervisor to have assumed that the plaintiff's induction training would have in-cluded instruction on single-handled lifting and advice – which would have been to go down with the patient, bending the knees.) Damages of £5,270 were awarded (1983, High Court, unreported).

HALL v EDINBURGH CITY COUNCIL
Council blacksmith carrying bag of cement; negligence case not made out; but breach of MHOR 1992; no thought given to risk

A council blacksmith was required in 1995 to a carry with a colleague a bag of ce-ment weighing 50kg; he was injured.

No liability in negligence. The case failed in negligence because the injury had to be reasonably foreseeable. Also, since the operation had been carried out for a con-siderable number of years without complaint, incident or injury, this meant that the defenders were not required to instruct that the cement should not be lifted – even though by 1995, a reasonably careful employer should have been aware of Health and Safety Executive guidance relating to manual handling. Nevertheless, guidance issued in the context of the *MHOR 1992* could not be incorporated into the common law as to what was reasonably foreseeable.

Liability under the MHOR 1992. However, the case was made out under the *MHOR 1992*, r.4. The judge was:

> not satisfied that the defenders have discharged the onus incumbent on them of showing that it was not reasonably practicable to avoid the need for the pursuer to undertake a manual handling operation which involved a risk of injury. It may well be that there would have been economic or practical objec-tions to equipping every pick-up truck with an on-board hoist. It may well be that in organisational terms there would be very great difficulty in making a forklift truck available whenever a bag of cement required to be loaded onto a pick-up. There may have been difficulties in manoeuvring the conveyor into the shed where the bags were kept. Some of the methods suggested might not have eliminated manual handling completely. None of the defenders' wit-nesses, however, appeared to have applied his mind in a comprehensive way to the question of how the manual handling operation on which the pursuer was engaged might have been avoided. In the absence of proper consider-ation having been given to the matter, and in the absence of any evidence of any reasonably practicable alternative, I am not prepared to hold that the ran-dom objections to individual proposals expressed in the evidence properly

support the conclusion that the avoidance of the need for the pursuer to undertake the operation in question was not reasonably practicable.

Damages of £9,600 were awarded ([1998] GWD 37–1935, Outer House, Court of Session, Scotland).

HALLIDAY v TAYSIDE HEALTH BOARD
Charge nurse; injury on ward; return to ward; heavy lifting

A charge nurse damaged her back in 1988 when a patient collapsed. She returned to work to the same ward, before being transferred to another ward which involved more frequent and heavy lifting. She told the assistant director of nursing that this work was damaging her back. A couple of weeks later she sustained a back injury, and was successful in her claim at first instance.

The court now overturned this decision, stating that the assistant director had not been obliged to remove her from the latter ward, in the absence of certification from her doctor of her unfitness for work or of the need for lighter work. Although the evidence was sufficient to show that the injury had been sustained during work on the latter wards, it was insufficient to show that she had a high risk of injury by remaining on that ward ((1996) SC 434, Inner House, Court of Session, Scotland).

HAMMOND v CORNWALL AND ISLES OF SCILLY HEALTH AUTHORITY
District nurse; home visit; lifting bedridden patient; training; system of work; negligence case

An accident occurred in 1980 to a district nurse on a home visit, who was lifting a severely disabled, bed-bound woman suffering from disseminated sclerosis who lived with her sister. The nurse had one arm under the small of the patient's back, and the other arm under the thigh. She had trained in 1955, and was appointed as a district nurse in 1978. During the case, the judge referred to statistics given in court – namely that in 1979 it was estimated that nearly 50 per cent of all nurses in the United Kingdom suffered back pain at least once – in order to emphasise the seriousness of the risk to nurses

Training. The judge considered what a safe system of work for district nurses required – a class of nurses whom he accepted were at particular risk, working alone in the community in people's homes. First, adequate training was required, and the plaintiff had not received this, due to the fact that there was no regular training or regular reminders about it.

Protection of district nurses. Second, there should have been some of way of protecting district nurses; yet despite a number of representations made to a nursing officer about the circumstances and risk implications of this particular patient, there was no follow-up.

Reassessing patients to protect nurses. Third, there was no proper system for assessing this patient's situation, in terms of review and reassessment; for instance, the patient did accept a hoist in 1982, but might have accepted it earlier had there been such a system. Such an earlier assessment might therefore have resulted in avoidance of the accident. On all the evidence, it was clear that 'in their anxiety to care for the patients, the defendants lost sight of their duty to take reasonable steps to protect their district nurses'. This was causative of the accident. Liability was established and damages of £40,500 awarded. There was no contributory negligence because the employer had allowed a system of work to grow up in which the plaintiff did not consider herself but only the comfort of the patient (1986, High Court, unreported).

HAWKES v SOUTHWARK LONDON BOROUGH COUNCIL
Council carpenter; hanging doors; low risk but low cost involved; MHOR 1992; negligence case

In 1993, a carpenter was hanging heavy doors in a block of flats. The doors weighed 72lb. There were no lifts. He lost his balance on a landing and fell down the stairs, injuring his foot. The judge at first instance dismissed the case, because although there had been no risk assessment under r.4(1)(b) of the *MHOR 1992*, even if there had been one, the evidence suggested that the supervisor would still not have sanctioned assistance.

Reasonable practicability. The Court of Appeal overturned the judge's decision, finding that a proper assessment would have concluded that the task of moving the doors was a two-man job and assistance would have been provided. The court accepted that 'reasonably practicable' in the Regulations bore the meaning generally accepted by the courts since 1938 (that is, a setting of risk against the cost of doing something about it: *Edwards v National Coal Board*). The court had:

> to assess the risk of the plaintiff falling down the stairs and hurting his foot. If there was a real risk, then the court must go on and decide whether that risk could have been reduced and if so, how it could have been done with the least sacrifice to the defendants. It is that step which can be taken for comparison as the lowest level of sacrifice to the defendants. The court then has to carry out the weighing operation… The amount of risk to the plaintiff by doing what he did has to be weighed against the measures involved in reducing the risk. If the risk was insignificant in relation to the sacrifice then the defendants discharged the onus on them.

Adequacy of assessment. The court held that the judge's finding at first instance, that a risk assessment would have made no difference (because no assistance would have been provided by the Works Department), would only hold good if the 'hypothetical assessment were "a suitable and sufficient" (or proper) risk assessment as required by the Regulations'. Yet, given his acceptance of the plaintiff's expert evidence – to the effect that an assessment would have concluded that there was a significant risk of injury and two men would have been needed for the work in order to reduce – the judge was wrong to hold that any assessment which had concluded that there was no risk could have been suitable and sufficient.

Did the failure to assess risk cause the injury? The court also accepted that a failure to carry out a risk assessment did not in itself establish liability, since the plaintiff could only succeed if he established that his injury was caused by the failure of the defendants to take appropriate steps to reduce the risk of injury to the lowest level practicable. Put another way, if the employers complied with their duty to reduce the risk in this way, 'it was immaterial whether they made an assessment'. Likewise, if they did not so reduce the risk, 'no amount of assessment would save them from liability. So, at least in the circumstances of the present case, I would regard [the risk assessment] as merely an exhortation with no sanction attached, although it is no doubt a very wise precaution in many manual handling operations'.

Slight risk but slight cost to reduce it. Thus although the risk of injury was relatively slight, so too would have been the cost of providing an assistant to help with the hanging of the doors – whom the council should therefore have provided, in order to reduce the risk of injury to the lowest level reasonably practicable:

> The evidence of past practice establishes that the risk of falling down the stairs was slight and, for my part, I do not believe that the reasonable man would believe that the defendants were at fault for not providing assistance. That does not mean that they complied with the regulations… In my view the risk was slight as was the sacrifice. There was no evidence to suggest that the defendants, with their workforce, could not have made available a second man to help carry the door upstairs. How many extra man-hours would have been needed over a year was not clear and I do not believe it appropriate to assume, in the defendants' favour, that they would be other than minimal in the context of the total number of hours worked by the relevant personnel employed by the [council]. If so, the risk was not in my view insignificant in relation to the sacrifice.

Risk assessment. The court observed that the works department of the council had introduced manual handling protection, since the employee responsible for allocating work did not know of the *MHOR 1992* (1998, Court of Appeal, unreported).

HEALTH AND SAFETY AT WORK ACT 1974 (HSWA 1974)
The Health and Safety at Work Act 1974 (HSWA 1974) is the umbrella under which more specific regulations – such as the *MHOR 1992* – are made. Therefore the *MHOR 1992* must be seen in the context of the 1974 Act, as well as other complementary regulations such as the *Lifting Operations and Lifting Equipment Regulations 1998 (LOLER 1998)*, the *Provision and Use of Work Equipment Regulations 1998 (PUWER 1998)*, and the *Management of Health and Safety at Work Regulations 1999*.

Duties towards employees. The duties in s.2 of the HSWA 1974 towards employees are clearly relevant to manual handling and associated equipment, referring as they do to *systems of work*; to *information, instruction, training* and *supervision*; and to the use, handling, storage and transport of articles (e.g. manual handling equipment). If the HSE wishes to serve an *improvement notice* in respect of manual handling and the *MHOR 1992*, it will do so under s.21 of the HSWA 1974. Section 6 of the HSWA 1974 places specific duties in relation to persons who design, manufacture or supply equipment for use at work (e.g. manual handling equipment).

Duties towards non-employees. In relation to manual handling, the 1974 Act remains of great importance. First, the *MHOR 1992* do not apply to non-employees, so that if the Health and Safety Executive (HSE) wished to take action in respect of manual handling policies, practices or injuries concerning non-employees – such as patients, clients, relatives, care agency staff or staff of another statutory body – then it would normally do so under s.3 of the 1974 Act (see below) or r.3 of the *Management of the Health and Safety at Work Regulations 1999*.

Under s.3 of the 1974 Act, NHS Trusts have been prosecuted for failing to maintain equipment (*Health and Safety Executive v Norfolk and Norwich Healthcare NHS Trust*). Likewise, for instance, if a local authority is contracting out services (e.g. personal care/manual handling) to the independent sector it must pay reasonable attention to the tendering process and monitoring of the contract; if a failure to do this jeopardises the safety of either clients or the employees of the agency, then the local authority may be in breach of s.3 of the 1974 Act (see e.g. *Health and Safety Executive v Barnet London Borough Council*).

1. **HSWA 1974: employers and employees**. 'It shall be the duty of every employer to ensure, so far as is reasonably practicable, the health, safety and welfare at work of all his employees.' The employer's duty includes 'in particular:

    (a) the provision and maintenance of plant and systems of work that are, so far as is reasonably practicable, safe and without risk to health;

    (b) arrangements for ensuring, so far as is reasonably practicable, safety and absence of risks to health in connection with the use, handling, storage and transport of articles and substances;

    (c) the provision of such information, instruction, training and supervision as is necessary to ensure, so far as is reasonably practicable, the health and safety at work of his employers;

    (d) so far as is reasonably practicable as regards any place of work under the employer's control, the maintenance of it in a condition that is safe and without risks to health and the provision and maintenance of means of access to and egress from it that are safe and without such risk;

    (e) the provision and maintenance of a working environment for his employees that is, so far as is reasonably practicable, safe without risks to health, and adequate as regards facilities and arrangements for their welfare at work' (s.2).

2.   **HSWA 1974: employers and non-employees**. 'It shall be the duty of every employer to conduct his undertaking in such a way as to ensure, so far as is reasonably practicable, that persons not in his employment who may be affected thereby are not thereby exposed to risk to their health and safety' (s.3).

3.   **HSWA 1974: self-employed persons**. 'It shall be the duty of every self-employed person to conduct his undertaking in such a way as to ensure, so far as is reasonably practicable, that he and other persons (not being his employees) who may be affected thereby are not thereby exposed to risks to their health and safety' (s.3).

4.   **HSWA 1974: employees**. 'It shall be the duty of every employee while at work – (a) to take reasonable care for the health and safety of himself and of other persons who may be affected by his acts or omissions at work ...' (s.7).

5.   **HSWA 1974: health and safety at work policy**. Every employer with over five employees must prepare and revise as often as is appropriate a written statement of general health and safety policy (including the arrangements for carrying it out) and bring it to the attention of employees (s.2).

6.   **HSWA 1974: domestic servants**. Nothing in Part 1 of the Act applies 'in relation to a person by reason only that he employs another, or is himself employed, as a domestic servant in a private household' (s.51).

7.   **HSWA 1974: design, manufacture, supply of equipment**. 'It shall be the duty of any person who designs, manufactures, imports or supplies any article for use at work or any article of fairground equipment –

   (a)   to ensure, so far as is reasonably practicable, that the article is so designed and constructed that it will be safe and without risks to health at all times when it is being set, used, cleaned or maintained by a person at work;

   (b)   to carry out or arrange for the carrying out of such testing and examination as may be necessary for the performance of the duty imposed on him by the preceding paragraph;

   (c)   to take such steps as are necessary to secure that persons supplied by that person with the article are provided with adequate information about the use for which the article is designed or has been tested and about any conditions necessary to ensure that it will be safe and without risks to health at all times as are mentioned in paragraph (a) above and when it is being dismantled or disposed of; and

   (d)   to take such steps as are necessary to secure, so far as is reasonably practicable, that persons so supplied are provided with all such revisions of information provided to them by virtue of the preceding paragraph as are necessary by reason of its becoming known that anything gives rise to a serious risk to health or safety' (s.6).

'It shall be the duty of any person who undertakes the design or manu-facture of any article for use at work...to carry out or arrange for the car-rying out of any necessary research with a view to the discovery and, so far as is reasonably practicable, the elimination or minimisation of any risks to health or safety to which the design or article may give rise.'

'It shall be the duty of any person who erects or installs any article for use at work in any premises where that article is to be used by persons at work...to ensure, so far as is reasonably practicable, that nothing about the way in which the article is erected or installed makes it unsafe or a risk to health at any such time as' it is being set, used, cleaned or main-tained by a person at work (s.6).

HEALTH AND SAFETY AT WORK LEGISLATION

Health and safety at work legislation includes the *Health and Safety at Work Act 1974, Management of Health and Safety at Work Regulations 1999, Manual Handling Operations Regulations 1992, Lifting Operations and Lifting Equipment Regulations 1998* and the *Provision and Use of Work Equipment Regulations 1998*. Mainly dealing with the duties of em-ployers toward employees, such legislation also contains some duties towards non-employees. Such legislation should be distinguished sharply from *welfare legisla-tion* which sets out the duties and powers of local authority social services depart-ments and the NHS to provide services and equipment for clients and patients.

The Health and Safety Executive can bring criminal prosecution under health and safety at work legislation; employees can bring personal injury, civil compensa-tion cases for breach of statutory duty under some of the legislation (e.g. under the *MHOR 1992*, but not under the 1974 Act or 1999 regulations); but clients and pa-tients cannot sue for compensation under this legislation, and so must use the com-mon law of *negligence.*

HEALTH AND SAFETY EXECUTIVE v BARNET LONDON BOROUGH COUNCIL

Contracting out services; refuse collection; Health and Safety at Work Act 1974; prosecution

This case concerned the contracting out by a local authority of a refuse collection service; however, the principle and law involved could apply equally well to the con-tracting out of personal care services involving manual handling.

The Health and Safety Executive successfully prosecuted the local authority un-der s.3 of the *Health and Safety Work Act 1974* on the grounds that it knew that the contract for its refuse collection service was potentially under-funded; did not check the safety credentials of the contractor; and failed to monitor the contract conditions. Bad practices flourished, unsafe working was endemic and two serious accidents to employees of the contractor occurred (1997, Crown Court, unreported).

HEALTH AND SAFETY EXECUTIVE v GLOUCESTERSHIRE AMBULANCE SERVICE NHS TRUST
Manual handling risk assessments; failure to carry out; MHOR 1992

The NHS Trust was successfully prosecuted for failure to comply with an improvement notice, which had required that assessments be carried out under the *MHOR 1992* (1997, unreported).

HEALTH AND SAFETY EXECUTIVE v TRAFFORD HEALTH AUTHORITY
Patient falling out of bed; multiple burns received; Health and Safety at Work Act 1974

The health authority was successfully prosecuted under s.3 of the *Health and Safety at Work Act 1974* for failure to take care that patients were not exposed to risk from hot pipes. The patient concerned had fallen out of bed and received burns from unprotected pipes (1997, unreported).

HEALTH AND SAFETY EXECUTIVE v NORFOLK AND NORWICH HEALTHCARE NHS TRUST
Cardio-angiography equipment; failure to check; introduction of air; death of patient; Health and Safety at Work Act 1974, s.3; prosecution

The case concerned cardio-angiography and the failure to check the equipment properly. As it happened, air had got into the syringe. This made the equipment lethal, since it was almost an inevitable consequence that a patient would die (which is what occurred).

The court found that there was a failure to have a reasonably safe *system of work* to provide for the safety of patients under s.3 of the *Health and Safety at Work Act 1974*, given that there was an obvious risk in respect of this equipment. The court asked the question: 'Why was it that there was no strict discipline and procedure in being which meant that it was a matter of axiomatic routine that those deployed and using the machine went through a process of thorough checking to ensure that before the equipment was used, the syringe did not contain air?'

The fact that such equipment had been in place since 1980 and that 30,000 procedures had been performed without incident was not the point as the court saw it. This was because the health service had a duty to have a reasonably safe *system of work* since the:

> purpose of the law in this field is to ensure that the employer does not rest upon the assumptions that those he employs will always do the obvious. It is no more appropriate for those who employ medical experts than it is for those who employ people in a factory, for them to assume that medical experts and medical staff will act invariably to prevent the consequences of an obvious risk (1998, Crown Court, unreported).

HEALTH SERVICE OMBUDSMAN

Under the Health Service Commissioners Act 1993, the health service ombudsman can investigate complaints about injustice or hardship sustained as a result of a failure in a service, failure to provide a service for which there is a duty to provide, or maladministration. Since April 1996, the health service ombudsman has been able to question the merits of professional decision-making by NHS staff. Maladministration could include, for instance, bias, neglect, inattention, delay, incompetence, ineptitude, perversity, turpitude, arbitrariness, or *fettering of discretion* (e.g. *Epsom and St Helier NHS Trust*). Decisions involving manual handling related services and equipment potentially come within the ambit of health service ombudsman investigations.

HEALTH SERVICES AND PUBLIC HEALTH ACT 1968

Under s.45 of this Act, local authorities in England and Wales have a general power to arrange in the homes of those older people deemed not to be disabled, practical assistance, home adaptations and equipment. However, it is probable that where there are significant manual handling needs, older people will often be treated as disabled and therefore come under the *Chronically Sick and Disabled Persons Act 1970*, which contains a duty rather than a power.

HEAVY PATIENTS

In both hospital and the community, health and social care staff are increasingly encountering very heavy patients and clients; if policies and practices are not in place for dealing with such people, then the safety and dignity of all may be at risk, and sometimes even the physical fabric of a building (for instance, the combined weight of a very heavy person and his or her electric wheelchair might test the capacity of some floors). In one situation, for instance, a district nurse was asked by a general practitioner to visit and 'sort out' an elderly woman who had fallen at home from her commode. The general practitioner failed to mention that she weighed 25 stone; eventually lifting her in a blanket required four ambulance staff, six fire officers, the district nurse and the woman's husband (Williams 1996).

Guidance states that the encountering of such heavy people is foreseeable; and that any large NHS Trust might expect to treat a number of patients each year weighing over 20 stone; and that therefore suitable equipment and procedures must be available (RCN/NBPA 1997, p.189; see also HSC 1998, p.44).

HILLHOUSE v SOUTH AYRSHIRE COUNCIL

Caretaker; moving tables; weight of tables; reasonable practicability of reducing risk; credibility of evidence; MHOR 1992

In 1996, a caretaker at a visitor attraction had been asked to move a number of tables weighing 30lb and measuring three by six feet. The judge found that he was not a credible witness and so dismissed his case on the basis that he was not prepared to find that the employee had suffered any back pain or strain as a result of moving the tables. However, the judge went on to consider what the position would otherwise have been under the *MHOR 1992*.

No duty of risk assessment. First, he found that the duty to carry out a risk assessment arose if there was a foreseeable risk of injury. But the tables were lightweight and fell well within the guidelines included in the Health and Safety Executive's guidance (HSE 1998). Given that the employer had been assured previously by the employee that he was fit for all his duties, the court found that there had been no duty of risk assessment.

Avoidance or reduction of risk. Second, just in case he was wrong in that conclusion, the judge went on to consider what the employer would have concluded following a risk assessment. He found that the conclusion would have been that there was no other practicable method of moving the tables. For instance, the employee had claimed that had he been allowed to drive his van closer to the building, he would not have had to walk so far with the tables. But this would have been impracticable because it would have meant walking through the cafeteria where customers were sitting at tables and moving about carrying hot food and liquids. Also, the tables were of such a shape and size that a barrow would have been of no assistance; and even two persons would not only have not reduced the risk of injury, but even possibly increased it – the tables were designed for carrying by one person. So there was anyway no breach of the *MHOR 1992* ([2000] GWD 31–1240, Outer House, Court of Session, Scotland).

HOISTS

Hoists are a key type of lifting equipment and their provision and use are subject to various *health and safety at work legislation*, including the *Lifting Operations and Lifting Equipment Regulations 1998*, and the *Provision and Use of Work Equipment Regulations 1998*. Some personal injury compensation cases have involved the failure either to provide hoists (e.g. *McGowan v Harrow Health Authority*) or to ensure that they are actually used (e.g. *Salvat v Basingstoke and North Hampshire Health Authority*): see under *equipment* for further cases.

Equipment stores in the NHS and social services constantly have to decide the extent to which they will 'mix and match' the hoists of one manufacturer with the slings of another. Strictly speaking, this might appear to be a form of what the Medical Devices Agency (MDA) has called 'cannibalisation' – that is, the mixing of parts from different manufacturers – and which it does not recommend for equipment in general (MDA DB9801, p.C12). Nevertheless, practicality means that many equipment stores do mix hoists and slings; and more specific MDA advice is to the effect that where this does happen, the following factors should be considered as part of a risk assessment: (a) guidance from the hoist manufacturer or supplier; (b) whether the sling has been designed for use with the specific hoist; (c) assurance from the sling manufacturer that the sling is suitable for use with the particular model of hoist; (d) advice from legal advisors and insurers; (e) professional assessment of compatibility;

and (f) whether the sling meets requirements of relevant standards (these points are drawn from a standard MDA letter used to answer enquiries concerning hoists and slings).

For more on hoists and other equipment, including notices issued by the Medical Devices Agency, see *equipment*.

HOME ADAPTATIONS

Home adaptations, like equipment, might be one way of meeting disabled people's mobility and manual handling needs, as well as preserving their *carers* from injury. Assistance with home adaptations is potentially available through the *Housing Grants, Construction and Regeneration Act 1996* (England and Wales), the *Chronically Sick and Disabled Persons Act 1970* (England, Wales and Scotland), the *Health Services and Public Health Act 1968* (England and Wales), and the *Housing (Scotland) Act 1987*.

It is beyond the scope of this book to set out the system of obtaining home adaptations, which is complex and is also different in England and Wales than in Scotland. However, obtaining major adaptations in timely fashion is not necessarily easy; apart from the practicalities involved in all major work to dwellings, the process within councils of assessment, decision-making and provision might be longwinded and arduous for clients. In order to illustrate this, a few (there are many which could be cited) local government ombudsman investigations are included in this book, in some detail, in order to give a flavour of the potential difficulties (see *Barking and Dagenham London Borough Council; Bristol City Council* (on rehousing); *Camden London Borough Council; Islington London Borough Council; Rotherham Metropolitan Borough Council*).

HOME AND FAMILY LIFE

The right to respect for home and family life is sometimes referred to in the context of the *Human Rights Act 1998* and the *European Convention on Human Rights*, as possibly applicable to manual handling decisions.

HOPKINSON v KENT COUNTY COUNCIL
Care assistant; standing resident up; bending and twisting; voluntary and unpaid induction programme; negligence case

The plaintiff was a care assistant at a residential home for older people. In 1982, she was dressing a heavy man suffering from multiple disabilities. With another care assistant, she had got the patient sitting on his bed with his pants and trousers round his ankles. As they stood him up, each with an arm under one of his arms, she bent down to pull up the trousers and pants and felt a terrible pain in her back. The evidence suggested that she must have bent and twisted, and so committed 'the cardinal sin of kinetics'. The plaintiff claimed that she was totally untrained in the potentially dangerous task of handling old, disabled and sometimes heavy patients.

There had been an induction programme for staff consisting of two sessions, one of 75 minutes and the other 80 minutes. The judge referred to two obvious flaws, namely that they were voluntary and unpaid; in any case the plaintiff had been on neither. The judge found that had the plaintiff received the appropriate training, she would have been specifically warned against bending and twisting. Damages of £33,750 were awarded (1987, High Court, unreported).

HOUSING (SCOTLAND) ACT 1987

Grants – known as improvement grants – for *home adaptations* for disabled people are available in Scotland, subject to various conditions, under the *Housing (Scotland) Act 1987* (as amended by the *Housing (Scotland) Act 2001*). As housing legislation, the Act represents an alternative to the social services route of s.2 of the *Chronically Sick and Disabled Persons Act 1970* for the provision of such adaptations. It is beyond the scope of this book to set out the details of the Act. For England and Wales, see the *Housing Grants, Construction and Regeneration Act 1996*.

HOUSING GRANTS, CONSTRUCTION AND REGENERATION ACT 1996

Grants – known as disabled facilities grants – for *home adaptations* for disabled people are in some circumstances mandatory for disabled people of all ages under the Housing Grants, Construction and Regeneration Act 1996. As housing legislation, the Act represents an alternative to the social services route of s.2 of the *Chronically Sick and Disabled Persons Act 1970* for the provision of such adaptations.

It is beyond the scope of this book to set out the details of the Act and its operation, but it should be borne in mind that (a) such adaptations might be crucial in relation to a person's mobility and access to rooms and facilities in the home (and therefore in relation also to manual handling issues); (b) the duty to approve such grants is in principle a strong one, though subject to a means test; and (c) the disabled facilities grants system is in some areas beset by practical difficulties and consequently is not always lawfully operated by local housing authorities.

For Scotland, see the *Housing (Scotland) Act 1987*.

HUMAN RIGHTS: see *European Convention on Human Rights; Human Rights Act 1998*

HUMAN RIGHTS ACT 1998

When public bodies such as local authorities and NHS Trusts make decisions and provide services, they must, since October 2000, comply not just with relevant domestic, United Kingdom legislation, but also with the Human Rights Act 1998 which has incorporated the *European Convention on Human Rights* into United Kingdom law. For an outline of how manual handling decisions might or might not be affected, see the entry *European Convention on Human Rights*.

HUNTER v HANLEY
Test of professional carelessness; negligence

A case (involving an injection) setting out the test for establishing professional care-lessness in *negligence* cases:

> To establish liability by a doctor where deviation from normal practice is alleged, three facts require to be established. First of all it must be proved that there is a usual and normal practice. Secondly it must be proved that the defender has not adopted that practice, and thirdly (and this is of crucial importance) it must be established that the course the doctor adopted is one which no professional man of ordinary skill would have taken if he had been acting with ordinary care ((1955 SC 200, Inner House, Court of Session, Scotland).

ILLEGALITY

Illegality is a ground on which the decision-making of public bodies such as the NHS and local authorities is sometimes challenged by clients and patients. Courts will strike decisions down if they are based on apparent contravention of legislation – as happened, for example, when a local authority's community care assessment of a disabled person failed to take account of his social, recreational and leisure needs, despite explicit reference to such matters in s.2 of the *Chronically Sick and Disabled Persons Act 1970 (R v Haringey London Borough Council, ex p Norton)*.

IMPROVEMENT NOTICES

Preceding possible criminal prosecution under *health and safety at work legislation*, the Health and Safety Executive may issue an improvement notice under s.21 of the *Health and Safety at Work Act 1974* demanding that an organisation carry out certain tasks – for instance, undertake risk assessments under the *MHOR 1992*. Failure to comply with an improvement notice might then result in prosecution (e.g. *Health and Safety Executive v Gloucestershire Ambulance Service NHS Trust*).

INDEPENDENT LIVING

Community care direct payments are aimed at giving greater choice and independence to disabled people, by allowing them, for example, to employ their own care assistants. This situation sometimes gives rise to disputes, when the disabled person maintains that it is safe for assistants to handle him or her in a certain way, but the local authority (provider of the payment) does not agree: see *community care direct payments*. More generally, it has been argued that the way in which the *MHOR 1992* have been implemented locally by the NHS and by local authorities has unreasonably restricted disabled people's lives (Cunningham 2000, p.1). See further in section 6 of the Overview in this book.

INDIVIDUAL CAPABILITY

Apart from identifying general risk existing in certain types of situation, risk assessments must also take account of individual capability – as is made clear in schedule 1 of the *MHOR 1992* and r.13 of the *Management of Health and Safety at Work Regulations 1999*.

In manual handling cases, the courts have considered the importance of this issue (often in relation to a pre-existing back injury and the role of medical certificates, to representations by employees about problems they were having with manual handling tasks, and to the extent that the employer should have checked the individual's ability to carry out the task), sometimes finding that employers did not take adequate steps (e.g. *Paramerissios v Hammersmith and Fulham London Borough Council; Seamner v North East Essex Health Authority; Wells v West Hertfordshire Health Authority*) and sometimes that they did (*Bowfield v South Sefton (Merseyside) Health Authority; Halliday v Tayside Health Board; Parkes v Smethwick Corporation; Rozario v Post Office; Slater v Fife Primary Care NHS Trust*).

In addition, the courts have recognised that a necessary implication of risk assessment, for both staff generally and for individual members of staff, is that individual needs of patients and clients too will need to be assessed, to identify particular or additional risk posed: see under *patient and client need*.

INFORMATION: see *instructions and information*

INSTRUCTIONS AND INFORMATION

Instructions, information and warnings are legally a crucial part of a safe *system of work* under the *Health and Safety at Work Act 1974, MHOR 1992, Management of Health and Safety Work Regulations 1999, Provision and Use of Work Equipment Regulations 1998*, and in the common law of negligence. Failure to provide them has resulted in liability in many cases for employers.

Such cases have included failure to instruct or inform: nurses about the use of hoists (*Edwards v Waltham Forest Health Authority*); nurses about how to perform a particular type of lift (*Fraser v Greater Glasgow Health Board; Hadfield v Manchester Health Authority*); hospital craft ladies about assistance for elderly patients (*O'Neill v Boorowa District Hospital*); hospital laundry workers (*Anderson v Lothian Health Board*); swimming pool attendants packing away slides (*Barnes v Stockton Borough Council*); social workers (*Colclough v Staffordshire County Council*); lorry or van drivers about unloading (*Blanchflower v Chamberlain*); electricians about the manufacturer's instructions (*McBeath v Halliday*); and road workers about laying pavement slabs (*Skinner v Aberdeen City Council*). In one case, a manual handling trainer was held not to have given adequate instructions to trainees on her course (*Beattie v West Dorset Health Authority*). Notably, the Court of Appeal has held that the duty to provide information about loads under the *MHOR 1992* does not depend on there having been a risk assessment first (*Swain v Denso Martin*).

Of course, sometimes the courts rule that information or instructions were not required – for a nurse aide experienced and knowing how to do the task which caused injury in handling geriatric patients (*Charnock v Capital Territory Health Commission*), for school staff moving cupboards (*Taylor v Glasgow City Council*) or scrap metal yard workers moving lumps of lead (*Chalk v Devizes*). Alternatively, the instructions might have been relatively clear; for instance, on the procedure for lifting nursing home residents (*McCaffery v Datta*).

IRRATIONALITY: see *unreasonableness*

ISLINGTON LONDON BOROUGH COUNCIL
Local government ombudsman investigation; manual handling; shower and stairlift; conflict between need and safety policy concerning stairlift installation; inaction of council; failure to resolve issue; maladministration

This was an investigation by the local government ombudsman illustrating, amongst other things, the manual handling implications for clients and *carers* of delay in dealing with applications for *home adaptations*.

The complainant was the mother of a man with motor neurone disease; she complained that the council had unreasonably (a) delayed in providing a shower, and (b) refused to provide a stairlift. The man had three children aged between 11 and 15 years; his wife had recently had heart surgery.

Range of options identified. The original assessment by an occupational therapist in July 1986 identified a number of options: transfer of accommodation, conversion of the basement, two internal stairlifts, through-floor lift, external shaft lift, and level access shower unit. The shower and internal stairlifts were the options preferred by the family. In addition, a number of minor adaptations were installed quickly: entry phone, cordless telephone and stair rail.

Unacceptable delay in installing shower. The shower took 18 months to install; part of the delay had been because of the workload on the surveyors within the council. However, the order had been marked urgent and did not appear to have received corresponding priority. This was maladministration.

Stairlift: conflict between a person's needs and safety policy. As to one of the stairlifts, the council stated that without an increase in the depth of the first floor landing, it would not achieve the recommended clearance (with safety in mind) at the top of the stairs as recommended in the council's design guide for people with disabilities. However, any such alteration would have involved setting back the man's bedroom wall; this was not acceptable to the family because of the fear of dust and draughts during the works, since colds or respiratory illness could be extremely dangerous for people with motor neurone disease.

Further options were considered but agreement could not be reached; for example, another type of stairlift with a swivel chair was considered, but the occupational therapy team leader expressed concern because the chair would block the staircase and constitute a risk for other members of the family.

Differing opinions within council, and the manual handling implications. Differences of opinion persisted on the safety ground – between the architects department (which was prepared to proceed) and the building works department, which was not. In the meantime, the man had offered to sign any disclaimer (in case of accident) which the council felt was appropriate. This offer was not taken up.

Family's perception of situation and danger involving manual handling. The family felt that the council's preoccupation with safety was somewhat 'hollow', since it appeared to disregard completely the daily risks to the family, when the children and elderly mother carried the man up and down the stairs.

The ombudsman pointed out that the family was in an unfortunate situation: both man and wife had serious health problems, and his mother, though in better health, was 76 years old. In the circumstances, it was inappropriate for 'others to quarrel with the family's perception of the situation' which led the family to reject the idea of setting the bedroom wall back. Furthermore, the man faced 'very real danger' every day; the family had tried to cope with the situation as far as possible without calling on social services; and the man had offered to sign a disclaimer.

Failure of council to resolve conflicting considerations. The ombudsman found these arguments 'compelling' and could not 'understand that the importance of the design brief must outweigh them all'. In the light of the council's policy of enabling people to remain at home, it needed 'to give very careful consideration to those cases where another aspect of their policy contradicts this'. The ombudsman did not believe that the council had thought through adequately the consequences of such a clash; and that it should 'put all the facts to Members who will then be in a position to come to a proper reasoned decision' as soon as possible (1988: case 88/A/303).

JONES v SOUTH GLAMORGAN HEALTH AUTHORITY
Home visit; auxiliary nurse; lifting patient up in bed; liability admitted; damages agreed, subject to causation; negligence case

An auxiliary nurse was in 1984 visiting a patient at home, who was lying in a double bed. In order to lift the patient up, with the assistance of another lady on the far side of the bed, she had to get onto the bed and was kneeling with her left hand on the headboard and her right arm under the patient's arm to pull him up. She rotated her lower back, so as to twist round the upper part of her body; something in her back 'gave'. In the decade since the accident, the pain and attendant problems had worsened. She was virtually never free from pain, had not worked and could not carry out everyday household tasks. Treatments had included traction, plaster jacket, physiotherapy, hydro-therapy, epidural injection into her back, a number of injections into the facet joints and various drugs. The judge noted that it was accepted that she was entirely honest and genuine in her claim.

The health authority admitted liability and also agreed £175,000 damages, subject to causation being shown between the accident and the extent of disability now claimed for. This causation was shown and that amount of damages awarded (1996, High Court, unreported).

JUDE v ELLIOTT MEDWAY LTD
Prefabricated wall panels; damaged jig; question of limitation of time for bringing action; manly attitude; negligence case

An injury was allegedly sustained by a 39-year-old employee in July 1992 (although he argued also cumulative injury prior to that particular incident) when he was removing a prefabricated wall panel from a damaged jig. At first instance, the court had dismissed the action because of breach of s.14 of the *Limitation Act 1980*, which required that it be brought within three years of the accident. However, the Court of Appeal now decided on balance that it should exercise its discretion to allow the case to progress. Amongst other points, it stated that although the plaintiff did not act promptly and reasonably, this did 'not prevent the court from having sympathy with the manly attitude to get on with work and not to rush to the lawyers. It would be a sad day if we were to penalise the plaintiff for not rushing to litigation when litigation is the thing that we strive to discourage' (1999, Court of Appeal, unreported).

JUDICIAL REVIEW
Judicial review is the type of legal action that can be brought by clients and patients to challenge the decision-making of public bodies, including the NHS and local authority social services departments. The courts apply a number of principles in order to test whether a public body is acting lawfully. For instance, they wish to see that it is: *taking account of all relevant factors* (and leaving aside irrelevant factors), not *fettering its discretion* (i.e. not applying a policy totally rigidly), not guilty of *illegality* (i.e. not blatantly contravening legislation), avoiding *unreasonableness* (i.e. taking leave of its senses in terms of irrationality), and not dashing people's *legitimate expectations*.

For instance, when a local authority reduced services to a woman with multiple sclerosis, it appeared to have paid attention to manual handling implications and to resources, but not to the woman's needs. The judge's striking down of the decision was in effect a finding of *illegality*, since community care legislation demanded that people's needs be properly assessed and reassessed. And in finding that relevant medical evidence had not been obtained and considered, the judge was in effect finding that not all relevant factors had been considered (*R v Birmingham City Council, ex p Killigrew*).

Judicial review cases should be sharply distinguished from personal injury compensation cases in *negligence* or under *health and safety at work legislation*; judicial review is primarily about changing decisions, not about financial compensation.

KELLY v FORTICRETE LTD
Investing in training; videos; adequacy; MHOR 1992

The plaintiff worked for architectural masons who manufactured concrete blocks; he had to remove the wooden side pieces; the particular piece involved in the 1993 accident could have weighed 50–95lb. He argued that he had received no proper training, although he had worked in the department for 14 years. At first instance, the Assistant Recorder had held the employer liable. He found that training had been given including theoretical instructions, video and practical demonstration. However, it was clear on the evidence that only 15 minutes were allocated for 35 minutes of video, and the fourth video would not necessarily be shown. Yet it was this fourth video that showed a labourer doing a routine job and how he should be alert to the need to ask for help.

Now the Court of Appeal held that it could not consider overturning the original court's finding of liability (and £4,500 damages). It had sympathy for the defendants who said that they had invested in appropriate training – but they had ignored other means of minimising risk:

> The Manual Handling Operations Regulations require the performance of a risk assessment. This requires employers to think about the ways in which they can reduce the level of risk to their operatives in the way required of them by Parliament. It is well-known that operatives can do silly things which expose them to significant risk of personal injury if appropriate steps are not taken to diminish the risk. The Assistant Recorder appears to have taken the view that if the defendants decided to place all their eggs in one basket (by investing in training without seeing what other comparatively straightforward steps might be taken to avoid the risk) then they would be at risk if the training which they had commissioned for one reason or another failed to come up to their expectations or to the contractor's contractual obligations, with the effect in the present case that within six months of going through one of those training courses the plaintiff did something which the training was designed to prevent him doing. (1999, Court of Appeal, unrecorded)

KEMPSEY DISTRICT HOSPITAL v THACKHAM
Casual nurse; bed rail negligently left down; injury when assisting patient who was trying to pull himself out of bed; negligence case

This was a case appealed on various points. However, the original injury and thus the root of the compensation claim rested on a bed rail having been left down, the patient then trying to pull himself out of bed, and the casual nurse, the plaintiff, coming to assist him, but sustaining an injury. This had occurred in 1981, but there was no trial until 1994, because it was many years before the seriousness and real consequences of the injury became apparent. At this trial, the judge found the employer vicariously liable for the negligence of the member of staff who had left the bed rail down and no contributory negligence; these findings were not challenged in this appeal (1995, Supreme Court of New South Wales Court of Appeal, Australia, transcript).

KENT v GRIFFITHS
Non-arrival of ambulance; injury suffered as a result; negligence case by patient against the NHS; relevance of resources and priorities

This was a negligence case against the NHS, illustrating the potential reluctance of the courts to find liability if the matter is, overall, one of lack of resources and the case has been brought by a patient (as opposed to an employee).

It was brought against the London Ambulance Service. At first instance, the judge awarded the plaintiff £362,377, after an ambulance had taken 40 minutes to respond to an emergency call for a woman who had suffered a severe asthma attack. This was despite several calls to the service, and a reassurance on each occasion that the ambulance's arrival was imminent. She suffered a respiratory arrest and substantial memory impairment, personality change and a miscarriage as a result. The Court of Appeal now upheld the finding of liability, noting that the case did not hinge on an argument about lack of resources – but that had this been the root cause, then the court's judgment might have been different:

> An important feature of this case is that there is no question of an ambulance not being available or of a conflict in priorities. Again I recognise that where what is being attacked is the allocation of resources, whether in the provision of sufficient ambulances or attendants, different considerations could apply. There then could be issues which are not suited for resolution by the courts. However, once there are available, both in the form of an ambulance and in the form of manpower, the resources to provide an ambulance on which there are no alternative demands, the ambulance service would be acting perversely...if it did not make those resources available. Having decided to provide an ambulance an explanation is required to justify a failure to attend within a reasonable time. ([2001] QB 36 2000, Court of Appeal).

KING v CARRON PHOENIX LTD
Work with spanner; repetitive tasks; whether coming under the MHOR 1992; negligence case

A case indicating court-imposed limits on the scope of the physical activities which can come under the *MHOR 1992*.

A 42-year-old mechanical maintenance engineer sought damages for tennis elbow, allegedly caused by the repetitive removing and replacing of bolts with a spanner on eight-hour shifts. The case was brought both in negligence and under the *MHOR 1992*.

The common law case failed on insufficient evidence both as to causation and as to what the employer might reasonably have done by way of alternative arrangements. The court held that the task did not come under the *MHOR 1992*: 'as a matter of ordinary language and in the context of the regulations, although the pursuer was no doubt involved in pushing and pulling when working with the spanner, it could not be said that he was involved in transporting or supporting a load' ([1999] GWD 9–437, Outer House, Court of Session, Scotland).

KING v RCO SUPPORT SERVICES AND ANOTHER
Laying grit; slipping on ice; whether coming under MHOR 1992; avoidance of risk

A case illustrating the potential scope of activities to which the *MHOR 1992* might be held to apply.

The court held that a 57-year-old employee laying grit in the icy yard of a steam cleaning concern in 1996 was undertaking an activity subject to the *MHOR 1992*, and that the employer ought to have avoided the risk of slipping, unless it was not reasonably practicable to do so. He had been gritting the yard, as he usually did on an icy morning, for nearly two hours when he inadvertently stepped off the gritted area on to the ice and was injured. He had failed in his County Court case and now appealed.

Foreseeability of risk, reasonable foreseeability or whether either is necessary. The claimant's case was that the underlying purpose of the framework European directive (89/391), which underlies the *European directive on manual handling* (and thus also the *MHOR 1992*), was to impose an absolute duty. Thus, in respect of the risk which there was a duty to avoid or reduce, there should be no qualification of reasonable foreseeability or even foreseeability. The Court of Appeal avoided answering this question, by stating that it was not necessary to decide whether the risk in r.4 of the *MHOR 1992* 'carries with it a necessary implication of foreseeability because I am entirely satisfied that whatever definition of risk that one applies, there was a risk here'. The court also dismissed the argument that the distribution of the grit had nothing to do with the transporting or moving or handling of any load within the meaning of the *MHOR 1992*.

No defence. Furthermore, as no defence was put forward that it was not reasonably practicable to avoid the risk, the court would assume that it was – namely by means of a mechanical gritter. The court accepted that there should be 50 per cent contributory negligence, since the claimant had suffered a lapse of concentration; however, 'the task was a long one and any prudent employer would have to recognise that [the employee's] concentration might wander over the prolonged spell of two hours that the task would take' ([2001] PIQR P15, Court of Appeal).

KINSELLA v HARRIS LEBUS LTD
Cabinet maker; Factories Act 1937; system of work; whether 145lb excessive weight

An older case, illustrating that what is considered to be a safe lifting weight has changed over time.

The case was brought under s.56 of the Factories Act 1937 (now obsolete). The employee, a cabinet maker, suffered a hernia injury when moving, single-handed in a constricted space, a large, unwieldy jig weighing 145lb. The court stated that the *system of work* was no system at all, since it put the onus on individual employees to decide whether or not to get assistance. However, the Act was designed to protect against excessive weight only, and 145lb was not likely to cause injury to a man of experience ((1963) 108 Sol Jo 14, Court of Appeal).

KOONJUL v THAMESLINK HEALTHCARE NHS TRUST
Care assistant; making beds; whether MHOR 1992 breached in respect of everyday tasks

The claimant was a 47-year-old care assistant who had worked for eight years in a residential home for children with learning disabilities, which also provided respite care for children with emotional and behavioural disorders. Previously she had been a care assistant in a hospital. She suffered injury in 1996 whilst making a bed, but her case under the *MHOR 1992* failed, the court referring to a number of matters including her experience, the reasons for the beds being arranged as they were, and the impracticality of conducting precise risk assessments for innumerable everyday tasks.

Injury whilst making bed. She injured her back on a Sunday when making an unusually low bed, some 18 inches high; the bar along the side, which she pulled, was some five inches off the ground. The beds were used for children who had epilepsy or other conditions which meant they might easily fall out of bed; hence the lowness of the beds. Likewise for safety reasons the bed had one side pushed against the wall; so that to make it, the assistant had to move a chest of drawers and chair out of the way and pull the bed away from the wall. The home had three beds like this; the two metal ones had castors on the bed-head legs but not on all four legs (again for safety reasons). The wooden bed may or may not have had castors on at the time. It was not clear now which bed she had been making when she was injured.

Risk of foreseeable but not probable injury. The Court of Appeal rejected her claim. It accepted that for the *MHOR 1992* to apply there had to be a 'real risk, a foreseeable possibility of injury; certainly nothing approaching a probability'. Furthermore:

> in making an assessment of whether there is such a risk of injury, the employer is not entitled to assume that all his employees will on all occasions behave with full and proper concern for their own safety. I accept that the purpose of regulations such as these is indeed to place upon employers obligations to look after their employees' safety which they might not otherwise have.

However:

[everyday tasks] 'The question of what does involve a risk of injury must be context-based. One is therefore looking at this particular operation in the context of this particular place of employment and also the particular employees involved. In this case, we have a small residential home with a small number of employees. But those employees were carrying out what may be regarded as everyday tasks, and this particular employee had been carrying out such tasks for a very long time indeed. The employer in seeking to assess the risks is entitled to take that into account.

[background and experience] Furthermore, when one comes to the question of whether there was indeed a risk in this case, one has to bear in mind that this particular employee accepted that she had been taught in the hospital that if she bent down she had to keep her knees bent and her back straight. She knew, therefore, as a result of her employment of long standing, how to go about tasks which involved pulling, pushing or lifting, for which it might be necessary to reduce her height. Furthermore, she had gone on a moving and handling course at the Faculty of Health at the University of Greenwich in June 1995 some ten months before the accident; the content of that course makes it plain that it entailed the principles involved in avoiding injury when carrying out manual handling tasks of the sort involved, in particular, in lifting patients; but those principles are of course applicable in other contexts as well...

[avoidance of risk] I am prepared to assume that some risk could be envisaged from such an operation... However, when it comes to whether or not there was a breach of the regulations, it seems to me that in the particular circumstances of the case there was no such breach. The first obligation is to avoid the need for employees to undertake such operations, as far as reasonably practicable. In this case, it is alleged that the bed did not need to be against the wall and has since been moved away from the wall. But the purpose of having the bed against the wall was to save children from risk of harm through falling out of bed, and it seems to be me that if there are children resident in the home for whom that is a risk, it is entirely appropriate that such beds should be against the wall and it is therefore not right to expect the employer to have the beds away from the wall in every circumstance.

[reducing risk] The other relevant obligation is to take appropriate steps to reduce the risk of injury to employees, arising out of their undertaking any such manual handling operations, to the lowest level reasonably practicable. [It was argued] that it was the simplest thing in the world to tell the claimant in this case that she had to kneel down or squat down when trying to pull this bed away from the wall. That has a superficial attraction to it. Nevertheless, if one again looks at it in the context of this particular employment, it is an employment involving a number of everyday tasks, any one of which could involve something which could be described as a manual handling operation – lifting bedding, moving beds around in order to make them, moving the chest of drawers, or moving the chair in order to make the bed. There are innumerable tasks around such a home, and the idea that the level of risk involved (which I have already said was very low) should be met by a precise evaluation of each of those tasks and precise warnings to each employee as to how each was to be carried out, seems to me to take the matter way beyond the realms of practicability.

[no breach of MHOR 1992] It has to be borne in mind throughout that this is an experienced employee who knew how she should be carrying out tasks of this sort. In those circumstances it does not seem to me that there is any breach of these regulations involved. ([2000] PIQR P123, Court of Appeal)

LAING v TAYSIDE HEALTH BOARD
Nursing auxiliary; home visit; lift from wheelchair to bed; bed moving; unsafe system of work; two staff required; training; modification of environment; negligence case

A nursing auxiliary aged 40 was injured in 1990. She worked two evenings a week, visiting sick or elderly people at home, and helping them undress, get into bed and settle down for the night.

Home visit and accident: moving bed. The patient in question was a 68-year-old man who had suffered a right-sided stroke depriving him of normal speech. He lived with his wife and weighed 10.5 stone. The court accepted that although he could be cooperative and able to assist in the mornings, in the evenings he could not give any substantial assistance when being transferred from wheelchair to bed. The pursuer had visited him previously without problem – she would pull him to the front of the wheelchair, and then lift him straight up vertically, at which point she would be supporting his entire weight. She would then twist or turn him to her left and put him on the bed. On the evening in question, as she was lifting, the bed moved (the cause was never established, although the suspicion had been that the bed had come off its raising blocks).

Injury and pain. The pursuer subsequently had an operation involving the grafting of bone from her hip. However, the pain returned for the next few years until in 1995 it got worse. The pain was so bad she was physically sick on many occasions and sometimes had to remain for up to two weeks in bed. She now had morphine tablets to relieve the pain; and had to stop having physiotherapy because it precipitated pain and was too distressing. Her condition was likely to remain the same for the foreseeable future.

System of work and whether two staff required for lift. The court held the employer liable. The *system of work* was held not to be safe, since the bed movement caused the accident – but if the pursuer had had assistance, the injury probably would not have occurred. There was nothing about the layout of the room that would have prevented two people lifting; and for some patients, arrangements were made for two staff members to lift. The question was therefore whether there should have been two people lifting this particular patient.

The court was unimpressed with the argument that up to 1990, the man's wife had managed to look after her husband single-handed, since the very reason why the health board was called on for assistance was precisely because the wife had hurt her back when assisting her husband out of the bath. The evidence was to the effect that a reasonable approach would have been to provide two people for lifting a fairly heavy patient who could not take his or her own weight – and the husband was just such a patient. Furthermore, the court was shown a 'nursing procedure book' from one of the health board's hospitals which stated that in 'the majority of lifting situations assistance should be obtained and the nurse should direct such assistance in the use of correct lifting techniques'. It also transpired that in the hospital, two nurses were always used to transfer a patient from a wheelchair. Thus, it was reasonably foreseeable that the pursuer would sustain an injury in such circumstances. Damages were awarded of some £79,100.

Training. Although the employer was in breach of the duty to provide training in lifting techniques for the pursuer, nevertheless, the court held that the training would not have taught her how to avoid injury in the situation of the bed moving.

Modifying the home environment. It was not clear whether the bed was on castors or blocks, but the court made the point that:

> there must be thousands of beds on castors and it is common knowledge that castors are often fitted in order to reduce the effort involved in moving a bed. Against that background I would not be prepared to hold, in the absence of any evidence on the point, that a reasonable health board would have had the castors on a bed in a private house put in cups or removed simply because a patient was to be transferred to the bed by a nurse working without assistance. ([1996] Rep LR 51 1996, Outer House, Court of Session, Scotland)

LANE v CAPITAL TERRITORY HEALTH COMMISSION
Trainee nurse aide; nursing home; lift of resident from wheelchair to bed; absence of wardsmen; negligence case

An older case, in which the plaintiff, a trainee nurse aide, was injured in 1978 when lifting a patient from wheelchair to bed, one nurse putting her arms underneath his armpits, and the plaintiff gripping his legs above his knees. The latter suffered an injury.

At first instance, the judge had concluded that the plaintiff had received adequate instruction about the lifting of patients from chair to bed. The plaintiff on appeal to the Supreme Court had alleged that the evidence showed a failure in the *system of work* in that no wardsman was available to assist, and in requiring the plaintiff to lift the particular patient at all. (This case might be decided differently today.)

The Federal Court now found that the original judge had sufficient evidence to reach the conclusion that he did in finding no liability. For instance the plaintiff was lifting the patient's legs (the lighter end) and by means of an accepted and widely used method; and the fact that wardsmen had been introduced into nursing homes, to reduce the risk of injury generally, was not enough to show that the absence of them was negligent in this particular situation. This decision was reached by two of the Federal Court judges and so the plaintiff's appeal was dismissed. However, the third judge dissented, finding on the evidence that the injury was foreseeable since she was lifting a difficult, heavy male patient who moved during the lift; that he probably would not have done so had a wardsman been involved; that she would then not have been injured; and that a wardsman should have been available (1985, Federal Court of Australia, on appeal from the Supreme Court of the Australian Capital Territory, transcript).

LANE v SHIRE ROOFING CO (OXFORD) LTD
Safety at work; whether worker employee or not; negligence case

A case concerning an ostensibly self-employed builder who was injured when he fell from a ladder. It illustrates that the courts may lean, in health and safety matters, toward regarding workers as employees and so afford them additional protection.

The builder sought to hold the company liable as his employer; the company argued that he was an independent contractor. The court ruled applied the 'control' test and also asked the question as to whose business it was; it concluded that although the builder was neither employee nor specialist subcontractor, he was nearer the former than the latter because the business was clearly that of the company ([1995] PIQR P417, Court of Appeal).

LANG v FIFE HEALTH BOARD
Ambulance driver; trolley; iced ramp; gritting; system of work; negligence case

The pursuer, a 40-year-old ambulance driver, was in 1986 pushing a trolley down the slope of a ramp leading out of the hospital. When he got to the ambulance he had to let go of the ramp's hand-rail in order to raise the rear of the trolley. He slipped on snow and ice on the ramp. He claimed that the employer should have had an effective system for checking and gritting the ramp during cold weather. The court found that there would have been no difficulty in doing so, since only two entrances to the hospital were used by ambulancemen and it would have taken five to ten minutes to grit each entrance. There was thus no reasonable system in place, and the health board was liable in negligence; damages were set at some £31,000 ((1990) SLT 626, Outer House, Court of Session, Scotland).

LEGAL LIABILITY

Legal liability may arise in various ways in relation to manual handling.

Criminal liability. Criminal liability may be incurred by employers under *health and safety at work legislation*, following prosecution by the Health and Safety Executive (HSE). Such prosecution does not require that harm has been suffered, unlike a civil personal injury claim; so the HSE can act with deterrent, as well as punitive, effect in mind.

Health and safety at work legislation: civil liability. Civil liability of employers in respect of employees may arise for breach of statutory duty by an employer under some (but not all) *health and safety at work legislation* – such as the *MHOR 1992* and the *Provision and Use of Work Equipment Regulations 1998*. However, employees cannot pursue a civil case under the *Health and Safety at Work Act 1974* (see s.47 of the Act), or under the *Management of Health and Safety at Work Regulations 1999* (see r.22).

Patients and clients anyway cannot use *health and safety at work legislation* to pursue civil claims and must instead use the common law of *negligence*; this is notwithstanding the fact that under s.3 of the *Health and Safety at Work Act 1974*, and r.3 of the *Management of Health and Safety at Work Regulations 1999*, duties are owed to non-employees and can give rise to criminal prosecution by the Health and Safety Executive.

Common law of negligence. The common law of *negligence* can be used by both employees and patients or clients to pursue a claim.

Employees may have a better chance of winning their case under *health and safety at work legislation*, which sometimes imposes stricter liability than *negligence*. For instance, some manual handling cases have failed in negligence but succeeded under the *MHOR 1992* (e.g. *Hall v Edinburgh City Council*). See section 3 of the Overview.

Patients and clients, as non-employees, have to sue in negligence alone.

Judicial review. When patients or clients are not seeking personal injury compensation, but instead wish to overturn NHS or local authority social services decisions (whether or not concerning manual handling) made under *welfare legislation*, they may seek to bring a *judicial review* case in order to establish whether the NHS or local authority has acted unlawfully.

LEGITIMATE EXPECTATIONS

Legitimate expectation is a ground on which the decision-making of public bodies such as the NHS and local authorities is challenged by clients and patients by means of *judicial review*. Courts might strike decisions down if they represent blatant dashing of people's reasonable expectations.

For instance, in *R v North and East Devon Health Authority, ex p Coughlan*, a promise by the health authority of a home for life carried such weight, that in the circumstances its breach amounted to a dashing of expectations, an abuse of power and a breach of article 8 of the *European Convention on Human Rights*. And in *R (Bodimeade) v*

Camden London Borough Council, the court found that the council had not paid due attention to the legitimate expectations of residents of a home, since it had failed to take proper account of the contents of the residents' handbook which referred to a 'home for life'.

LIFTING OPERATIONS AND LIFTING EQUIPMENT REGULATIONS 1998

Very clearly complementing *MHOR 1992*, the Lifting Operations and Lifting Equipment Regulations 1998 (LOLER 1998) apply to equipment used at work for lifting people or loads. They impose a range of duties covering such matters as strength and stability, positioning and installation, marking of safe working load, organisation of lifting operations, examination and inspection. A number of questions have arisen about the application of LOLER 1998 in the health and social care context concerning the definition of lifting equipment, the meaning of 'use at work', and the duty of examination and inspection.

Is it lifting equipment? One way of identifying lifting equipment is to apply the test of primary purpose or principal function. On this basis, hoists and bath lifts would be lifting equipment, but electric riser-recliner chairs or adjustable height beds would not be, on the grounds that primarily they are chairs and beds respectively. This is the test apparently favoured by the Health and Safety Executive (HSE SIM 7/1999/18), although ultimately it would be for a court to decide. However, for practical purposes, it should be left to the lawyers to logic chop this matter; for those working in the health or social care field, the answer is to try to ensure that equipment is used safely, since even if a particular item were not defined as lifting equipment, it would still be covered by the detailed provisions of the *Provision and Use of Work Equipment Regulations 1998*, which cover all equipment used at work (including lifting equipment).

Is it being used at work? The HSE considers that equipment is being used at work if it is provided primarily for employees to use. For instance, lifting equipment provided for use in the homes of patients and clients would be covered by LOLER 1998 if it is used by employees, but not covered if used only by clients, patients, relatives, friends and so on. Similarly, the HSE believes that even in an institution such as a residential care home, equipment such as stairlifts, bath lifts or toilet riser seats which is used only by residents should not be considered to be equipment used at work. Once again, undue concern about exact definitions is not necessary, since even if LOLER 1998 do not apply, the duty toward non-employees under s.3 of the *Health and Safety at Work Act 1974* would. Indeed, the HSE has suggested that this s.3 duty under the 1974 Act 'should be applied, where necessary, to require a similar standard of safety as LOLER would require, by reference to existing standards' under the approved code of practice and guidance for LOLER 1998 (HSE SIM 7/1999/18).

It should also be noted that LOLER 1998 cover not just employers but also persons who have control to any extent of lifting equipment used at work; so it is arguable that the regulations would apply, for instance, to a local authority that provides and maintains lifting equipment used by the employees of a care agency (rather than by its own employees).

Frequency of examination. The duty to examine equipment thoroughly every six months, or in accordance with an examination scheme specifying an alternative interval, arises in the case of lifting equipment which is exposed to conditions causing deterioration liable to result in dangerous situations. The HSE points out that a dangerous situation is one 'which presents a significant risk liable to result in a major injury, or worse'; that thorough examination 'will not be necessary for lifting equipment which only presents a low risk in the event of its failure'; and so a 'risk assessment of an item such as an inflatable lifting cushion may conclude that the risk is not sufficient to warrant a thorough examination, provided the equipment is adequately maintained as required' by the *Provision and Use of Work Equipment Regulations 1998* (HSE SIM 7/1999/18).

Where the duty of thorough examination is triggered, the six-monthly period applies by default; however, the employer is free to draw up an alternative examination scheme, which may specify longer or shorter periods. The examination scheme cannot simply be plucked out of the air; it must be drawn up by a 'competent person'. In drawing up such a scheme, relevant information clearly needs to be taken into account; for instance, in the case of hoists, advice from the Medical Devices Agency is that hoist attachments should be inspected at least every six months (MDA SN9929).

Selected extracts. LOLER 1998 include the following provisions:

1. **LOLER 1998: lifting equipment used at work**. Lifting equipment is defined as work equipment for lifting or lowering loads and includes attachments for anchoring, fixing or supporting it. Work equipment in turn is defined as any machinery, appliance, apparatus, tool or installation for use at work (r.2).

2. **LOLER 1998: self-employed people**. As well as to employers, the regulations apply to self-employed people in respect of lifting equipment they use at work (r.2).

3. **LOLER 1998: people having control of equipment**. The requirements imposed on employers extend also 'to a person who has control to any extent of —

   (i)   lifting equipment;

   (ii)   a person at work who uses or supervises or manages the use of lifting equipment;

   or

   (iii) the way in which lifting equipment is used,

   and to the extent of his control' (r.2).

4.   **LOLER 1998: sale, agreement for sale, hire purchase**. The regulations do not apply to persons who supply equipment in any of these ways (r.2).

5.   **LOLER 1998: strength and stability**. Every employer must ensure that (a) lifting equipment is of 'adequate strength and stability for each load, having regard in particular to the stress induced at its mounting or fixing point'; (b) every part of a load and anything attached to it and use in lifting is of adequate strength' (r.4).

6.   **LOLER 1998: lifting people**. In the case of equipment for lifting people, employers must ensure that it (a) 'is such as to prevent a person using it being crushed, trapped or struck or falling from the carrier'; (b) prevents 'so far as is reasonably practicable a person using it, while carrying out activities from the carrier, being crushed, trapped or struck or falling from the carrier'; (c) has suitable devices to prevent the risk of a carrier falling'; (d) 'is such that a person trapped in any carrier is not thereby exposed to danger and can be freed' (r.5).

7.   **LOLER 1998: positioning and installation**. Employers must ensure that lifting equipment is positioned and installed so as 'to reduce to as low as is reasonably practicable the risk' (a) of the lifting equipment or load striking a person, or (b) the load drifting, falling or being released unintentionally, and is otherwise safe. They must also ensure there are suitable devices to stop a person from falling down a shaft or hoistway (r.6).

8.   **LOLER 1998: marking**. Employers must ensure that machinery and accessories for lifting loads are clearly marked with safe working loads. If this depends on the configuration of the machinery, then the machinery must be clearly marked to indicate its safe working load with each configuration – and the information about this must be kept with the machinery. Accessories for lifting must also be marked so as to identify the 'characteristics necessary for their safe use'. Lifting equipment designed for lifting people must be clearly marked as such. Conversely, lifting equipment not so designed but which could be so used in error must be appropriately and clearly marked that it is not for lifting people (r.7).

9.   **LOLER 1998: organisation of lifting**. Employers must ensure that every lifting operation is properly planned by a competent person, appropriately supervised and carried out safely (r.8).

10. **LOLER 1998: examination and inspection**. Employers must ensure that lifting equipment is thoroughly examined for any defect when it is put into service for the first time, unless (a) it has not previously been used; *and* (b) in the case of lifting equipment for which an EC declaration of conformity could have been drawn up, the employer has received such a declaration not more than 12 months before the equipment is put into service. Alternatively, if the equipment has been obtained from another undertaking, no such examination is necessary if it is accompanied by physical evidence that the 'last thorough examination required to be carried out under this regulation has been carried out' (r.9).

Where the safety of equipment depends on its installation, employers must ensure that it is thoroughly examined 'after installation and before being put into service for the first time; and after assembly and before being put into service at a new site or in a new location – to ensure that it has been installed correctly and is safe to operate' (r.9).

Employers must ensure that 'lifting equipment which is exposed to conditions causing deterioration which is liable to result in dangerous situations is –

(a)   thoroughly examined

   (i)   in the case of lifting equipment for lifting persons or an accessory for lifting, at least every 6 months;

   (ii) in the case of other lifting equipment, at least every 12 months; or

   (iii) in either case, in accordance with an examination scheme; and

   (iv) each time that exceptional circumstances which are liable to jeopardise the safety of the lifting equipment have occurred; and

(b)   if appropriate for the purpose, is inspected by a competent person at suitable intervals between thorough examinations,

to ensure that health and safety conditions are maintained and that any deterioration can be detected and remedied in good time' (r.9(3)).

Employers must ensure that

(a)   no lifting equipment leaves his or her undertaking; or

(b)   equipment obtained from another undertaking is not used in his or her own undertaking, 'unless it is accompanied by physical evidence that the last thorough examination required to be carried out under this regulation has been carried out' (r.9).

11. **LOLER 1998: examination scheme**. '… means a suitable scheme drawn up by a competent person for such thorough examinations of lifting equipment at such intervals as may be appropriate for the purpose described in regulation 9(3)' (r.2).

12. **LOLER 1998: thorough examination**. In relation to regulation 9, this:

(a)   'means a thorough examination by a competent person;

(b)   where it is appropriate to carry out testing for the purpose described…includes such testing by a competent person as is appropriate for the purpose' (r.2).

13. **LOLER 1998: report of examination.** Various information must be contained in a report of a thorough examination including:

– sufficient particulars to identify the lifting equipment including (where known) date of manufacture;

– date of last thorough examination;

– safe working load of equipment;

– if it is the first thorough examination since installation or assembly at new site/location, that it is such a thorough examination and that the equipment has been installed correctly and would be safe to operate;

– where it is not such a first thorough examination, whether it is a thorough examination within the specified 6-month or 12-month interval, in accordance within an examination scheme, or in connection with exceptional circumstances (see above for all of these) – and whether the lifting equipment would be safe to operate;

– identification of part with a defect which is or could be a danger;

– particulars of repair, renewal, alteration to remedy defect;

– where a defect is not yet a danger but could become so, the time when it could become such a danger and particulars of repair, renewal, alteration required;

– latest date for next thorough examination;

– particulars of any testing used;

– date of thorough examination (schedule 1).

14. **LOLER 1998: reports and defects**. A person thoroughly examining lifting equipment for an employer under r.9 must:

   (a) 'notify the employer forthwith of any defect in the lifting equipment which in his opinion is or could become a danger to persons;

   (b) as soon as is practicable make a report of the thorough examination in writing authenticated by him or on his behalf by signature or equally secure means and containing the information specified in Schedule 1' to the employer and any person from whom the equipment has been hired or leased;

   (c) 'where there is in his opinion a defect in the lifting equipment involving an existing or imminent risk of serious personal injury send a copy of the report as soon as is practicable to the relevant enforcing authority'.

An employer who has been so notified must ensure that the lifting equipment is not used before the defect is rectified, or not used later than a time identified at which a defect could become a danger to people.

A person inspecting under r.9 must notify the employer about a defect which is or could become a danger, and as soon as practicable make a written record of the inspection (r.10).

15. **LOLER 1998: information**. Employers must keep any EC declaration of conformity for so long as they operate the equipment. Various rules apply to the keeping of examination and inspection reports (r.11).

LIMITATION ACT 1980: see *limitation of actions*

LIMITATION OF ACTIONS

The *Limitation Act 1980* in England and Wales, and the *Prescription and Limitation (Scotland) Act 1973* in Scotland, place time limits on the bringing of legal actions for personal injury.

The question of limitation is particularly important in the manual handling context because of the potentially insidious nature of back injury. For example, employees, whether working in hospital or factory, might assume that a painful back injury will get better in a few days, weeks or months. It might only be some years later that they realise that it has become a chronic injury which may terminate prematurely, or at least permanently hinder, their work, and also affect aspects of home life such as lifting babies and small children, gardening, sport and sitting still for any length of time (e.g. *Coad v Cornwall and Isles of Scilly Health Authority; Kempsey District Hospital v Thackham; Murray v Healthscope*).

Three year limit. In the case of personal injury, the normal limit is three years. For children in England and Wales, time does not 'start to run' until the child is 18 years old, so that he or she can bring a personal injury case up to the age of 21. However, in Scotland, because of the effect of the Age of Legal Capacity (Scotland) Act 1991, time starts to run when the child reaches the age of 16 years. In addition, if an adult does not have legal (mental) capacity to bring an action, then time does not start to run until he or she does.

These capacity issues apart, time only starts to run from (a) the date on which the accident occurred; or (b) if later, the date of knowledge of the person who has been injured (s.11 of the 1980 Act). Knowledge means knowing (a) that the injury was significant; (b) that it was attributable wholly or partly to an act or omission which is the subject of the personal injury claim; (c) the identity of the defendant (i.e. who did it); and (d) if it is alleged that the act or omission was the responsibility of a person other than the defendant, the identity of that other person and of additional relevant facts (s.14 of the 1980 Act). For Scotland, the rules are roughly the same although stated slightly differently (see s.17 of the 1973 Act). Even if the injured person has consulted health care professionals, the courts acknowledge the difficulties in recognising the seriousness of an injury – for instance, if conflicting advice from general practitioners (*Pacheco v Brent and Harrow Area Health Authority*) or chance remarks from chiropractors (*Anderson v Associated Coop Creameries*) are received.

Waiving the time limit. However, in addition, the courts have the power to waive the time limits, if it would be equitable to do so, having regard to various factors such as prejudice to the claimant or to the defendant, all the circumstances of the case generally, length of and reasons for delay, cogency of evidence in the light of delay, conduct of the defendant in responding to requests for information by the claimant, how reasonably and promptly the claimant acted once aware that the act or omission could give rise to an action, steps taken to obtain legal, medical or other expert advice and the nature of any advice received (s.33). Similarly, in Scotland, a power of waiver is available under s.19A of the 1973 Act.

For manual handling case examples, see *Coad v Cornwall and Isles of Scilly Health Authority* and *Pacheco v Brent and Harrow Area Health Authority*, where s.33 discretion was exercised; *Weston v South Coast Nursing Homes* where it was not; and *Jude v Elliott Medway Ltd* where the discretion was exercised, partly because the court had 'sympathy with the manly attitude to get on with work and not to rush to the lawyers'.

LOADS

Manual handling might be of animate or inanimate loads. Manual handling injuries might be connected not just with the weight of loads (see e.g. *Cullen v North Lanarkshire Council*), but also the conditions in which they are handled, their shape, the ease with which they can be gripped, the repetition of a handling task, the length of time a weight is supported, the speed of the work – indeed all the factors listed in schedule 1 to the *MHOR 1992*. Loads need not even be freely moveable but could be attached to something else (e.g. *Divit v British Telecommunications*).

However, as far as weight is concerned, guidance from the Health and Safety Executive suggests a way of identifying situations in which a risk assessment will be necessary. It includes a 'risk assessment filter' in the form of a diagram, indicating for men and women weights of load that will not necessitate risk assessments – although this will vary depending on the height, and also distance from the body, that the weight is being handled. One stated purpose of this guidance is to exclude an excessive number of risk assessments covering trivial risk; so that organisations do not carry out assessments of the risk in lifting a tea cup (HSE 1998, pp.42–3).

LOCAL GOVERNMENT OMBUDSMEN

Under the Local Government Act 1974 for England and Wales, and the Local Government (Scotland) Act 1975, the local government ombudsmen (Commissioners for Local Administration) independently investigate – normally once social services complaints procedures have been exhausted or otherwise baulked before formal exhaustion – maladministration causing injustice. There are three such ombudsmen in England, one in Wales and one in Scotland.

They can investigate a very wide range of matters, from breach of legal duty to rudeness, poor communication with clients, arbitrary decision-making, delays in assessment and provision, and so on. One lengthy investigation concerned a protracted dispute over manual handling for a person in a residential home (*Redbridge London Borough Council*). There have also been many investigations into delays in provision of home adaptations by local social services and housing authorities; when this occurs there might be severe manual handling implications for clients and their *carers* (see e.g. *Barking and Dagenham London Borough Council; Bristol City Council; Camden London Borough Council; Islington London Borough Council; Rotherham Metropolitan Borough Council*).

LOGAN v STRATHCLYDE FIRE BOARD
Fireman; power pack; lack of thought given to reducing risk; MHOR 1992

In 1993, a fireman sustained an injury using a power pack weighing 83kg, which clearly exceeded Health and Safety Executive guidelines of 25kg for one man and 33kg for two. Breach of r.4(1)(a) of the *MHOR 1992* – avoidance altogether of manual handling with risk – could not be made out because some manual handling would have been necessary even if a trolley had been used.

However, as to r.4(1)(b)(ii) – reduction of risk – there was evidence that the power pack could have been split into two components, that this was in fact done at other fire stations, and that the operation of making the hose connection would not have been in any way time consuming – and there was not generally a shortage of staff at such incidents to carry the components. No real thought had been given as to whether to separate the power pack components, and thus the employer had not shown that it was not reasonably practicable to reduce the risk. As to other steps which could have been taken, the argument for a non-slip surface on the tailgate was not made out, but consideration had not been given to a sack barrow which could have been used to transport the power pack. In addition, training could have been given to train the pursuer and colleagues in appropriate manual handling techniques, and there was no evidence of risk assessment. Thus liability was established under the *MHOR 1992*; and had it been necessary to do so, the court would have been inclined to find fault also in common law ((1999) Rep LR 97, Outer House, Court of Session, Scotland).

MacGREGOR v SOUTH LANARKSHIRE COUNCIL
Assessment of need; nursing home place/funding; delay of several months; breach of duty; community care

This is a case serving as a warning that once a council has identified that it has a duty to provide crucial services for clients, it must provide those services within a reasonable period of time.

A Scottish council had concluded that a person needed nursing home care under s.12 of the *Social Work (Scotland) Act 1968*, following a community care assessment under s.12A of that Act. The court found that it was a breach of duty for the council to fail to provide funding for several months ([2001] SC 502, Outer House, Court of Session, Scotland).

MANAGEMENT OF HEALTH AND SAFETY AT WORK REGULATIONS 1999 (MHSWR 1999)

These regulations cover a number of basic matters including *risk assessment*, principles of prevention, duties on host employers, *cooperation and coordination in a shared workplace*, taking account of *individual capability, training, employee duty to report and use equipment safely*, and so on. Selected extracts include the following:

1. **MHSWR 1999: risk assessment**. 'Every employer shall make a suitable and sufficient assessment of:

    (a) the risks to the health and safety of his employees to which they are exposed whilst they are at work; and

    (b) the risks to the health and safety of persons not in his employment arising out of or in connection with the conduct by him of his undertaking,

    for the purpose of identifying the measures he needs to take to comply with the requirements and prohibitions imposed upon him by the relevant statutory provisions' (r.3).

    Every self-employed person must likewise carry out a suitable and sufficient assessment in relation to his or her own health and safety, and also to that of people not in his/her employ, but arising out of the conduct of his/her undertaking (r.3).

2. **MHSWR 1999: review of risk assessment**. There is a duty to review the assessment if there is reason to believe it is no longer valid or there has been a significant change to which it relates – and where changes to the assessment are required, the employer or self-employed person must make them (r.3).

3. **MHSWR 1999: principles of prevention to be applied**. Employers must implement preventive and protective measures on the basis of specific principles. These are:

    (a) avoiding risks;

    (b) evaluating risks that cannot be avoided;

    (c) combating risks at source;

    (d) adapting work to the individual, especially as regards the design of workplaces, the choice of work equipment and the choice of working and production methods, with a view, in particular, to alleviating monotonous work and work at a pre-determined work-rate and to reducing their effect on health;

    (e) adapting to technical progress;

    (f) replacing the dangerous by the non-dangerous or the less dangerous;

(g)   developing a coherent overall prevention policy which covers technology, organisation of work, working conditions, social relationships and the influence of factors relating to the working environment;

(h)   giving collective protective measures priority over individual protective measures; and giving appropriate instructions to employees (r.4 and schedule 1).

4.   **MHSWR 1999: appropriate arrangements**. 'Every employer shall make and give effect to such arrangements as are appropriate, having regard to the nature of his activities and the size of his undertaking, for the effective planning, organisation, control, monitoring and review of the preventive and protective measures... Where the employer employs five or more employees, he shall record the arrangements...' (r.5).

5.   **MHSWR 1999: health surveillance**. The employer must ensure that employees are provided with such health surveillance as is appropriate having regard to the risks to their health and safety identified by the assessment (r.6).

6.   **MHSWR 1999: information**. 'Every employer shall provide his employees with comprehensible and relevant information on:

(a)   the risks to their health and safety identified by the assessment;

(b)   the preventive and protective measures';

(c)   the serious and imminent danger procedures and persons nominated in relation to them;

(d) any risks notified to him by other employers (see below) (r.10).

7.   **MHSWR 1999: cooperation and coordination in shared workplace**. 'Where two or more employers share a workplace (whether on a temporary or permanent basis) each such employer shall:

(a)   cooperate with the other employers concerned so far as is necessary to enable them to comply with the requirements and prohibitions imposed upon them by or under the relevant statutory provisions...;

(b)   (taking into account the nature of his activities) take all reasonable steps to coordinate the measures he takes to comply with the requirements and prohibitions imposed upon him by or under the relevant statutory provisions with the measures the other employers concerned are taking to comply with the requirements and prohibitions imposed upon them by or under the relevant statutory provisions ...; and

(c)   take all reasonable steps to inform the other employers concerned of the risks to their employees' health and safety arising out of or in connection with the conduct by him of his undertaking'.

The above applies also as between the self-employed and between employers and the self-employed (r.11).

8.   **MHSWR 1999: host employers**. 'Every employer and every self-employed person shall ensure that the employer of any employees from an outside undertaking [or self-employed persons] who are working in his undertaking is provided with comprehensible information on:

(a)   the risks to those employees' health and safety arising out of or in connection with the conduct by that first-mentioned employer or by that self-employed person of his undertaking;

(b)   the measures taken…'.

'Every employer shall ensure that any person working in his undertaking who is not his employee and every self-employed person (not being an employer) is provided with appropriate instructions and comprehensible information regarding any risks to that person's health and safety which arise out of the conduct by that employer or self-employed person of his undertaking'. The above applies as between self-employed people, and between self-employed people and employers (r.12).

9.   **MHSWR 1999: capabilities of individual: risk to self and others**. 'Every employer shall, in entrusting tasks to his employees, take into account their capabilities as regards health and safety' (r.13).

10.   **MHSWR 1999: training**. Every employer 'shall ensure that his employees are provided with adequate health and safety training

(a)   on being recruited into the employer's undertaking; and

(b)   on their being exposed to new or increased risk because of

(i)   their being transferred or given a change of responsibilties within the employer's undertaking,

(ii)   the introduction of new work equipment into or a change respecting work equipment already within the employer's undertaking,

(iii) the introduction of new technology into the employer's undertaking, or

(iv) the introduction of a new system of work into or a change respecting a system of work already in use within the employer's undertaking'.

The training 'shall

(a)   be repeated periodically where appropriate;

(b)   be adapted to take account of any new or changed risks to the health and safety of the employees concerned; and

(c)   take place during working hours' (r.13).

11. **MHSWR 1999: employees' duties**. 'Every employee shall use any machinery, equipment, dangerous substance, transport equipment, means of production or safety device provided to him by his employer in accordance both with any training in the use of the equipment concerned which has been received by him and the instructions respecting that use which have been provided to him by the said employer in compliance with the requirements and prohibitions imposed upon that employer by or under the relevant statutory provisions' (r. 14).

12. **MHSWR 1999: informing employer about danger to health and safety**. 'Every employee shall inform his employer or any other employee of that employer with specific responsibility for the health and safety of his fellow employees:

(a)   of any work situation which a person with the first-mentioned employee's training and instruction would reasonably consider represented a serious and immediate danger to health and safety;

(b)   of any matter which a person with the first-mentioned employee's training and instruction would reasonably consider represented a shortcoming in the employer's protection arrangements for health and safety,

insofar as that situation or matter either affects the health and safety of that first-mentioned employee or arises out of or in connection with his own activities at work, and has not previously been reported to his employer or to any other employee of that employer in accordance with this paragraph' (r 14).

MANUAL HANDLING OPERATIONS REGULATIONS 1992: CASE LAW

The following is a summary of legal case law included in the book which has considered the *MHOR 1992*, particularly in relation to risk assessment, avoidance of risk, reduction of risk, reasonable practicability and provision of information, and the scope of manual handling tasks covered.

Risk assessment. The courts regularly find breaches of the *MHOR 1992*, insofar as employers put forward no evidence that they have carried out risk assessments, leaving courts relatively free to draw their own conclusions (based on evidence presented) about what solutions by way of equipment or otherwise were reasonably practicable, and so impose liability in cases such as *Cullen v North Lanarkshire Council, Hall v Edinburgh City Council, King v RCO, Logan v Strathclyde Fire Board, Hawkes v Southwark London Borough Council, Wilson v British Railways Board*. By the same token, the courts were quick to reject the attempt to argue that a failure to carry out a risk assessment under the *MHOR 1992* meant that the duties to reduce risk or provide information were never triggered (*Swain v Denso Martin*).

However, lack of risk assessment is not enough in itself to demonstrate liability for injury, if it cannot be shown that this was the cause of the accident. For instance, the court might doubt the credibility or reliability of the evidence (see immediately below), or it might consider the overall question of whether, had a risk assessment been undertaken, it would have made any difference (*Hawkes v Southwark London Borough Council*).

The duty to assess risk generally might be discharged by manual handling training, and specifically by an individual patient's care plan (*Brown v East Midlothian NHS Trust*). Risk assessments need not necessarily be formal (*Rowe v Swansea City Council*), but the courts would expect them to be competent since, as the *MHOR 1992* state, they must be suitable and sufficient (*Hawkes v Southwark London Borough Council*). For instance, a firm's health and safety officer, rather than a production fitter, would have been the 'natural person' to carry out a risk assessment of a manual handling task of an unknown nature (*Swain v Denso Martin*).

Foreseeability of risk. The courts have stated that the risk referred to in the *MHOR 1992* is foreseeable risk, and not the weaker notion of reasonably foreseeable risk (*Anderson v Lothian Health Board, Cullen v North Lanarkshire Council, Koonjul v Thameslink Healthcare NHS Trust*) and have had asked of them the question (which they did not answer) of whether even foreseeability is required – or whether the duty is stricter still (*King v RCO*). Emergency situations are clearly covered (*Purvis v Buckinghamshire County Council, Fleming v Stirling Council* – though see the almost certainly erroneous view in *Fraser v Greater Glasgow Health Board*).

Avoidance of risk. Breach of this duty was established when the courts held that it was reasonably practicable to avoid manual handling with risk in a hospital laundry (*Anderson v Lothian Health Board*). Equally, there was no breach of this duty when the *system of work*: simply did not involve the manual handling of equipment (*Gordon v British Airways*); involved carrying a a 35lb cupboard up stairs (*Taylor v Glasgow City Council*); or involved only lightweight tables – which fell within the Health and Safety Executive's guidelines as to weights (30lb) and method of carriage, and so did not trigger a risk assessment under the *MHOR 1992 (Hillhouse v South Ayrshire Council)*. Likewise there was no breach when it was not reasonably practicable to avoid the risk associated with patient handling (*Brown v East Midlothian NHS Trust*), with beds which were low and against the wall to prevent injury to the children (*Koonjul v Thameslink Healthcare NHS Trust*), or with lifting and laying pavement slabs (*Skinner v Aberdeen City Council*).

Taking appropriate steps to reduce the risk to the lowest level reasonably practicable. This duty has been breached when word-of-mouth, but not written, instructions about laundry loads were given (*Anderson v Lothian Health Board*), when adjustable height beds and hoist were not provided (*Commons v Queen's Medical Centre*) or when a hose was not provided to avoid the lifting of a bucket (*Warren v Harlow District Council*). A lack of adequate training may breach this duty (*Kelly v Forticrete; Logan v Strathclyde Fire Board; Skinner v Aberdeen City Council*); likewise the failure to provide instructions (*McBeath v Halliday*). However, this might depend on the circumstances; a failure to train will not necessarily result in breach (*Purvis v Buckinghamshire County Council*).

However, a five-day training course for a care assistant satisfied the duty (*Rowe v Swansea City Council*). The duty might also be satisfied in the form of individual care plans (*Brown v East Midlothian NHS Trust*), or where lightweight tables could not be more safely carried by two people rather than one, and carrying them on a shorter route would have created its own hazards (*Hillhouse v South Ayrshire Council*). Likewise, precise evaluation of everyday, innumerable tasks carrying a very low risk of injury was held to be way beyond the realms of practicability and simply not demanded by the *MHOR 1992 (Koonjul v Thameslink Healthcare NHS Trust)*.

Reasonable practicability. The nature of reasonable practicability was considered in *Hawkes v Southwark London Borough Council*.

Cumulative strain. It has always been difficult to argue cumulative strain in manual handling cases, whether in negligence or under the *MHOR 1992*, but see *Black v Wrangler; Commons v Queen's Medical Centre; Stone v Commissioner of Police for the Metropolis; Wells v West Hertfordshire Health Authority*.

Scope in terms of injury. The courts have clearly accepted that it is not merely back injury which is covered by the *MHOR 1992*; for instance, cases have been heard relating to a cut hand (*Divit v British Telecommunications*), an injured shoulder (*Cullen v North Lanarkshire Council*) and an injured foot (*Hawkes v Southwark London Borough Council*).

Treating manual handling operations as a whole. The courts have not generally been receptive to arguments by employers which attempt to break down a manual handling operation into component parts, and then to exclude the part which caused injury from coming under the *MHOR 1992*. Such unsuccessfully argued exclusions have been in respect of falling patients and clients when they have been taken to the lavatory, on the basis that the falling and subsequent staff reaction and injury was not part of the manual handling operation of taking people to the toilet (*Fleming v Stirling Council; Wiles v Bedfordshire County Council*); and also the hitting of a nurse by a trolley, on the grounds that she was not pushing the trolley at the time (*Postle v Norfolk and Norwich Healthcare NHS Trust*).

Scope in terms of manual handling tasks. Manual handling has a wide range of application to work situations and goes beyond the weight of a *load* (animate or inanimate itself), extending to matters such as how a load is held, its shape, grips on it, sharp surfaces, frequency or prolongation of handling, floor surfaces, space constraints, lighting, temperature, individual capabilities, and so on (see *MHOR 1992*, schedule 1).

In this respect, the many manual handling cases speak for themselves, involving as they do the unloading of relatively light fencing from a truck (*Cullen v North Lanarkshire Council*), the cutting of an engineer's hand on a telephone kiosk roof flap (*Divit v British Telecommunications*), slipping while gritting an icy yard (*King v RCO*), the moving of demonstrators by police (*Peck v Chief Constable of Avon and Somerset*) and dancing (*Woods v Barry Clayman Concerts*). Even so, some tasks have been held not to come under the *MHOR 1992*, including removing bolts with a spanner (*King v Carron Phoenix*), packing crisp boxes (*Gissing v Walkers Smith*), or using a grass mower (*Mitchell v Inverclyde District Council*).

Credibility of witnesses. Just as with cases under the common law of *negligence*, so under the *MHOR 1992*, a claimant or pursuer whose *evidence* lacks credibility or reliability may fail for this very reason (*Aitken v Board of Management of Aberdeen College; Callaghan v Southern General Hospital NHS Trust*) even if there was a clear breach of the *MHOR 1992 (Boyd v Lanarkshire Health Board)*.

MANUAL HANDLING OPERATIONS REGULATIONS 1992: LEGISLATION

At the heart of the Manual Handling Operations Regulations 1992 (MHOR 1992) lies the duty to avoid, so far as is *reasonably practicable*, the need for employees to undertake manual handling which involves a risk of injury. Failing this, the duty is at least to take appropriate steps to reduce the risk of injury to the lowest level reasonably practicable, and to provide information. Underpinning these duties is risk assessment, under r.3 of the *Management of Health and Safety at Work Regulations 1999* to identify manual handling with risk of injury in the first place; and then under the MHOR 1992 with a view to reducing the risk to the lowest level reasonably practicable.

The MHOR 1992 themselves are transposed from a *European directive on manual handling*, and the courts may sometimes refer to this original directive (e.g. *Cullen v North Lanarkshire Council*); indeed, in case of any judicially identified discrepancies in meaning between the directive and the MHOR 1992, the former would trump the latter.

1. **MHOR 1992: avoiding or reducing the risk of injury.** 'Each employer shall

    (a) so far as is reasonably practicable, avoid the need for his employees to undertake any manual handling operations at work which involve a risk of their being injured;

    (b) where it is not reasonably practicable to avoid the need for his employees to undertake any manual handling at work which involves a risk of their being injured

        (i)   make a suitable and sufficient assessment of all such manual handling operations to be undertaken by them, having regard to the factors which are specified…and considering the questions which are specified…'

        (ii) take appropriate steps to reduce the risk of injury to those employees arising out of their undertaking any such manual handling operations to the lowest level reasonably practicable;

(iii) take appropriate steps to provide any of those employees who are undertaking any such manual handling operations with general indications and, where it is reasonably practicable to do so, precise information on –

(aa) the weight of each load, and

(bb) the heaviest side of any load whose centre of gravity is not positioned centrally (r.4(1)).

2. **MHOR 1992: review of assessment.** 'Any assessment such as is referred to in paragraph (1)(b)(i) of this regulation shall be reviewed by the employer who made it if –

(a) there is reason to suspect that it is no longer valid; or

(b) there has been a significant change in the manual handling operations to which it relates;

and where as a result of any such review changes to an assessment are required, the relevant employer shall make them' (r.4(2)).

3. **MHOR 1992: employees.** 'Each employee while at work shall make full and proper use of any system of work provided for his use by his employer in compliance with r.4(1)(b)(ii)' (r.5).

4. **MHOR 1992: self-employed.** 'Any duty imposed by these Regulations on an employer in respect of his employees shall also be imposed on a self-employed person in respect of himself' (r.2).

5. **MHOR 1992: definitions.** 'In these Regulations, unless the context otherwise requires –

"injury" does not include injury caused by any toxic or corrosive substance which – (a) has leaked or spilled from a load; (b) is present on the surface of a load but has not leaked or spilled from it; or (c) is a constituent part of a load…;

"load" includes any person and any animal;

"manual handling operations" means any transporting or supporting of a load (including the lifting, putting down, pushing, pulling, carrying or moving thereof) by hand or bodily force' (r.2).

6. **MHOR 1992: factors to which regard must be had for assessment of manual handling operations.**

'1. The tasks. Do they involve:

– holding or manipulating loads at distance from trunk?
– unsatisfactory bodily movement or posture, especially twisting the trunk, stooping, reaching upwards?
– excessive movement of loads, especially excessive lifting or lowering distances, excessive carrying distances?

      – excessive pushing or pulling of loads?
      – risk of sudden movement on loads?
      – frequent or prolonged physical effort?
      – insufficient rest or recovery periods?
      – rate of work imposed by a process?'

'2.   The loads. Are they

– heavy, bulky or unwieldy, difficult to grasp, unstable or with contents likely to shift?
– sharp, hot or otherwise potentially damaging?'

'3.   The working environment. Are there

– space constraints preventing good posture?
– uneven, slippery or unstable floors?
– variations in level of floors or work surfaces?
– extremes of temperature or humidity?
– conditions causing ventilation problems or gusts of wind?
– poor lighting conditions?'

'4.   Individual capability. Does the job:

– require unusual strength, height etc?
– create a hazard to those who might reasonably be considered to be pregnant or to have a health problem?
– require special information or training for its safe performance?'

'5.   Other factors. Is movement or posture hindered by personal protective equipment or by clothing? (schedule 1)'

MANUAL HANDLING TASKS: see *Manual Handling Operations Regulations: case law*

MANUAL HANDLING TECHNIQUES

As pointed out in the Introduction to this book, ideas about manual handling techniques change over time, and the reader wishing to grasp what is considered reasonable practice in 2001 and beyond should consult relevant national *guidance*.

It should be noted that when such *guidance* – such as that published by the Royal College of Nursing and National Back Pain Association, as it was then (RCN/NBPA 1997) – strongly criticises a particular technique, the courts will often place considerable weight on that fact. However, this is not the same as saying that the particular technique is legally 'banned' – and sometimes the courts have accepted alternative expert evidence to the effect that in all the circumstances, the lift condemned by the guidance was in fact acceptable.

McBEATH v HALLIDAY
Electrician; failure to issue manufacturer's instructions; MHOR 1992

A case illustrating the importance, practically and legally, of issuing instructions to employees.

An electrician sustained injuries when fitting electrical wiring to a floodlighting column. The court held that a failure to carry out a suitable and sufficient assessment would not necessarily lead to liability in damages under the *MHOR 1992*. However, it was enough to ask whether appropriate steps had been taken to reduce the risk to the lowest level reasonably practicable. The employer's failure to issue the manufacturer's instructions had contributed materially to the accident, since (a) the employee would probably have acted on them, and (b) this signified a failure to reduce the risk to the lowest level reasonably practicable. However, the plaintiff was 30 per cent contributorily negligent for not applying his mind to the situation ([2000] GWD 2–75, Outer House, Court of Session, Scotland).

McCAFFERY v DATTA
State enrolled nurse; inadequate training of care assistant; advice to avoid heavy lifting; arranging resident's bed; contributory negligence

A state enrolled nurse, 39 years old at the time of the accident in 1989 and working in a nursing home, was injured when a care assistant, who had not been sufficiently trained, failed to take the full weight of her share of the patient. They had been attempting to lift a patient up the bed; the patient was 60 years old, weighed about 12 stone and had hemiplegia.

Training of care assistant. The employer was therefore liable in negligence for not training the care assistant.

Medical advice not to undertake heavy lifting. However, a finding of one-third contributory negligence had been made on the part of the nurse. This was based on the fact that she had suffered a previous back injury, that she had been given medical advice not to undertake heavy lifting, and that she had not arranged the patient's bed so as to optimise the effectiveness of the lifting method. The judge had not considered the first issue so significant, since she was only working one night a week at the time – and had perhaps felt reasonably reassured, since the 1982 warning not to undertake heavy lifting, that now her back was safe after all for this type of work.

Arranging of bed. However, the second issue involved more significant contributory negligence. The judge referred to written instructions in use at the nursing home which covered the importance of thinking and planning the lift, arranging the room beforehand, and ensuring that there was sufficient space in which to perform a lift. The judge went on to find that the way in which the plaintiff had in fact moved the bed prior to the lift meant that she did not have a full, clear area in which to move. Second, it also reduced the area in which the care assistant could move. Third, the plaintiff knew the care assistant was inexperienced and untrained and that it was particularly important for her to have adequate room in which to lift. Fourth, the bed could have been moved elsewhere to provide sufficient room.

Appeal. The plaintiff's appeal against this finding of contributory negligence was now dismissed in the Court of Appeal ([1997] CL 97/3768, Court of Appeal).

McGOWAN v HARROW HEALTH AUTHORITY
Nurse; negligence of porters in team lift; failure of risk assessment at senior level; supervision

The plaintiff, a state enrolled nurse, was injured in 1984 when lifting, with three porters, a sixteen-and-half-stone patient with multiple injuries. The so called 'orthodox lift' was used so that an X-ray plate could be placed underneath him. At the word of command, two of the porters lifted fractionally late; the plaintiff suffered a back injury. Liability was established.

Orthodox lift, porters' negligence, failure to consider risk at senior level. The court accepted that the orthodox lift should not normally be used, that there had been a failure to consider risk at a senior level in the hospital, and that there was no consideration of alternatives such as hoists and slings. Yet the plaintiff 'who, apart from this man [i.e. the patient], had never lifted or been part of a team lifting such a heavy person before was left to take the whole of the responsibility and decided what should be done. There was no supervision at all or consideration given to what should happen'. The plaintiff therefore succeeded on both of the following grounds: (a) that the porters failed to respond properly and coordinate the lift; and (b) the failure at senior level to consider the risks and alternatives. Damages of £184,600 were awarded.

Effect of injury. The plaintiff was considerably disabled; her nursing career had been wrecked; and her life as a mother and in her house and in her pastimes much handicapped. Her two pregnancies were difficult, and her handling of her children – including providing love and affection by lifting them up – together with household activities, was affected (1991, High Court, unreported).

McILGREW v DEVON COUNTY COUNCIL
Care assistant; drag lift; appeal on damages; effect of injury

The plaintiff was a care assistant at a residential home for older people, and was 23 years old at the time of the accident. Together with another care assistant, she was using the 'drag lift' to help stand a resident up from a sitting-up position on her bed. The resident wished to use her commode but was now so frail that she could not weight-bear. The plaintiff leant forward, placing her right arm under the right arm of the resident; the other care assistant did likewise on the other side. As they lifted the resident out of the bed and swivelled her around to place her on the commode, the plaintiff felt a sharp pain in her back. The case now concerned an appeal by the council on the amount of damages of £205,000 awarded in the High Court; the appeal was dismissed by the Court of Appeal.

Effect of injury. The plaintiff had not worked since the accident and was now severely disabled. Now aged 29 years, she walked with a stick. She could not sit for longer than an hour without moving; she could stand for somewhat longer. Her sleep pattern was disturbed and she had to sleep during the day. She used a shower because of potential difficulty in using a bath. She wore flat, slip-on shoes, since she could probably not do up shoelaces, and in any case this would be painful. She could manage light housework, but nothing that involved stooping or lifting. She could load a washing machine but not unload it or hang washing on the line. She could cook, but not lift heavy pots and pans; she had had to have her kitchen modified. She needed help with the shopping. She had given up disco dancing, aerobics and hiking.

She felt she was a wet blanket in the company of her friends, and both she and her husband acknowledged that their sexual life had been severely interfered with – as the judge put it, a grave disadvantage in a young couple. An unsightly scar, from a necessary operation, ran 21cm across her stomach. Wishing to become pregnant, she was reluctant to take analgesics or pain-killers as much as she otherwise would have. If successful in having children, she would need assistance at least until they were capable of getting out of the bath unaided. Delivery by Caesarian section might be necessary (1994, Court of Appeal, unreported).

McLEAN v PLYMOUTH HEALTH AUTHORITY
Nurse; turning a patient; expert view differing from guidance; negligence case

A pupil nurse aged 43 was in 1983 assisting a registered nurse to lift a 10-stone woman aged 62, four feet high and obese. The patient had to be turned every two hours to prevent pressure sores; the nurses used the 'orthodox lift' to lift the patient up the bed. They also used the same lift to move the patient laterally six inches to the side before rolling her over. The claim failed.

The plaintiff argued that the orthodox lift should not have been used. However, the judge stated that the opinion in the Royal College of Nursing *guidance*, 'The handling of patients – a guide for nurses', that the orthodox lift should not be used, was only one view (and was that strongly expressed only in the 1987 edition, after the date of the accident). He accepted conflicting expert opinion that the orthodox lift was safe if performed competently and that it should be used when the Australian lift could not be (1988, High Court, unreported).

McLEOD v ABERDEEN CITY COUNCIL
School auxiliary; handling unruly pupil; training in restraint techniques; negligence case

In 1995, a school auxiliary was repeatedly kicked and head-butted by a pupil, whilst she was attempting to remove him from a room where he was not supposed to be. Part of her claim alleged that she should have been trained in restraint techniques.

The council attempted to have the case dismissed, partly on the grounds that the pursuer could not establish (a) that there was a generally recognised body of training which the council would have been aware of; and (b) that the techniques she referred to were recognised techniques which any reasonable employer would have taught. In addition it was clear, the council argued, that such training was in a development stage and there was no evidence submitted of any education authority providing such training.

The court decided that the case should proceed. It found that the claim was ample, given the existence of techniques to prevent or minimise violence; furthermore such training was provided for the teachers in the school and had been requested by the pursuer, and there clearly was a developing practice in providing such training ([1999] GWD 23–1115 1999, Outer House, Court of Session, Scotland).

McMENAMIN v LAMBETH, SOUTHWARK AND LEWISHAM AREA HEALTH AUTHORITY (TEACHING)
Porter; pushing food trolley; whether two-man job; simple instructions needed; negligence case

The plaintiff, a member of the portering staff, claimed for a back injury sustained in 1968 when pushing a food trolley down a walkway from a hospital kitchen to ward. He alleged that the trolley was either defectively designed or unsuitable. It weighed 440lb.

The judge concluded that there was nothing defective about the trolley, which was supplied by a manufacturer specialising in hospital equipment; nor was there anything wrong with the walkway, since the camber down which the trolley had veered was necessary unless the walkway was to be permanently wet in rainy weather. However, there was undisputed evidence from a large number of people that one person would find the trolleys difficult to manoeuvre and that there was foreseeable risk of strain and injury. Given that the employer itself agreed that really this was a two-man job, the judge concluded that there 'was a foreseeable risk of injury which by the simple instruction that [the trolleys] were not to be pushed down that walkway except by two men...would have been avoided'. There was thus liability; damages amounted to £19,500.

Accident on physiotherapy traction couch. A second accident which subsequently occurred to the plaintiff was not considered in depth because it added little to the overall claim, but even so the judge found liability established. The porter attended hospital for physiotherapy treatment for the first injury, and he fell through the traction couch. The judge concluded that either the couch was insufficiently strong (the porter weighed some 19 stone) and he should not have been on it at all; or it was defective. Whilst accepting that there was an adequate system of inspection generally, nevertheless the employer's inability to explain the defect did not defeat the negligence claim, since they 'have proved a perfectly adequate system, but unless it be known what the defect was, and nobody does, but there must have been one, and unless there has been some careful investigation and examination afterwards, the necessary evidence is simply lacking to show that…the system in this case was carried out' (1982, High Court, unreported).

MILETIC v CAPITAL TERRITORY HEALTH COMMISSION
Cleaner/housemaid; nurses' home; making beds; jammed castors; falling onto floor; negligence case

A 36-year-old cleaner/housemaid worked at a nurses' home and made the beds. As she was pushing a bed back one day in 1978, the castors jammed, she pushed harder – and as she did so, she fell forward onto the floor. She apparently suffered significant pain and injury which had persisted for over twelve years.

The court dismissed her claim on the grounds that although the jamming of castors from time to time was foreseeable (although no particular defect was identified), there was not an obvious risk of injury by falling unless the floor was slippery, she was wearing the wrong footwear, or the castors had jammed and suddenly released themselves. However, there was no evidence that any of these three conditions was satisfied. If, alternatively, there was a foreseeable risk of falling from jamming castors, there was nothing to suggest that the defendant should have done anything more than it had done to reduce or eliminate the risk. (Normally if the castors were jammed, the beds would not be moved out from the wall at all and a maintenance man would be called) ([1992] ACTSC 57, Supreme Court of the Australian Capital Territory).

MITCHELL v INVERCLYDE DISTRICT COUNCIL
Grass cutting; slipping causing injury; negligence case; MHOR 1992; Provision and Use of Work Equipment Regulations 1992; Personal Protective Equipment at Work Regulations 1992

This case illustrates the breadth of law potentially applicable to some manual handling type situations. The 42-year-old pursuer suffered an injury in 1993 when he slipped using a powered, rotary grass mower on a wet embankment. He was wearing safety boots provided by the employer.

Negligence. The pursuer's case in negligence succeeded; the chargehand could not explain why, if it was too dangerous to cut the embankment when it was raining, it was safe immediately after the rain had stopped. He was also aware that the footwear provided did not in fact prevent the risk of slipping.

MHOR 1992. As for the *MHOR 1992*, the court concluded that the mower was not to be regarded as a load being transported or supported, so the *MHOR 1992* did not apply.

Provision and Use of Work Equipment Regulations 1992. Under r.5 (now r.4 of the 1998 regulations of the same name), equipment had to be suitable for both the operation and the conditions in which it was used. This claim succeeded; the wet grass made the mower more difficult to push.

Personal Protective Equipment at Work Regulations 1992. The employers led no evidence that the boots they had provided were suitable to avoid risk of injury; thus a breach of r.4 of the 1992 regulations was established. Regulation 4 required that employers ensure that suitable protective equipment is provided for employees, unless any relevant risk was adequately controlled by other means ([1998] SCLR 191 1997, Outer House, Court of Session, Scotland).

MOORE v NORFOLK AREA HEALTH AUTHORITY
Nursing auxiliary; duty on employer to safeguard nurses; negligence case

A 36-year-old nursing auxiliary with four years' experience, some previous back trouble, and no training, was injured in 1974 when turning a 12-stone, paraplegic, uncooperative patient using the 'orthodox lift'. This entailed the patient being rolled from his side onto his back, then to his other side, then moved back to the centre of the bed by the staff standing on opposite sides of the bed, linking arms under the patient and lifting him. Liability was established.

Duty on employers to remind nurses of dangers. The court pointed out that because staff naturally underestimate dangers, the employer has a high degree of duty to safeguard them from injury, by laying down a regime which reminds nurses of the dangers. This was because nurses in their enthusiasm to treat their patients to the best of their ability would otherwise take unwarranted risks. Even so, it was also important to keep in mind that hospital authorities did not have unlimited resources – they had to do the 'best they can with the staff and equipment which they have available'.

Asking for assistance. It was true that the position of a nurse was not comparable to that of an employee in a factory and that a certain amount of discretion had to be left with nurses when they were handling patients. In emergencies, immediate decisions had to be taken by nursing staff in circumstances which could not be anticipated by health authorities. However, leaving to the nurse the decision about whether assistance was required applied perhaps more readily to a trained nurse than to an auxiliary nurse. In this case it would have been setting an 'unrealistic standard' to have expected the nurse to ask for help. Damages of £7,775 were awarded (1982, High Court, unreported).

MORAN HEALTH CARE SERVICES v WOODS
Nursing assistant; mobile lifting equipment used in shower; locking wheels; back injury

This was a workers' compensation claim case in Australia, concerning the extent of a nursing assistant's incapacity arising from an accident in 1993 when she was 45 years old. It involved the showering of a patient with a 'Henry lifter', which was manoeuvred by two members of staff. As they were coming out of the shower, the wheels locked and the nursing assistant felt a sharp pain in her back. The court found that this caused permanent, total incapacity for work, and now dismissed the appeal of the employer against the finding of the judge at first instance ((1997) Supreme Court of New South Wales Court of Appeal, transcript).

MUNROW v PLYMOUTH HEALTH AUTHORITY
State enrolled nurse; lifting patient up the bed; hoist use; negligence case

In 1986, a state enrolled nurse was using the 'Australian lift' with another nurse to lift an obese woman weighing over 16 stone up the bed; the latter had a hip dislocation and skin sores. The woman jerked back, causing the injury.

Balancing patient comfort and nurse safety. The court accepted, as did the health authority's handbook on manual handling, that the authority had to balance the comfort of patients with the safety of nurses.

Patient's care plan. The patient's care plan specified that three nurses would be required for getting the patient on to a bed pan, but did not explain how the patient was to be handled.

Training. The judge accepted that she had been adequately trained and had no doubt whatsoever that she knew how to carry out the 'Australian lift'.

Hoist use. The judge appreciated that hoist use was not without problems, especially because of patients' dislike of them generally, the necessity of finding the right sling given this patient's hip problem and skin sores, and nurses' own traditional reluctance to use them. But for a patient so short, obese, great in girth and heavy, special consideration was required. If the patient had demurred, she could have been told that if she wanted continued care she would have to put up with a hoist, if she did not want the nurses injured. On the evidence, the judge found that the hoist would not have injured the patient any more than the manual handling.

Responsibility at senior level for care plan: liability. The judge stated that the patient's care plan needed a senior mind to apply itself to a patient with a special problem. A senior person needed to 'devise and authenticate a plan for a patient whom it was appreciated was liable to injure herself perhaps, and also injure the very nurses who were caring for her'. The health authority maintained that the plaintiff had chosen one of four methods of lifting patients, and it was up to her to decide. The judge felt that was not good enough. She chose the second best method, but 'she should have been told that she had to use a hoist'. The court was not looking for perfection but for reasonable steps. Hoists constituted a reasonable step as confirmed by the Royal College of Nursing *guidance* 'The handling of patients'. Even on the accepted knowledge of 1986, it was well known that there was a case for using the hoist in difficult situations. The health authority did not sufficiently apply its mind. Damages of £172,000 were agreed.

Background of nurse. The nurse was twenty-five years old at the time of the accident:

> She had always been keen on nursing; she was enthusiastic from her school-days onwards; she was a thoughtful, willing, competent, pleasing nurse who was ambitious to spend her life in a nursing career till she was over 60. She put this above having children and though she married last year, says – and I believe her – that she had no wish to have children and would have put her nursing career first, so that I am not speaking of any lackadaisical type of nurse; I am speaking of an enthusiastic and competent one. One has only to look at her references and acceptance by hospitals to recognise this.' (1991, High Court, unreported)

MURRAY v HEALTHSCOPE LIMITED TRADING AS NORTH WEST PRIVATE HOSPITAL
Auxiliary nurse; lift of patient into wheelchair; injury; whether arguable case; time limits on bringing case; breach of statutory duty (Australian legislation); negligence case

The plaintiff was an auxiliary nurse. She alleged that in 1995 she was called by a patient who wanted to go the lavatory; there was a danger she would soil herself. Of two other nurses, one was on the telephone and the other at lunch. The patient was sitting in a very low chair. Placing a wheelchair beside the chair, the nurse used a body hug to lift the patient to an upright position and then tried to turn her; however, the patient became a dead weight, fell back into the armchair, and the nurse injured her back.

She further alleged that although there was lifting equipment, (a) it required two staff to manage it; (b) the doorways between the patient's chair and the lavatory were too narrow to accommodate the lifting equipment; and (c) the patient's arthritis made it impossible for her to use the equipment anyway.

Her claim in negligence therefore centred on failure to organise staff such that assistance would be available; failure to instruct the plaintiff that she should not lift without assistance; and failure to provide suitable lifting equipment. She also made a claim for breach of health and safety at work legislation.

Breach of time limits. However, the plaintiff was now bringing the case slightly outside of the legal time limit of three years (the same as in the United Kingdom). The court found, first, that there was an arguable case on the basis of the above allegations. Second, it concluded overall that – despite having consulted a doctor and solicitor initially – she had had some initial expectation that the injury would resolve itself and believed that she could continue in her hospital employment, albeit with a transfer of duties (however, she was subsequently made redundant). Once she realised the full position, she then acted expeditiously through a third solicitor (after a second solicitor had improperly served a writ); and the court felt that the employer would not be unduly prejudiced by the delay ([2000] TASSC 162, Supreme Court of Tasmania).

NATIONAL ASSISTANCE ACT 1948 (NON-RESIDENTIAL SERVICES FOR DISABLED PEOPLE)

The National Assistance Act 1948 is a key piece of *welfare legislation* underpinning the provision of community care services by local authority social services departments in England and Wales. Under s.29, a local authority has in some circumstances a general *duty*, and in others a *power*, to arrange non-residential welfare services for disabled people, following an assessment of need under s.47 of the *NHS and Community Care Act 1990*.

Of the services listed under s.29, a number might be relevant to manual handling. For instance, there is (a) the general duty 'to provide a social work service and such advice and support as may be needed for people at home or elsewhere'; (b) the general duty 'to provide, whether at centres or elsewhere, facilities for the social rehabilitation and adjustment to disability including assistance in overcoming limitations of mobility or communication'; and (c) the power to 'give instruction to people at home or elsewhere in methods of overcoming effects of their disabilities'. Indeed, it was this last power that the judge in *R v Cornwall County Council, ex parte Goldsack*, identified as underlying the assistance with mobility (including manual handling) provided for a disabled woman at a day centre.

NATIONAL ASSISTANCE ACT 1948 (RESIDENTIAL ACCOMMODATION)

The National Assistance Act 1948 is a key piece of welfare legislation underpinning the provision of community care services by local authority social services departments in England and Wales. Under s.21, a local authority has in some circumstances a specific duty, and in others a power, to arrange residential or nursing home accommodation for people deemed by the local authority to be in need of such accommodation following an assessment under s.47 of the *NHS and Community Care Act 1990*. Manual handling needs and issues might sometimes be material (a) to a decision about whether residential care is required or not; and (b) to the nature and type of accommodation arranged.

The key condition that needs to be satisfied under s.21 is that the person be somebody aged 18 years or over who by reason of age, illness, disability or any other circumstances is in need of care and attention which is not otherwise available to him or her. Local authorities must give effect to people's choice of residential accommodation subject to its suitability, availability and its coming within the usual cost that the authority would pay for that type of accommodation (LAC(92)27).

NEEDS: see *patient and client needs*

NEGLIGENCE

The common law of negligence remains highly relevant to manual handling law. It is called common law because its rules are not to be found in legislation, but in legal judgments. In England and Wales, it is part of the law of torts, and in Scotland part of the law of delict.

Employees. Employees bringing cases might well sue both under the *MHOR 1992* and in negligence (see section 3 of the Overview for a comparison). There is no problem in principle for employees in bringing manual handling cases against the NHS – witness the many nursing cases cited in this book – or against social services (see e.g. *Colclough v Staffordshire County Council*).

Non-employees. Non-employees, such as patients and clients, are unable to use the *MHOR 1992* to bring a compensation claim and so must use the law of negligence instead.

Given the amount of litigation brought by patients against the NHS, it is clear that in principle, a patient could argue a claim against the NHS if he or she has been injured because of a poor manual handling decision or practice. It should be noted, however, that where the alleged negligence is directly attributable to general policy and resources issues, the courts might shy away from imposing liability (see e.g. *Kent v Griffiths*).

Likewise on the social services side, there has been a pronounced reluctance by the courts to entertain certain types of negligence case, for example, involving policy, resources and complicated child care and child protection decisions made under children's legislation (*X v Bedfordshire County Council*). However, this reluctance, which has anyway been put in question to some extent by recent human rights considerations (see e.g. *Z v United Kingdom*), has not prevented the courts from being prepared to consider relatively straightforward situations involving alleged negligence and non-employees – such as a failure to provide training or information to a foster parent about manual handling (*Beasley v Buckinghamshire County Council*), the dropping of a client by a home care assistant through careless handling (*Wyatt v Hillingdon London Borough Council*), a failure to identify dyslexia in a child (*Phelps v Hillingdon London Borough Council*), and failure to provide reasonably careful information or advice (*Vicar of Writtle v Essex County Council; T (A Minor) v Surrey County Council*).

Standard negligence test. The test for negligence is commonly referred to as comprising three main questions: (a) was there a duty of care between the alleged perpetrator of the accident (e.g. an employer in the case of employee injury, or service provider in the case of non-employee); (b) was that duty breached through carelessness or lack of reasonable competence; and (c) was the harm directly caused by that breach of duty?

Professionals involved in manual handling – whether making decisions, formulating care plans, delegating, instructing, guiding, advising, training, demonstrating or actually manually handling – should be aware that the test of carelessness concerns whether they can show that they made a reasonably competent decision.

This does not mean they have to show that they possessed the 'highest expert skill' in their field of work, but that they acted competently (*Bolam v Friern Hospital*). Thus, for a case to have a chance of succeeding, it would have to be shown that the professional acted in such a way as no other professional of ordinary skill in that field would have done (*Hunter v Hanley*). This further means that it is not necessary even to decide which of two professional practices was the better practice, as long as what the defendant professional did was in accordance with a practice accepted by at least some responsible professionals (*Bolam v Friern Hospital*). Nevertheless, the court would need still to satisfy itself that any expert view put forward on behalf of a professional could be justified on an objective, logical basis (*Bolitho v Hackney Health Authority*).

This test for carelessness therefore makes it absolutely necessary for professionals to base their manual handling decisions on clear, informed reasoning which is then *documented* – if they are to be in a position to defend their decisions and actions at a later date. It is also of course fundamental that professionals should not undertake tasks beyond their competence. (This might be particularly relevant in manual handling when, for instance, therapists are asked to make complex decisions, and give advice, demonstration and training. This is sometimes on the assumption that all therapists are automatically competent to do so, when in fact this is not necessarily the case – and in practice in some organisations, such staff might even themselves be denied the relevant, specialist training because of a lack of resources to pay for it.)

Vicarious or direct liability. An employer organisation might find itself both vicariously liable on behalf of the individual negligent acts of its employees/staff, and/or directly liable for its failure as an organisation. For instance, in one manual handling case (*McGowan v Harrow Health Authority*), the nurse involved won her case against her employer both in respect of the porters failing to lift when they should have (this is straightforward vicarious liability), but also because there had been a failure at senior level to consider risks and alternatives (this is moving toward direct liability, for a failure in a system of work). Another example of vicarious liability was when one of the nurses in a team of three failed to lift at the right time thus causing injury to the plaintiff nurse (*Page v Enfield and Haringey Health Authority*).

Contributory negligence. Even when an employer is found to be responsible overall for an accident in negligence and thus liable, the courts sometimes find that an employee has contributed to his or her own misfortune, in which case a finding of contributory negligence is made and damages payable are reduced accordingly. For example, in *McCaffery v Datta*, the nurse was found contributorily negligent in respect of not following medical advice about lifting and not arranging the patient's bed optimally for the lifting operation.

Independent contractors. Where a local authority or NHS Trust has contracted with a third party agency to deliver care, including manual handling related services and equipment, an injured client or patient might seek to sue both the agency and the Trust or local authority. Assuming the agency or its staff were negligent, the chances of success against either the Trust or the local authority also – as opposed to the agency – will probably depend on how carefully the contract was first placed and then monitored and reviewed. Alternatively, to the extent that any accident was due not to the agency, but anyway to the negligence of the Trust or local authority, then either might simply be liable in its own right.

NHS ACT 1977
Ultimately, health services – including manual handling related services – are provided under ss.1 and 3 of the NHS Act 1977 in England and Wales (for the equivalent in Scotland, see the *NHS (Scotland) Act 1978).*

The duties contained in these sections are vague, and judicial review challenges to rationing and waiting lists – which mean that some people do not get the services they need either at all or in time – tend to fail, although there are some exceptions: see section 6 of the Overview of this book.

1. **NHS Act 1977: comprehensive health service**. The Secretary of State has a duty 'to continue the promotion in England and Wales of a comprehensive health service designed to secure improvement (a) in the physical and mental health of the people of those countries, and (b) in the prevention of, diagnosis and treatment of illness, and for that purpose to provide or secure the effective provision of services in accordance with this Act' (s.1).

2. **NHS Act 1977: medical, nursing and other services**. The Secretary of State must provide throughout England and Wales 'to such extent as he considers necessary to meet all reasonable requirements' various services including (a) medical, dental and nursing services, (b) hospital or other accommodation, and (c) 'such facilities for the prevention of illness, the care of persons suffering from illness and the after-care of persons who have suffered from illness as he considers are appropriate as part of the health service' (s.3).

NHS (SCOTLAND) ACT 1978
Sections 1, 36 and 37 of the NHS (Scotland) Act1978 apply roughly the same general duties to the NHS in Scotland, as apply to England and Wales under the *NHS Act 1977.* For these and a discussion of their import, see immediately above and the Overview of this book.

NHS AND COMMUNITY CARE ACT 1990
Section 47 of the NHS and Community Care Act 1990 is a key piece of *welfare legislation* underpinning community care in England and Wales (for Scotland, see the same duty contained in s.12A of the *Social Work (Scotland) Act 1968).*

It places a strong duty on a local authority social services department to assess any person, if it appears that he or she might possibly be in need of community care services. In deciding whether the person's needs call for such services – whether in a residential or nursing home or in a person's own home – the local authority will have to consider whether there are manual handling issues and how to resolve them.

Under the umbrella of the s.47 assessment, the manual handling related provision of equipment, adaptations and personal assistance in a disabled person's own home will come under s.2 of the *Chronically Sick and Disabled Persons Act 1970* (or, in the case of adaptations, a referral may be made to the local housing authority, to exercise its functions under the *Housing Grants, Construction and Regeneration Act 1996*). If, instead, residential or nursing home care is arranged under s.21 of the *National Assistance Act 1948*, manual handling will remain an issue in terms of a home's suitability to cope with an individual's manual handling needs (see e.g. *Redbridge London Borough Council*).

1.   **NHS and Community Care Act 1990, s.47: assessment**. 'Where it appears to a local authority that any person for whom they may provide or arrange for the provision of community care services may be in need of any such services, the authority (a) shall carry out an assessment of his needs for those services; and (b) having regard to the results of that assessment, shall then decide whether his needs call for the provision by them of any such services'.

2.   **NHS and Community Care Act 1990, s.47: special consideration for disabled people** 'If at any time during the assessment of the needs of any person under [the above subsection] it appears to a local authority that he is a disabled person, the authority (a) shall proceed to make such a decision as to the services he requires as is mentioned in section 4 of the Disabled Persons (Services, Consultation and Representation) Act 1986 without his requesting them to do so under that section; and (b) shall inform that they will be doing so and of his rights under that Act'.

3.   **NHS and Community Care Act 1990, s.47: involving the NHS and housing authorities**. If it appears to the local authority that there may be a need for NHS or housing services, it must notify the health or housing authority and invite them to assist in the assessment to such extent as is reasonable in the circumstances. In coming to a decision about services, the local authority must take into account any services likely to be made available by the health or housing authority.

4.   **NHS and Community Care Act 1990, s.46: definition of community care services**. Defines community care services as falling within a number of other Acts: *National Assistance Act 1948, Chronically Sick and Disabled Persons Act 1970, Health Services and Public Health Act 1968, NHS Act 1977* (schedule 8), Mental Health Act 1983 (s.117).

5.   **NHS and Community Care Act 1990, s.47: urgency**. 'Nothing in this section shall prevent a local authority from temporarily providing or arranging for

the provision of community care services for any person without carrying out a prior assessment of his needs...if, in the opinion of the authority, the condition of that person is such that he requires those services as a matter of urgency...as soon as practicable thereafter, an assessment of his needs shall be made.'

NO LIFTING POLICIES

So-called 'no lifting' or 'no manual handling with risk' policies are not referred to in legislation, but are arguably implied by the *MHOR 1992* in some health and care situations – although clarity about what either of those terms actually means is clearly required. For discussion, see section 3 of the Overview to this book.

NURSES

As a profession, nurses and nursing auxiliaries are heavily involved in manual handling and have unfortunately been involved in a stream of compensation cases both in the common law of *negligence* and under the *MHOR 1992*. This seems clearly to indicate their vulnerability to manual handling injury. One feature in many cases has been the relative inexperience of the injured nurse; and it is easy to see why the Royal College of Nursing has produced extensive and forthright guidance on manual handling (RCN/NBPA 1997). It is also notable that in many cases the courts are slow to be persuaded by the customary argument of the NHS that the nurse is to blame.

O'NEILL v BOOROWA DISTRICT HOSPITAL
Craft lady at hospital; left to help patient go to the lavatory; whether contributory negligence in not asking for assistance; negligence case

A craft lady was employed by the hospital at its day centre. At the time of the accident in 1985, neither the sister in charge nor the other nurse was present. The client involved was an elderly person in her late seventies, confined to a wheelchair with one leg partially amputated, who needed to get to the lavatory. The craft lady asked the assistance of another client to help her assist the first client. There was no lifting equipment in the centre, nor had the craft lady received any training; she now ruptured a disc.

At first instance, the jury had found the employer liable, but reduced the damages by 35 per cent on grounds of contributory negligence. The craft lady now claimed that either the trial judge should not have left such a finding to the jury, or alternatively the jury's decision in this respect was perverse.

Instructions and training. The Court of Appeal now found that there was indeed no contributory negligence. The craft lady had not been given any instruction regarding treatment or caring of disabled clients – but equally she had not been instructed not to undertake particular tasks. Furthermore, she had in the past assisted nursing staff in such tasks; and the court felt that it was reasonable for her to understand that they were an ancillary or subsidiary part of her function, in the absence of other staff. Yet she had received no training, and there were inadequate facilities to assist her to perform such a function.

Asking for assistance. As to whether she should have asked for further assistance, the court accepted that the sister in charge and nurse could have been anywhere in the hospital, and that there was no evidence as to how quickly any other nursing assistance could have been found – and of course elderly people needing to get to the lavatory would not wish to wait. The court went on:

> Once it is appreciated that the only evidence before the jury was that the tasks which it was the function of the [craft lady] to perform, as she understood them, included helping persons who were in some situation or emergency, be it great or small, to do whatever was required or needed at the time in the absence of nursing staff; and once it is recognised that there was in truth no system in place whereby the hospital ensured that there were adequate facilities or adequate assistance to enable the appellant to carry out those tasks, it seems to me that it cannot be said that there was in truth any question of contributory negligence to go the jury ((1996) Supreme Court of New South Wales Court of Appeal, transcript).

OCCUPATIONAL THERAPISTS

Occupational therapists, in common with physiotherapists, are involved in *rehabilitation* and independence activities with patients and clients, and are frequently called on to make decisions about, and give instructions on, manual handling. Their professional body has issued guidance on manual handling (COT 1995). This makes a number of particular basic points including the need to avoid hazardous manual handling where reasonably practicable, to assess risks to both staff and patients, and to reduce risk as far as reasonably practicable. It refers to the importance of training in order to ensure the competency of staff in respect of manual handling generally – but also emphasises that professional staff 'responsible for training other staff must ensure that they have the necessary knowledge, experience and competence in the specialist subject of the handling of people and loads, and have the required teaching skills. Competency should be gained by undertaking a validated and/or accredited post registration course' (p.5). A notable negligence case in the manual handling field involved an occupational therapy assistant who was injured (*Stainton v Chorley and South Ribble NHS Trust*).

The following example shows how occupational therapists might in practice have to consider in depth how manual handling affects their work. A hospital occupational therapy department initially identified no less than 63 different risks. These were then simplified into the following areas and types of activity: patient handling, access to the department and room layout, equipment storage, changing rooms, delivery and fitting of equipment in the community, home visits, getting equipment in and out of cars, splinting at school, use of suspended sensory equipment, moving equipment in the children's centre (Hignett 2001).

OFFICES, SHOPS AND RAILWAY PREMISES ACT 1963

Section 23 of this Act, rendered obsolete by the *MHOR 1992*, stated that: 'no person shall in the course of his work, in premises to which this Act applies, be required to lift, carry or move a load so heavy as to be likely to cause injury to him'.

PACHECO v BRENT AND HARROW AREA HEALTH AUTHORITY
State enrolled nurse; lifting patient from wheelchair to bath; time limits on bringing case; back injury advice; negligence case

The court allowed a manual handling case to proceed on the grounds that either it was in fact within the time limits, or those limits should be waived. It also recognised the difficulty of obtaining clear advice about back injuries.

The plaintiff – a state enrolled nurse in a hospital, 37 years old at the time of the accident – allegedly sustained an injury on 13 March 1978, when assisting a nursing sister to bathe an elderly patient, and lifting her from wheelchair to bath. She claimed that the *system of work* was unsafe because the construction of the bathroom meant that mechanical aids could not be used; and also that the nursing sister was negligent in allowing a large part of the patient's weight to fall upon the plaintiff. The case now hinged on whether the plaintiff could proceed with the legal action at all, because it had been brought two months, over the three year time limit specified in the *Limitation Act 1980*.

Date of knowledge; individual circumstances. In deciding when the plaintiff had, under ss.11 and 14 of the Act, knowledge enough to bring the case, the court accepted that individual circumstances had to be considered. These included the fact that the plaintiff was of Spanish origin, and her English was not perfect; that she was a state enrolled, not a state registered, nurse; that she had received conflicting advice from general practitioners (the judge accepted that back injuries often attracted conflicting advice); and that she did not appreciate the significance of her injury and her rights until 26 May 1979. This brought her within the three year time limit.

Waiving the time limits. In case the judge was wrong about that, he considered also whether the s.33 discretion to waive the time limits could be exercised by the court. He found that it would be just and equitable to do so. Even though the employer would be deprived of its 'splendid shield', he asked why not – after all, 'if they have no or little answer to the plaintiff's claim, I do not see why they should not be deprived of their shield. If they have a complete answer, then they will succeed…' (1984, High Court, unreported).

PAGE v ENFIELD AND HARINGEY HEALTH AUTHORITY
Nurse; team lift; negligence case

In 1977, a newly qualified 23-year-old nurse was moving a terminally ill patient weighing eight stone in order to wash her and relieve her pressure sores. She got backache from stooping. Later that day, she was part of a team of three nurses lifting the same patient into a chair. At the command to 'lift', one of the other nurses did not lift. The plaintiff took the full weight of the patient and felt a sharp, lower back pain like an electric shock. Liability was established, given that all members of the team had to lift together; it was foreseeable that if this did not happen, injury might occur. Damages were awarded at £17,238 (1985, High Court, unreported). On appeal, they were reduced by £4,000 (1986, Court of Appeal, unreported).

PAINTER v BARNET COMMUNITY HEALTHCARE NHS TRUST
Nursing auxiliary; assisting patient to the toilet; patient falling; no training; patient's assessment and needs for mobility; negligence

The plaintiff was a nursing auxiliary who at the time of the accident in 1991 was 38 years old, and who had had a long nursing career.

Absence of training. When she started working at the hospital, she participated in a one-day induction course; the employer could provide no evidence that it included any manual handling training. The judge was shown the contents of a three-day induction course at the same hospital; this did not include manual handling training. On this basis the judge concluded, in line with the plaintiff's contention, that the one-day course did not either.

In 1990, she suffered a manual handling injury to her arm and was off work for six weeks. At this time, the senior nurse manager decided that the plaintiff needed manual handling training, along with all staff on the ward. Physiotherapy training was arranged but took place before the plaintiff returned to work.

Assessment ward to gauge independence of patients. The ward on which she worked contained patients who were admitted for an assessment of their abilities to cope without institutional care; it was the 'laudable aim of the ward that patients should be encouraged to be as independent as possible; the nursing staff were aware of and worked towards that aim, as they were expected to'.

Accident: not letting the patient go down. The accident involved an 85-year-old patient, physically well, but suffering from dementia and from a reversed sleep pattern. She was often confused and needed prompting in matters of hygiene and toileting; she was ambulant but needed accompanying to the toilet in case assistance was required. She probably weighed ten stone. Following the level of care deemed appropriate for this patient, the plaintiff walked with her; the patient held on to her left arm. The patient sat down on the lavatory, but the plaintiff realised that her underpants were still on, and she told her to remove them. As the patient stood up to do so, she started to fall toward the plaintiff and her head fell against her chest. Unable to get free, the plaintiff decided instinctively to raise the patient back on to the toilet seat; as she did so, she felt a sharp pain.

Injury because of lack of training. This reaction of the plaintiff was contrary to what was stated in the guidance published by the Royal College of Nursing and Back Pain Association in 1987, 'The handling of patients' – namely that the nurse should let the patient go down slowly to the floor. However, the plaintiff claimed that it was her lack of training which led her to act as she did; the judge quite accepted that the instinctive reaction of untrained nurses would be to prevent the indignity and perhaps serious physical effects for the patient of a nasty fall onto the floor of a toilet. It appeared that the senior nurse manager recognised that by 1991 proper training was required, but had been overruled by higher management. The failure to train the plaintiff – whose only training otherwise had been twenty years earlier in Iran – amounted to negligence which caused the plaintiff's accident. Damages of £131,571 were awarded.

Assessment of patient and need for independence. It was also argued that the patient's condition meant that it was unsafe for the plaintiff to escort her to the toilet and to stand back and observe her; and that either she should have been transferred onto a commode or sanichair first, or the plaintiff should have been instructed physically to help and support the patient. However, the judge noted that an important part of the patient's assessment was that she should be allowed to do as much for herself as she reasonably could; this was the general aim of the ward. There was no evidence that she had any physical as opposed to organisational and mental difficulties; and she had not previously fallen on the ward or posed a problem during toileting. Thus, the assessment of how the patient should go to the toilet was not negligent (1997, High Court, unreported).

PARAMERISSIOS v HAMMERSMITH AND FULHAM LONDON BOROUGH COUNCIL
Recreation assistant; swimming pool; buckets of water; negligence case

The plaintiff was a recreational assistant, 38 years old, who worked at a swimming pool. There was a daily routine of washing down the five pool surrounds using commercial three-gallon plastic buckets. On this particular day in 1985 she was detailed by the duty manager to do it alone; something that happened occasionally. She said it would be too much for her, but she was told that she was a 'strong girl' and would manage. For an hour she had to bend to lift water (from the pool) amounting to a load of about 25lb, turn through ninety degrees and throw the water onto the surrounds vigorously. She strained her spinal joints in the lower cervical and dorsal regions.

The court found liability. The employer knew her physical characteristics and also that the water level in the pools varied, and that this meant there was a greater degree of bending in some pools than others. Even one of the employer's witnesses gave evidence that he had found the task physically demanding. The management should have anticipated such an injury. The judge had sympathy for the management because of the shortage of staff and its policy not to discriminate between men and women in doing particular jobs. However, a heavy responsibility was placed on the management to consider the situation, when a person specially said that the job would be too much for her (1993, Mayor's and City of London Court: reported in PMILL, November 1993).

PARKES v SMETHWICK CORPORATION
Ambulance worker; equipment; employee's existing back problem; system of work; negligence case

An older case. An ambulance worker suffered a hernia injury in 1956, when moving backwards up the steps of an ambulance carrying a stretcher. He argued that a more suitable stretcher should have been supplied. It was proved that the ambulance drivers had complained that their work was awkward and heavy and had suggested that retractable stretcher gear be fitted to all ambulances. The County Court judge had found negligence in respect of the corporation's failure to check that the plaintiff was fit for that type of work, to provide proper equipment and to arrange a proper system of work.

The Court of Appeal now dismissed the case on the grounds that the corporation was not under a duty (a) to examine the plaintiff's capacity to undertake the work (he already suffered from a hernia); (b) to fit all ambulances with retractable stretcher gear, despite representations in the past by ambulance men about their awkward and heavy work; and (c) to lay down an exact system of working for ambulance men. This was on the basis that the work of ambulance men required strength and agility and the employer had no reason to suspect the plaintiff was particularly susceptible to injury. Also, the retractable stretchers could only be used in the vicinity of the ambulance; but the plaintiff could easily have suffered his injury on the stairs of a house. Lastly, the decision of what to do with particular patients had to be left to the ambulance men on the spot; such decisions were 'not of any great difficulty; they really involve the mere application of common sense to the situation and the circumstances of the moment' ([1957] 121 JP 415, Court of Appeal).

PATIENT AND CLIENT NEED
This entry considers how the courts view patient and client need, in the context of *negligence* cases and cases brought under the *MHOR 1992*, under NHS *welfare legislation* and under social services *welfare legislation*.

Patient and client need: negligence and MHOR 1992. In manual handling cases brought by injured employees, the courts quite accept that patients and clients have needs which have to be met – including the 'laudable aim' of assessment for independence (*Painter v Barnet Community Healthcare NHS Trust*), and maintaining mobility because of obesity (*Stainton v Chorley and South Ribble NHS Trust*) or osteo-arthritis (*Sommerville v Lothian Health Board*) – but still examine whether the employer, for example, took reasonable steps to maintain the correct balance between meeting patient need and preserving staff from injury.

This has meant judicial consideration of: a proper system for assessing the risk involved for staff such as student nurses and thus routinely having thought-out care plans (*Clarke v Oxfordshire Health Authority*) involving a senior mind (*Munrow v Plymouth Health Authority*); the drawing up of an adequate individual care plan (*Brown v East Midlothian NHS Trust*); ensuring that staff are familiar with it (*Dewing v St Luke's*);

the keeping of it up to date (*Bowfield v South Sefton (Merseyside) Health Authority*) and changing manual handling practices accordingly (*Stainton v Chorley and South Ribble NHS Trust*); and whether it has been followed (*Gysen v St Luke's; Sommerville v Lothian Health Board*). Thus, nurses needed to be protected through training when a particular patient's care plan entailed additional risks because of the need to give the patient one last chance of independence by encouraging her mobility (*Bayley v Bloomsbury Health Authority*).

Equally, the courts have accepted that some manual handling solutions might not be acceptable if they would result in pain (*Clarke v Oxfordshire Health Authority*) or the shearing action of a sling (*Fitzsimmons v Northumberland Health Authority*). Even so, this does not sanction the putting of nurses at undue risk; in one case, despite the possible adverse effect of hoist and sling on a patient's hip problem or skin sores, the court held that the patient's shortness, obesity, girth and weight would have justified insistence on hoist use – which anyway on the evidence would have not injured the patient any more than the manual handling (*Munrow v Plymouth Health Authority*). Nevertheless, where an important part of a patient's care plan was that she should do as much as she could for herself – and there was no evidence of previous physical difficulties or falling – it was not negligent to allow her walk to the toilet with one member of staff as escort and observer (*Painter v Barnet Community Healthcare NHS Trust*).

Patient and client need: NHS welfare legislation. A number of *judicial review* cases have explored how far the meeting of patients' needs can be enforced, or assessment decisions challenged at the outset (as opposed to suing in *negligence* after harm has occurred). Basically, it is difficult:

(a)   **Lack of NHS resources.** For instance, challenges have failed involving orthopaedic patients not getting the treatment they required (*R v Secretary of State for Social Services, ex p Hincks*), babies with a hole in the heart not receiving operations (*R v Central Birmingham Health Authority, ex p Collier*, and *R v Central Birmingham Health Authority, ex p Walker*) and a 10-year-old being denied potentially lifesaving leukaemia treatment (*R v Cambridgeshire Health Authority, ex p B*). And even when a child came into the highest category of need for various therapy services, an NHS Trust could lawfully argue that it would not make full provision because it did not have enough resources (*R v Brent and Harrow Health Authority, ex p Harrow London Borough Council*). This was in response to a request for assistance by an education authority under s.322 of the *Education Act 1996*.

Thus, generally speaking, where the NHS declines to provide a service – either at all, or to the extent and nature arguably required – on properly argued grounds of lack of resources, it will be almost impossible to upset that decision legally in a judicial review case, so long as the decision has a veneer of clinical assessment and the application of clinical priorities. The implications of this position can even be seen in a different type of case – one brought in *negligence* (*Stainton v Chorley and South Ribble NHS Trust*), in which the judge in effect ruled that in the absence of two adequately trained staff (i.e. an absence of sufficient human resources) to walk an obese woman, she should have been in a wheel-chair because of the risk she posed, even though this would not have been conducive to her need for mobility.

(b)   **Fettering of discretion by the NHS**. It is true that recently the NHS did lose a significant judicial review case when it imposed a blanket policy respecting the availability of gender reassignment surgery (*R v North West Lancashire Health Authority, ex p G, A and D*); this meant that it was *fettering its discretion* and so offending against a key principle applied by the courts in judicial review. Clearly, if the NHS can lose a case concerning such a specialist service, it could in principle do so just as easily in respect of any other service (including manual handling related services) where a blanket, rigid policy is imposed without exceptions ever being considered.

(c)   **NHS taking account of all relevant factors**. Similarly, another health authority lost a case when it refused beta-interferon treatment to a particular person with multiple sclerosis, because it had failed at least to take account of (though not necessarily to follow) central government guidance on the subject (*R v North Derbyshire Health Authority, ex p Fisher*). The authority had thus failed to *take account of all relevant factors*, another key test used in judicial review to identify unlawful decision-making.

(d)   **Health service ombudsman**. The *health service ombudsman* is able to consider complaints about NHS decision-making, including (since April 1996) the adequacy of professional judgement. The ombudsman, for instance, has over the years upheld a significant number of complaints about inadequate arrangements – which might include mobility and manual handling related arrangements – for the provision of services and equipment when elderly or disabled patients are discharged home from hospital.

Patient and client need: social services legislation. The following sums up how clients might challenge manual handling decisions made under such social services *welfare legislation*. It considers matters such as assessment of need, eligibility criteria, *taking account of relevant factors* and *fettering of discretion*. It will be seen that local authorities are more amenable to *judicial review* than the NHS, since their decision-making is viewed as more 'administrative', and so more open to judicial interference, than what is thought of as 'clinical' decision-making in the NHS.

(a)   **Duty to meet manual handling needs**. First, and generally speaking, once a local authority has identified that it is necessary for it to meet a person's needs under s.2 of the *Chronically Sick and Disabled Persons Act 1970*, and under some other community care legislation, then it must do so irrespective of its resources (*R v Gloucestershire County Council, ex p Barry*; see also *MacGregor v South Lanarkshire Council*).

It can then only subsequently withdraw or reduce services if there is an individual reassessment which identifies one of the following conditions: (a) the person's needs have lessened; (b) the eligibility criteria governing service provision have become stricter since the previous assessment; or (c) there is an alternative way of meeting the need. In the absence of any of these three conditions being present, a reduction in service will be unlawful. So, when a manual handling assessment indicated that two carers rather than one would be required for staff safety, and the local authority subsequently reduced the client's services, the decision was struck down by the High Court because in effect the authority was unable to show that any of these three conditions applied (*R v Birmingham City Council, ex p Killigrew*).

This duty and rule will generally apply to both adults and children under s.2 of the 1970 Act; to adults under legislation dealing with residential and nursing home care (s.21 of the *National Assistance Act 1948* and s.12 of the *Social Work (Scotland) Act 1968)*; but not apparently to children in need, including disabled children, under s.17 of the *Children Act 1989* (see *A v Lambeth London Borough Council*) and perhaps also, by extension, under the similar s.22 of the *Children (Scotland) Act 1995*.

(b) **Different ways of meeting a manual handling related need?** However, the courts have emphasised that if there is more than one way of meeting a need, then the final say on how it will be met rests with the local authority – so long as the option chosen does genuinely meet the need – even if this is against the wishes of the client. For example, it was lawful to offer to an elderly woman a placement in a nursing home, rather than support at home, because the former was cheaper (*R v Lancashire County Council, ex p RADAR*); and likewise to take into account cost-effectiveness when offering an elderly couple residential accommodation, rather than fully supporting them in the community (*R (Khana) v Southwark London Borough Council*).

From the client's point of view, the way to challenge this last aspect of social services decision-making would be to argue that the option chosen by social services does not in fact meet the need, and therefore is not a lawful option at all (for instance, the dispute might be about whether provision of a hoist as opposed to manual handling assistance would really meet the assessed need of a person: see e.g. *Redbridge London Borough Council*). In some circumstances it may even be possible for the client to argue, on the basis of all the evidence, that what the local authority had classed as a mere preference was in fact a need and therefore triggered a duty to provide the service desired by the client (e.g. *R v Avon County Council, ex p M*).

(c) **Taking account of health and safety of employees**. It was lawful to take into account the health and safety of staff (in respect of manual handling) when considering whether to provide a wheelchair or walking aid for a client at a day centre, instead of human walking assistance, in order to meet the client's need for general mobility (*R v Cornwall County Council, ex p Goldsack*).

(d) **Taking account of relevant factors**. Where a local authority can demonstrate that it has carried out a balanced assessment and taken into account all relevant factors, then challenging the assessment and offer of service will be difficult, since the courts in judicial review will often hesitate to dictate the precise weight to be given to each of these factors for fear of otherwise wholly taking over local authority decision-making. Thus in one case, the court was clear that manual handling safety was a material consideration, when the local authority was deciding how to meet a client's need for mobility at a day centre (*R v Cornwall County Council, ex p Goldsack*).

Conversely, a failure to take account of all relevant factors, whether information from a general practitioner in a community care assessment involving manual handling issues (*R v Birmingham City Council, ex p Killigrew*) or an apparent promise of a home for life for residents in a care home (*R (Bodimeade) v Camden London Borough Council*), will be unlawful. However, the legislation itself places the duty to make a final decision on the local authority; and there is no obligation to go along with the wishes of a person, so long as their preferences are taken into account (*R v North Yorkshire County Council, ex p Hargreaves*). Finally, where the assessment process appears blatantly incomplete or inadequate and to lack a reasoning process, then the courts might strike it down (*R v Ealing London Borough Council, ex p C*).

(e) **Eligibility criteria**. In determining whether there is a need in the first place and whether it is necessary that it be met, the courts have ruled that the local authority may apply eligibility criteria, which in turn may be formulated (at least partly) with resources in mind. Thus, a local authority which is short of resources may from time to time reformulate its criteria and make them stricter.

A client with manual handling needs apparently falling outside the criteria will have limited chances of challenging the decision, but could succeed if it can be shown that (a) the criteria were not drawn up in a balanced fashion – that is they took account of resources only and were not based also on a consideration of local needs (*R v Gloucestershire County Council, ex p Barry*); (b) that the criteria, though lawful in themselves, have been misapplied in his or her particular case (*R v Ealing London Borough Council, ex p C*, at the High Court stage of that case); (c) that the assessment of the client was flawed and overlooked certain factors (see immediately above); or (d) that the criteria allowed of no possible exceptions and so represented a *fettering of discretion*.

PATIENT AND CLIENT PREFERENCES

In the legal context, the NHS and social services are ultimately dealing in people's needs, in the sense that the fact that a person wants or prefers a particular type of service or treatment does not mean ultimately that they are legally entitled to that service (e.g. wanting manual handling instead of a hoist). This is more fully explained immediately above, under *patient and client need*. Even so, in the health and safety context, it is clear that in practice neglecting the views of the patients or clients being handled might simply result in the failure of manual handling systems of work, thus increasing risk to staff (RCN 2001, p.5). There is also the danger of professionals sometimes not listening to patients and clients properly, and simply dismissing their views – even when those views are in fact as expert as any. For instance, a disabled person might have considerable insight into his or her manual handling needs and the associated risks; insight which might subsequently be backed up by more formal professional assessment (e.g. *Redbridge London Borough Council*).

PEARSON v EASTBOURNE AREA HEALTH AUTHORITY
Nursing auxiliary; cot side related injury; reliability of evidence; maintenance; history of back trouble; negligence case

A 38-year-old nursing auxiliary claimed to have suffered back injury when she pulled up a jammed cot side. The judge found no liability on the grounds that on all the evidence there was no such defect likely to cause such an injury. In reaching this decision, the judge was impressed with the maintenance system in place in the hospital, which included emergency repairs being dealt with in an hour; others within 24 hours; and six-monthly maintenance plans for beds. The hospital engineer gave evidence that the cot sides were easy to manipulate and that he was not aware of any such problems with the relevant beds. The judge also concluded that even had there been a fault with the cot side, it would have been impossible to infer danger for an ordinary person going about their daily tasks – as opposed to the plaintiff who already suffered from a serious degenerative condition (1984, High Court, unreported).

PECK v CHIEF CONSTABLE OF AVON AND SOMERSET
Police officer; moving protestor; MHOR 1992; negligence case

A case illustrating the potential scope of the *MHOR 1992*, in terms of work situations covered and also their application to a situation not apparently involving a direct employer-employee situation.

A police officer claimed damages under the *MHOR 1992* and in *negligence* for injuries sustained when he was trying to move a person (sitting on the ground) taking part in a peaceful protest at a power station. The claim succeeded both under the regulations and in common law because he was allowed to lift on his own, had not been instructed to lift only with a fellow officer and had received no training in lifting in such situations. Considering the *European directive* underlying the *MHOR 1992*, the court held that the directive applied even though the plaintiff was not employed by the chief constable; the directive was intended to have wide effect and to apply in favour of all kinds of workers who were effectively controlled when on duty and acting under the instruction of other senior workers ([1999] CL 00/May, County Court).

PHELPS v HILLINGDON LONDON BOROUGH COUNCIL
Educational psychologist; failure to identify dyslexia; negligence case

A major negligence case, the potential impact of which will be to increase the vulnerability of local authorities in respect of negligent professional decisions (including those which are manual handling related) by employees. In this case, the local authority was held vicariously liable for the failure of an educational psychologist to apply a standard test for the identification of dyslexia ([2000] 3 CCLR 156, House of Lords).

PHYSIOTHERAPISTS

Chartered physiotherapists constitute a key group of NHS staff heavily involved in the manual handling of patients, both directly and through advice and instruction to other staff. Since effective rehabilitation of some patients requires manual handling, they might take a different approach from other professions, and believe that guidance on basic caring and nursing tasks is not necessarily appropriate to the physiotherapist's situation. This is spelt out in current guidance which sets out a 'position statement' to the effect that:

> Physiotherapy is an autonomous profession concerned with the rehabilitation of patients.

> Manual handling is integral to the practice of the profession of physiotherapy.

> It is not always reasonably practicable to avoid manual handling in physiotherapy without abandoning the goal of the rehabilitation of patients.

> A risk assessment must always be undertaken prior to handling any patient and appropriate steps taken to minimise any risk to the patient and to those delivering the physiotherapy intervention (CSP 2002, p.4).

The guidance goes on to point out that the principles of risk assessment extend not only to decisions physiotherapists make for themselves and their patients, but also to matters such as delegation to, advising or guiding others such as physiotherapy assistants and students, other professions, or informal carers. As the guidance points out, such matters are routine aspects of physiotherapy practice (CSP 2002, p.26).

Indeed, in a case involving an injured occupational therapy assistant, a physiotherapist and the walking of an obese patient, the court in effect made precisely this latter sort of point. The judge noted that the participation in a manual handling task of two chartered physiotherapists (or staff equivalently expert) would have reduced the risk to an acceptable level; whereas the participation of an inadequately trained, less skilled occupational therapy assistant with only one chartered physiotherapist did not so reduce the risk in all the circumstances (*Stainton v Chorley and South Ribble NHS Trust*).

Even so, questions still remain about the extent to which even physiotherapists are in fact able to carry out manual handling without exceeding an acceptable level of risk; for instance, a 1998 survey found a 73 per cent incidence of lower back pain in physiotherapists working with neurology patients, and a positive correlation between such pain and the length of time spent working in neurology. The authors conclude, unsurprisingly, that neuro-physiotherapists work in a potentially high risk environment – and that it is essential for them to be critical of their own handling techniques (ACPIN 2001, p.6).

POLICIES: see *manual handling policies*

POLLITT v OXFORDSHIRE HEALTH AUTHORITY
Nursing auxiliary; poles and sheeting; moving trolley; taking dead weight; liability agreed; negligence case

A 46-year-old nursing auxiliary was lifting a patient with two other colleagues (another nurse and a porter) in 1992. The patient weighed 18 stone and was semi-conscious, lying on his back on a bed. Using poles and sheeting they were attempting to transfer him from the bed to a trolley. On two occasions, as they tried to do this, the trolley moved. On the second occasion, the nurse bore some of the dead weight of the patient, because they were anxious not to drop the patient, and wanted to return him to the bed without incident. This produced unexpected stress on her back. There was a prior compromise on liability, with the health authority agreeing 80 per cent liability for the accident; the trial was now about the amount of damages appropriate for the extent of injury caused by the particular incident, which were set at £10,000 (1998, High Court).

POSTLE v NORFOLK AND NORWICH HEALTHCARE NHS TRUST
Nurse hit by trolley; artificial division of manual handling operation; MHOR 1992 applicable; but no liability

The plaintiff was a nurse employed in an accident and emergency department, when a patient collapsed in the waiting area and was placed on a hospital trolley. He was standing toward the foot of the trolley but not actually holding or pulling it. Another nurse pulled the trolley from the front and to the left; it swung round and struck the plaintiff. The defendant maintained that the *MHOR 1992* did not apply because the duty was owed to the employee involved in the manual handling operation, not the plaintiff.

Defining a manual handling operation. The court held that the *MHOR 1992* were applicable, since otherwise it would mean treating what was really a single operation as if it consisted of artificially distinct component parts, and each nurse would then only be involved for the purpose of the regulations at the precise moment that he or she was physically active in handling a load.

No liability. However, the judge did not impose liability, finding that a suitable and sufficient assessment would not have recognised the risk of injury to one nurse from the pulling of a trolley by another; nor would steps to reduce the risk have involved giving instructions which would have led the other nurse to pull the trolley forward rather than to the left, or to tell the other nurses that she was about to move ([2000] CL 00/2970, County Court).

PRESCRIPTION AND LIMITATION (SCOTLAND) ACT 1973: see *limitation of actions*

PRICE v UNITED KINGDOM

Human rights; disabled woman; detention in police station and prison; adequate facilities; manual handling

This case illustrates a breach of article 3 of the *European Convention on Human Rights*, in terms of the degrading treatment suffered by a disabled woman when sent to prison, because of the lack of facilities available to meet her needs – including those involving manual handling.

The applicant was a severely disabled person as a consequence of phocomelia due to Thalidomide. During civil proceedings in a County Court for debt, she refused to answer questions about her financial position; she was committed to prison for seven days for contempt of court. She spent the night in a police station, before moving to prison the next day. Her account of what happened was disputed by the United Kingdom government, but the court held as follows:

> **[Cold cell]** During her first night of detention the applicant was kept in a cell in local police station because it was too late in the day to take her to prison. The custody record shows that she was complaining of cold every half hour – a serious problem for the applicant who suffered from recurring kidney problems and who, because of her disability, could not move around to keep warm. Finally, a doctor was called, who noted that the applicant could not use the bed and had to sleep in her wheelchair, that the facilities were not adapted to the needs of a disabled person and that the cell was too cold. The Court notes, however, that despite the doctor's findings no action was taken by the police officers responsible for the applicant's custody to ensure that she was removed to a more suitable place of detention or released. Instead, the applicant had to remain in the cell all night, although the doctor did wrap her in a space blanket and gave her some pain killers.

> **[Manual handling]** The following day the applicant was taken to Wakefield prison, where she was detained for three days/two nights. During her first night's detention, the nursing record states that the duty nurse was unable to lift the applicant alone and thus had difficulty in helping her use the toilet. The applicant submits that as a result, she was subjected to extremely humiliating treatment at the hands of male prison officers. The Government deny her account, but nonetheless it seems clear that male officers were required to assist in lifting the applicant on and off the toilet.

> **[Inability to meet her needs]** The Court observes that there are notes in the applicant's admission records by a doctor and staff nurse expressing concern over the problems that were likely to be encountered during her detention, including reaching the bed and toilet, hygiene and fluid intake, and mobility if the battery of her wheelchair ran down. Such was the concern that the

prison governor authorised staff to try and find the applicant a place in an outside hospital. In the event, however, they were unable to transfer her because she was not suffering from any particular medical complaint. By the time of her release the applicant had to be catheterised because the lack of fluid intake and problems in getting to the toilet had caused her to retain urine. She claims to have suffered health problems for ten weeks thereafter, but has supplied no medical evidence in support.

[Degrading treatment] There is no evidence in this case of any positive intention to humiliate or debase the applicant. However, the Court considers that to detain a severely disabled person in conditions where she is dangerously cold, risks developing pressure sores because her bed is too hard or unreachable, and is unable to go to the toilet or keep clean without the greatest difficulty, constitutes degrading treatment contrary to Article 3.

Damages of £4,500 were awarded ((2001) TLR, 13 August, 2001 European Court of Human Rights).

PRIVACY

Privacy is sometimes referred to in the context of the *Human Rights Act 1998*, article 8 of the *European Convention on Human Rights*, and manual handling decisions.

PROVISION AND USE OF WORK EQUIPMENT REGULATIONS 1998 (PUWER 1998)

These regulations cover all equipment used at work, including manual handling and lifting equipment (see also the *Lifting Operations and Lifting Equipment Regulations 1998*). They impose a range of duties concerning matters such as the initial state of the equipment, purpose and suitability of the equipment, working conditions, maintenance, information, instructions and training. The regulations apply only to equipment used at work; the implications of this requirement are discussed under *LOLER 1998*.

It should specifically be pointed out that the duty of maintenance in regulation 5 is a strict one, and is not qualified by the term 'reasonably practicable'. Furthermore the courts have held that this strict duty is not just to have a maintenance system, but actually to have the equipment 'in an efficient state, in efficient working order and in good repair' (*Stark v Post Office*). The effect of this case would seem clear: an employee who is injured by a defective item of manual handling equipment will normally have a very strong case against the employer under this regulation. Indeed, the postman in that case failed in his argument based on the common law of *negligence*, because carelessness on the part of the Post Office in its system of maintenance could not be demonstrated; but he succeeded under regulation 5 which carries no connotation of carelessness or moral fault, but instead imposes strict liability.

Extracts from PUWER 1998 include:

1. **PUWER 1998: equipment used at work:** 'any machinery, appliance, apparatus or tool or installation for use at work' (r.2).

2. **PUWER 1998: use of equipment:** '…in relation to work equipment means any activity involving work equipment and includes starting, stopping, programming, setting, transporting, repairing, modifying, maintaining, servicing and cleaning' (r.2).

3. **PUWER 1998: persons covered**. Employers generally, self-employed people and also any person who 'has control, to any extent, of

    (i) work equipment;

    (ii) a person at work who uses or supervises or manages the use of work equipment; or

    (iii) the way in which work equipment is used at work,

    and to the extent of his control' (r.4). (But the regulations do not apply to suppliers of equipment by way of sale, agreement for sale or hire-purchase agreement.)

4. **PUWER 1998: purpose of the equipment.** 'Every employer shall ensure that work equipment is so constructed or adapted as to be suitable for the purpose for which it is used or provided' (r.4).

5. **PUWER 1998: working conditions** 'In selecting work equipment, every employer shall have regard to the working conditions and to the risks to the health and safety of persons which exist in the premises or undertaking in which that work equipment is to be used and any additional risk posed by the use of that work equipment' (r.4).

6. **PUWER 1998: suitability**. 'Every employer shall ensure that work equipment is used only for operations for which, and under conditions for which, it is suitable.' Suitability means: 'suitable in any respect which it is reasonably foreseeable will affect the health or safety of any person'. Where machinery has a maintenance log, the employer must ensure it is kept up to date (r.4).

7. **PUWER 1998: maintenance**. 'Every employer shall ensure that work equipment is maintained in an efficient state, in efficient working order and in good repair…shall ensure that where any machinery has a maintenance log, the log is kept up to date' (r.5).

8. **PUWER 1998: inspection**. 'Every employer shall ensure that, where the safety of work equipment depends on the installation conditions, it is inspected –

    (a) after installation and before being put into service for the first time; or

    (b) after assembly at a new site or in a new location,

    to ensure that it has been installed correctly and is safe to operate.'

'Every employer shall ensure that work equipment exposed to conditions caus-ing deterioration which is liable to result in dangerous situations is inspected –

(a)   at suitable intervals; and

(b)   each time that exceptional circumstances which are liable to jeopardise the safety of that work equipment have occurred,

to ensure that health and safety conditions are maintained and that any deterio-ration can be detected and remedied in good time.'

'Every employer shall ensure that the result of an inspection made under this regulation is recorded and kept until the next inspection under this regulation is recorded.'

'Every employer shall ensure that no work equipment –

(a)   leaves his undertaking; or

(b)   if obtained from the undertaking of another person, is used in this un-dertaking, unless it is accompanied by physical evidence that the last in-spection required to be carried out under this regulation has been carried out' (r.6).

9.   **PUWER 1998: inspection, definition**. In relation to r.6, inspection:

(a)   'means such visual or more rigorous inspection by a competent person as is appropriate for the purpose described in the paragraph;

(b)   where it is appropriate to carry out testing for the purpose, includes test-ing the nature and extent of which are appropriate for the purpose'.3

10.   **PUWER 1998: specific risks**. 'Where the use of work equipment is likely to involve a specific risk to health or safety, every employer shall ensure that

(a)   the use of that work equipment is restricted to those persons given the task of using it; and

(b)   repairs, modifications, maintenance or servicing of that work equipment is restricted to those persons who have been specifically designated to perform operations of that description (whether or not also authorised to perform other operations).

The employer shall ensure that the persons designated for the purposes of sub-paragraph (b)…have received adequate training related to any operations in respect of which they have been so designated' (r.7).

11.   **PUWER 1998: information and instructions**. 'Every employer shall en-sure that all persons who use work equipment have available to them adequate health and safety information and, where appropriate, written instructions per-taining to the use of the work equipment.'

'Every employer shall ensure that any of his employees who supervises or manages the use of work equipment has available to him adequate health and safety information and, where appropriate, written instructions pertaining to the use of the work equipment.'

The 'information and instructions…shall include include information and, where appropriate, written instructions on:

(a)   the conditions in which and the methods by which the work equipment may be used;

(b)   foreseeable abnormal situations and the action to be taken if such a situation were to occur;

(c)   any conclusions to be drawn from experience in using the work equipment.

Information and instructions…shall be readily comprehensibe to those concerned' (r.8).

12.   **PUWER 1998: training**. 'Every employer shall ensure that all persons who use work equipment have received adequate training for purposes of health and safety, including training in the methods which may be adopted when using the work equipment, any risks which such use may entail and precautions to be taken.'

'Every employer shall ensure that any of his employees who supervises or manages the use of work equipment has received adequate training for purposes of health and safety, including training in the methods which may be adopted when using the work equipment, any risks which such use may entail and precautions to be taken' (r.9).

13.   **PUWER 1998: conformity with European Community requirements**. 'Every employer shall ensure that an item of work equipment has been designed and constructed in compliance with any essential requirements, that is to say requirements relating to its design or construction in any of the instruments listed in Schedule 1 (being instruments which give effect to Community Directives concerning the safety of products)' (r.10).

To the extent that relevant Directives do not apply, rr.11–24 apply in respect of various matters including dangerous machinery parts, specified hazards, temperature, controls and control systems, isolation from energy sources, stability, lighting, maintenance operations (re manufacture or adaptation), markings, and warnings.

PURVIS v BUCKINGHAMSHIRE COUNTY COUNCIL
School welfare assistant; restraining five-year-old pupil; MHOR 1992

The plaintiff was employed as a welfare assistant in a department of a school for children with moderate learning difficulties. In May 1993, she was left alone with a five-year-old pupil whose first day this was at the department; the pupil persisted in trying to run away. At one point, when the child was in danger of escaping from the building, the assistant grabbed her under the armpits with both hands and injured her back. She claimed that she had not received training or instruction in safe handling techniques, that she had not been warned about the particular pupil, that the *MHOR 1992* had been breached – and that, given the pupil's history, she should have been in a special school.

The claim failed. The court found that the pupil's behaviour had improved after her first day, and there was no evidence that she had been inappropriately placed or that such running away was unusual for children of that age. The plaintiff had had two years' experience in the department, and it was difficult to see what training she could have had, nor how it would have prevented the injury. The council was entitled to regard her as adequately trained. The *MHOR 1992*, r.4(1)(b) had been breached because of a failure to assess the nature of such an emergency situation (the court disagreed with the case of *Fraser v Greater Glasgow Health Board* which had excluded emergencies from the *MHOR 1992*). However, this was a technical breach only and not causative of the accident ([1999] ELR 231, High Court).

R (BODIMEADE) v CAMDEN LONDON BOROUGH COUNCIL
Human rights; closure of residential home; importance of existing law; legitimate expectations; judicial review

This is a case indicating that, even with the introduction of the *Human Rights Act 1998*, existing domestic law might be effective in protecting human rights (whether or not manual handling related) without having to resort to the 1998 Act, when flawed decisions are made by public bodies such as local authorities.

The case involved a challenge to the proposed closure of a residential home. The court found that the local authority had failed to demonstrate that it had considered all material considerations (i.e. *taken account of all relevant factors*), including a statement in the home's handbook referring to a 'home for life', the legitimate expectations of the residents and the fact that 'best value reviews' did not render 'nugatory the well-established policy of a needs-led approach to the provision of accommodation'. The court ruled that the local authority should reconsider its decision, and come to a fresh conclusion. The judge noted that it was unnecessary to 'visit the Human Rights Act for resolving any remaining dispute between the parties. As is so often the position, the common law by its adaptability has demonstrated that it is capable of meeting human rights standards unaided' ([2001] EWHC Admin 271; [2001] 4 CCLR 247, High Court).

R (HEATHER, WARD AND CALLIN) v LEONARD CHESHIRE FOUNDATION AND HM ATTORNEY GENERAL

Human rights; whether charity was public body under the Human Rights Act 1998

The Leonard Cheshire Foundation, as a charity and company limited by guarantee, provided residential accommodation for residents placed and funded by the local authority or health authority. The court ruled that in respect of such residents, it was a public body neither for the purposes of *judicial review,* nor under s.6 of the *Human Rights Act 1998* ([2001] EWHC Admin 429; [2001] 4 CCLR 210, High Court).

R (KHANA) v SOUTHWARK LONDON BOROUGH COUNCIL

Community care; couple's wish to stay at home; residential care offered; human rights; judicial review

This is a case indicating that, even with the introduction of the *Human Rights Act 1998,* it is not necessarily legally incumbent on local authorities to give effect to people's wishes about the services (whether or not manual handling related) or assistance they should receive.

An elderly Iraqi-Kurdish couple had sought assistance from the local authority in obtaining suitable ground-floor accommodation under s.21 of the *National Assistance Act 1948* so that their family could continue caring for them; the current second-floor flat in which they were living was both inappropriate and overcrowded. The local authority instead offered first one and then both of the couple places in a residential home. They refused the offer, arguing a number of grounds including family, language, isolation and emotional well-being. They argued the case under both community care legislation and the *Human Rights Act 1998* – namely the right to respect for privacy, home and family life (under article 8 of the *European Convention on Human Rights*).

Balanced assessment. The couple failed both at first instance in the High Court, and then on appeal in the Court of Appeal. Both courts found that the local authority had carried out a proper assessment under community care legislation, taking account of various needs and preferences of the couple; and that it would also have been entitled to take account of cost-effectiveness in deciding what option to offer (i.e. residential home or care in the wider community). The Court of Appeal made the point that the reason, as it seemed to it, that Southwark was offering residential care under s.21 of the 1948 Act, was simply that the provision of services elsewhere would not meet the couple's needs. Nevertheless, it did accept that in the light of the couple's refusal, the local authority would still come under an obligation to do the best it could under s.29 of the *National Assistance Act 1948* and provide non-residential services such as meals on wheels and clean laundry.

Human rights. As to the human rights argument, the judge in the High Court had found that a balanced assessment under community care legislation and guidance – weighing up various factors including cost-effectiveness – not only conformed to that legislation but also to the *Human Rights Act 1998*. She made the point that 'the guidance and legislation, as far as this area of law is concerned, is very broad, very humane, and takes account of the needs and the respect for the family, home and private life referred to in article 8'. Thus any potential breach of article 8 would turn on whether the community care legislation had been breached – which here it had not. The human rights point was not further pursued in the Court of Appeal ([2001] EWCA Civ 999, Court of Appeal).

R (ROWE) v WALSALL METROPOLITAN BOROUGH COUNCIL
Community care; closure of residential home; human rights; judicial review

This is a case indicating that, even with the introduction of the *Human Rights Act 1998*, it is not necessarily incumbent on local authorities to give effect to people's wishes about the services (whether or not manual handling related) or assistance they should receive. The judge refused permission for the case to proceed to a full judicial review, in the following circumstances.

Two residents of a residential home for older people in Walsall challenged its proposed closure, arguing that they had been promised a home for life and that the closure would breach article 8 of the *European Convention on Human Rights* – namely their right to respect for their private and family life. The court rejected this argument, stating that there was no clear evidence of such a promise, and that there had been thorough consultation prior to the decision to close the home. Furthermore, even if there had been a breach of article 8.1, it would surely have been justified under article 8.2 as 'required for the economic well-being of the council and of those in need of its services' (2001, High Court, unreported).

R v AVON COUNTY COUNCIL, ex p M
Person with learning disabilities; whether request for more expensive residential home was preference or need; psychological need; judicial review

A case demonstrating the legal and practical importance of distinguishing client need from preference for services (whether or not manual handling related).

The local authority argued that the wish of a young man (with Down syndrome) to enter a more expensive residential home under s.21 of the *National Assistance Act 1948* was a mere preference; therefore it was instead offering an alternative, cheaper home. However, the judge concluded from all the evidence and expert opinion given to the local authority that it amounted to a psychological need, and therefore triggered a duty to arrange the more expensive accommodation ([1999] 2 CCLR 185, High Court).

R v BEXLEY LONDON BOROUGH COUNCIL, ex p B
Disabled child; meeting of needs; Children Act 1989; Chronically Sick and Disabled Persons Act 1970; judicial review

A case demonstrating that for the meeting of a disabled child's needs (whether or not manual handling related), s.2 of the *Chronically Sick and Disabled Persons Act 1970* might be more effective than s.17 of the *Children Act 1989*, given the stronger duty it contains.

The case concerned a mother's dispute about the withdrawal of support services to assist her in caring for her severely disabled son. Amongst other considerations the judge noted that the duty under the 1970 Act was specific toward disabled persons and therefore stronger than the general duty under s.17 of the 1989 Act toward children in need (including disabled children). With this in mind, he took exception to the local authority's artificial position that only s.17 was in play. In all the circumstances, it must have been clear to the local authority that the child came under the 1970 Act. (For other reasons, the mother's case was, overall, unsuccessful) ([2000] 3 CCLR 15, High Court).

R v BIRMINGHAM CITY COUNCIL, ex p KILLIGREW
Community care assessment; manual handling assessment; reduction of care; resources; unlawful decision; judicial review

A judicial review case involving a manual handling assessment and illustrating how, in attempting to balance the safety of employees, available resources and client need, a local authority appeared to neglect the last of these – client need – and so made an unlawful decision.

Background. A woman aged 40 had had multiple sclerosis from the age of 17. Her condition had worsened. She shook uncontrollably, had been registered blind for seven years, had deep vein thrombosis, had epilepsy which could give rise to extended seizures, and was incontinent but physically unable to tolerate a catheter. She could not undertake any personal task unaided, such as getting in and out of bed, dressing or moving from the chair. She lived with her husband who had arthritis of the hips and a chronic back condition. He was registered disabled and able to move his wife only at great risk both to her and to himself. Under a care plan dated 11 December 1997, the woman had 12 hours' continuous care every day, seven days a week, starting at 8.00am.

Manual handling assessment and general reassessment. In January 1998, the local authority undertook a manual handling risk assessment (by making use of a manual handling adviser employed by the local community NHS Trust) and advised the husband that he was liable to suffer permanent injury if he continued to lift his wife; that they should move accommodation; and that his wife should no longer be moved by one carer. Following a more general reassessment requested by the couple under s.47 of the *NHS and Community Care Act 1990* in April 1998, the local authority wrote that it could 'provide an assessed package of care which we believe would meet both [your] needs as well as the Manual Handling Regulations. However, this would involve a substantial change to the care package that you had previously, and would involve two carers coming on five occasions during the day and evening…'.

New care plans. Subsequently, there was a meeting involving the wife and husband; part of the minutes of that meeting read that there 'was a discussion around the current care package…and how this would be affected by the reassessment of need…to take into account the manual handling requirements'. The judge found that this showed that 'the reassessment of need was being carried out "to take account" of the need for two carers to assist in the lifting process'. A new care plan in July entailed a total of three and a half hours' care per day with some additional care at the weekend, and envisaged the presence of two carers at the times when lifting would be necessary. A further revision to the new care plan in October allowed for six hours' help per day.

Situation of informal carer. The manual handling risk assessment had concluded that the husband could suffer permanent injury which would stop him caring for his wife, if he continued to lift her. The subsequent community care assessment had identified significant issues about his ability to continue to care; his wife was also very concerned about this.

Unlawfulness of decision. The judge criticised the local authority's decision and ruled that it must reconsider the woman's needs and come to a fresh decision. The grounds were as follows:

> What was needed was a very careful assessment of why, if that was the case, 12 hours' care was no longer needed. The importance of the [local authority] satisfying itself that this was the case is obvious. The applicant and her husband were asking for the 12 hours' care to continue. Her condition was inevitably and steadily deteriorating. Not continuing the 12 hours' care could, it was being said, have serious consequences… The decision to reduce was made at a time when it had been decided that two carers were needed for lifting. It was important that the reduction to six hours' care was not driven by the need to have two carers to carry out the task. On the evidence available before me, the reduction to six hours' care could only be justified if there was no continuing need for 12 hours' care and not simply because two carers were needed when only one had sufficed earlier.

> Do we find that care assessment in the October care plan…? Making all allowances for the fact that this is not a legal document and should not be construed as such, I have no doubt that we do not. There is no proper analysis of why the 12-hour care plan had been originally adopted. What were the perceived advantages of that plan at the time of its implementation? Why are those perceived advantages no longer seen as advantages, if such be the case…'.

Medical evidence. The court also found that the failure to obtain, from a general practitioner, relevant medical evidence about the woman's condition and needs, also meant the council's decision had been legally flawed (in effect it had failed to *take into account all relevant factors*) ([2000] 3 CCLR 109, High Court).

R v BOULDSTRIDGE
Withdrawal of manual handling; refusal to accept hoist; attempted suicide and attempted murder of wife; prosecution for attempted murder

This case was reported in *The Guardian* newspaper; however, the full background to the circumstances of the case was not included. It highlights the need for the NHS or social services to be sensitive and cautious when withdrawing services from vulnerable people, particularly if there are mental health problems (the very point made in *R v Kensington and Chelsea Royal Borough Council, ex p Kujtim*).

Withdrawal of carers. The case concerned an elderly couple. The wife had been suffering from Alzheimer's Disease and was now doubly incontinent, completely immobile and required assistance from carers three times a day, seven days a week. She had received manual handling assistance in the past, but now represented an increasing risk to staff. For this reason, the social services department reportedly stated that unless her husband agreed to have a hoist installed, the carers would be withdrawn; this was after carers refused to lift her manually. He then attempted to kill both himself and his wife by leading a hose from the exhaust of his car into the bedroom; however, a neighbour heard the car engine running, saw the hose and intervened. The husband had left a note blaming a social worker and the owner of a private care company, stating that those evil people had deemed that services should be withdrawn and his wife left unattended.

His wife died a month later in a care home from an unrelated chest infection; on release from hospital he was arrested and charged with attempted murder. He pleaded guilty. The judge sentenced him to a year's probation but also criticised the Crown Prosecution Service for bringing the case at all, stating that it was not in the public interest to have done so (reported in: Kelso 2000).

R v BRENT AND HARROW HEALTH AUTHORITY, ex p HARROW LONDON BOROUGH COUNCIL
Occupational therapy; physiotherapy; speech and language therapy; special educational needs; whose duty to provide

A case with implications for the meeting of needs (whether or not manual handling related) of children with statements of special educational needs under the *Education Act 1996*.

Need for therapy. The education authority had placed provision of physiotherapy (at least 45 minutes a week), occupational therapy (one hour a week) and speech and language therapy (one hour a week) in the 'educational' part of the child's statement of special educational needs, but then asked the NHS to provide this therapy. The NHS refused; a refusal which the judge found justified.

NHS priorities. The health authority had developed priority categories under which it considered each individual case. This particular child came within its highest category, but the health authority still had insufficient resources available to meet all the identified needs, and so stated that it would meet only half of the assessed needs for the speech and language therapy and the occupational therapy. The judge found this to be an impeccable approach, given the terms of s.166 of the Education Act 1993 (now s.322 of the *Education Act 1996*) which stated that a health authority was obliged to comply with a request for assistance from the education authority, unless in the light of its resources it was not reasonable so to comply ([1997] 3 FCR 765, High Court).

Education authority's duty. At the same time, the child's mother successfully brought a parallel case against the education authority, since the court ruled that the authority had the overall obligation to arrange provision deemed educational as opposed to non-educational (*R v Harrow London Borough Council, ex p M* [1997] 1 ELR 62, High Court).

R v CAMBRIDGESHIRE HEALTH AUTHORITY, ex p B
NHS decision-making; rationing; leukaemia treatment; human rights; healthcare rationing; judicial review

A case illustrating the difficulty of challenging rationing by the NHS of services, whether or not manual handling related.

The Court of Appeal refused to interfere with the health authority's refusal to provide potentially lifesaving treatment for a 10-year-old girl suffering from leukaemia. The High Court had ruled that the health authority should think again, and at the very least give a more detailed explanation for their decision; it also thought that article 2 (right to life) of the *European Convention on Human Rights* potentially came into play. The Court of Appeal overturned the High Court's decision, making it clear that it was for health authorities to decide how to allocate limited resources for the greatest good of the greatest number – and effectively ignored the human rights argument ([1995] 6 MLR 250, Court of Appeal).

R v CENTRAL BIRMINGHAM HEALTH AUTHORITY, ex p COLLIER
NHS decision-making; rationing; child; heart operation; healthcare rationing; judicial review

A case illustrating the difficulty of challenging rationing by the NHS of services, whether or not manual handling related. It involved a challenge under the *NHS Act 1977* to the health authority which had failed to carry out an operation on a child's heart. The Court of Appeal indicated that, unless there was evidence of extreme circumstances suggesting legal unreasonableness in the allocation of resources, it could not possibly intervene. It was not for the courts to arrange hospital waiting lists (1988, unreported, Court of Appeal).

R v CENTRAL BIRMINGHAM HEALTH AUTHORITY, ex p WALKER

NHS decision-making; rationing; baby; heart operation; healthcare rationing

A case illustrating the difficulty of challenging rationing by the NHS of services, whether or not manual handling related.

It involved a challenge under the *NHS Act 1977* to the health authority which had failed to carry out an operation on a baby's heart. The Court of Appeal indicated that, unless there was evidence of legal unreasonableness in the allocation of resources, it could not possibly intervene. It was not for the courts to investigate staffing, facilities, or funding; these were questions of enormous public interest and concern but questions to be raised, answered and dealt with outside of the courts ([1987] 3 BMLR 32, Court of Appeal).

R v CORNWALL COUNTY COUNCIL, ex p GOLDSACK

Local authority day centre; mobility need of client; manual handling; health and safety; resources; community care; judicial review

A case in which the court concluded, amongst other things, that it was lawful for a local authority to take into account health and safety when deciding which option (including a manual handling option) to offer for meeting a person's community care needs.

The case concerned a 21-year-old woman with physical and learning disabilities who attended a day centre run by the local authority social services department. Initially she had received human walking assistance at the centre, but now a wheelchair and rollator (a wheeled walking frame) were being used. The authority had also at one stage said that she could walk unaided if she agreed to wear a crash helmet.

The local authority argued that its staff suffered back pain when they walked with her. The judge concluded that the primary assessed need under community care legislation (i.e. *NHS and Community Care Act 1990* and s.29 of the *National Assistance Act 1948*) was that of mobility, and that in deciding how to meet that need, the local authority was entitled (a) to take account of its resources; and (b) to regard health and safety as a material consideration when deciding what assistance to provide (1996, High Court, unreported).

R v EALING LONDON BOROUGH COUNCIL, ex p C

Disabled child; adequacy of social services assessment; assertions with no reasons; unreasonableness and unlawfulness; judicial review

This case demonstrates that the courts will interfere with what might appear to be professional aspects of local authority assessment of clients (whether or not manual handling related) – and thus normally beyond the purview of the courts in *judicial review* – if that assessment blatantly fails to *take account of relevant factors,* or is simply *irrational.*

The Court of Appeal struck down the decisions and actions of the local authority in relation to the assessment of an 8-year-old boy with profound eyesight problems, dyspraxia, severe asthma, incontinence and clumsiness. He lived with his mother and older brother; an initial assessment identified that he needed assistance with all tasks and daily living activities (e.g. washing, bathing, showering, dressing, continence or incontinence, mobility, picking things up, getting in or out of a chair, bed, bath, toilet or commode, outdoor mobility, and so on) and was at high risk because of falls in the house. After considerable delay, a subsequent assessment was carried out, which concluded that no alternative accommodation was required, but that aids and adaptations would suffice.

Inadequate assessment. However, this assessment was carried out without the assessor going upstairs to see the very significant problems associated with the bedroom, where the boy shared a bed with his mother. The court could not

> accept that it was sufficient to provide anyone with a full understanding of either the full practical implications of day and night living for this particular mother and this particular boy, or whether the aids and adaptations proposed would in reality ameliorate the situation to the extent that the accommodation could then reasonably be described as acceptable for this boy. There was, as I have already indicated, a good deal of assertion in the decision letter; there was very little, if any reasoning.

Assertions but no reasons: not asking the right questions.

> The council has not contended that it lacks resources, or that there were others in greater need whose interests have to be put first… The decision is stark and simple; it is asserted, and repeatedly asserted that fresh accommodation is not needed for this boy. In my judgment, both the decision and the decision-making process were flawed. Unless the repetition of an assertion is to be regarded as a proper manifestation of a reasoning process, there was none here… Certainly there was no analysis of the accommodation problems faced by this disabled boy and his mother.

The decision was therefore susceptible to judicial review on the basis that the local authority did not ask itself the right questions and take reasonable steps to acquaint itself with the relevant information.

Decision about boy's level of disability: irrationality of council's decision. A further aspect of the case was that the mother had sought respite care, but was refused on the grounds that her son's disabilities did not have a substantial and long-term adverse effect on his day-to-day activities. The High Court had found that this was *irrational*, given the local authority's own assessment of the boy's severe difficulties with daily living (see above); this finding was not contested in the Court of Appeal ([2000] 3 CCLR 122, Court of Appeal).

R v GLOUCESTERSHIRE COUNTY COUNCIL, ex p BARRY
Community care; withdrawing services or equipment; resources; extent of duty; judicial review

This major community care case (applying directly to England, Wales and Scotland) concerned the withdrawal from, or reduction of services to, significant numbers of social services clients in Gloucestershire. The rules set out by the House of Lords in the case are directly relevant to the provision of manual handling related services by local authorities. Indeed, one of the original applicants in the case was a lady who had been assessed by the council as needing a hoist as part of her hospital discharge; the council had now rescinded the decision, so that she was unable to leave hospital.

Absolute duty to meet need. The case established that local authorities could withdraw or reduce services to clients under s.2 of the *Chronically Sick and Disabled Persons Act 1970*, even if those clients' actual needs had not changed – so long as this was on the basis of both individual reassessments and changed eligibility criteria. Councils were free to alter eligibility criteria from time to time and could take account of their resources in so doing, so long as resources were not the only factor taken into account. Thus, such criteria could be used in deciding (a) whether people were in need, and (b) whether it was necessary for the local authority to meet that need. However, once clients had hurdled such criteria, then the local authority would be under an absolute duty to meet their needs within a reasonable time irrespective of resources (until such time as their needs, or the eligibility criteria, changed, and they received a reassessment). Nevertheless resources could again be taken account of in deciding how to meet the need, if there was more than one option available; i.e. the cheaper could be chosen ([1997] 2 All ER 1, House of Lords).

People at severe physical risk. At the High Court stage of this case, the judge suggested that if eligibility criteria resulted in disabled people at severe physical risk being left unassisted, this could constitute legal unreasonableness on the part of a local authority (*R v Gloucestershire County Council, ex p Mahfood* (1995) LGRR, 27 April 1996).

R v GLOUCESTERSHIRE COUNTY COUNCIL, ex p MAHFOOD:
see *R v Gloucestershire County Council, ex p Barry*

R V HARINGEY LONDON BOROUGH COUNCIL, EX P NORTON
Community care assessment; disregard of social, recreational and leisure needs; unlawfulness of assessment; NHS and Community Care Act 1990; Chronically Sick and Disabled Persons Act 1970

A case in which the court found that the local authority had acted unlawfully (or *illegally*) by failing at least to take account of a disabled man's social, recreational and leisure needs during his reassessment. The case could easily be relevant to a manual handling assessment, given the breadth of implications for people's lives of manual handling decisions. The judge simply referred to s. 2 of the *Chronically Sick and Dis-*

abled Persons Act 1970, which lists these very matters; the authority was clearly in breach of the legislation and the considerations it demanded of the local authority ([1998] 1 CCLR 168, High Court).

R v HARROW LONDON BOROUGH COUNCIL, ex p M: see *R v Brent and Harrow Health Authority, ex parte Harrow London Borough Council*

R v HILLINGDON AREA HEALTH AUTHORITY, ex p WYATT
Disabled woman at home; district nurses; husband rude and aggressive; withdrawal of service; judicial review

The courts in this case indicated when it would be reasonable for the NHS to withdraw a service, in the light of unreasonable patient behaviour.

District nurses provided assistance to a woman who was very sick with disseminated sclerosis, by visiting her at home. However, the husband was aggressive, abusive and threatening toward the nurses. He was asked to give an undertaking that he would cease to be so, but he refused. The health authority subsequently sent a solicitor's letter to the effect that the service would be withdrawn; this was now challenged. The Court of Appeal found the legal challenge misconceived, since the

> health authority is doing everything that it could reasonably be expected to do. It had made all reasonable arrangements for the securing and the attendance of nurses. Husband and wife cannot be separated for this purpose. So long as [the husband] behaves in this unreasonable and aggressive way, there is no duty on the area health authority to secure the attendance of nurses. (1977, Court of Appeal, unreported)

R v KENSINGTON AND CHELSEA ROYAL BOROUGH, ex p KUJTIM
Violent and disruptive behaviour by client; whether local authority could withdraw services; community care; judicial review

The courts in this case indicated when it would be reasonable for a local authority to withdraw a service, in the light of unreasonable client behaviour. Although it involved an allegedly violent asylum seeker, the principles identified by the court are potentially of wider application – in terms generally of clients refusing to accept a service (e.g. a manual handling related one) on the reasonable terms offered by a local authority.

An asylum seeker was assessed to be in need under s.21 of the *National Assistance Act 1948* and provided with accommodation, but was allegedly violent and disruptive in two hotels. He had received a warning from the local authority after the first incident. The local authority then withdrew its assistance after the second. The Court of Appeal held that the duty on the local authority was very strong but not absolute, and that if a client unreasonably refused to accept the accommodation, or in terms of behaviour failed to observe the reasonable requirements of the local authority, then it could treat its duty as discharged. However, before doing so, it would need to consider, where fundamental needs were at stake, the nature of the client's conduct, its causes and surrounding circumstances – in this case issues such as his depressive condition and the ill-treatment that had led him to seek refuge in England ([1999] 2 CCLR 341, Court of Appeal).

R v LAMBETH LONDON BOROUGH COUNCIL, ex p M

Special educational needs; access requirements; lift; not a special educational need; no duty to provide; Education Act 1993

This was a case with implications (including manual handling) for the meeting of children's mobility needs in school under the Education Act 1993 (now *Education Act 1996*). The girl's mother argued that her daughter's need for a lift so that she could access a particular classroom constituted – under her statement of special educational needs – educational provision, which therefore triggered a duty to provide it. The judge held that in law, a lift could not be educational provision but could only be non-educational, and thus would not trigger a duty to provide. (See s.324 of the *Education Act 1996* for the statutory context) ((1995) LGRR, 27 January 1996, High Court).

R v LANCASHIRE COUNTY COUNCIL, ex p RADAR

Community care; 24-hour care required; local authority entitled to offer cheaper option for meeting that need; judicial review

A case establishing that a local authority can offer the cheaper of two options to meet a person's need (whether or not manual handling related), so long as that option does genuinely meet the need.

The Court of Appeal held that the local authority, having assessed that an elderly woman's need was for 24-hour care every day under s.47 of the *NHS and Community Care Act 1990*, was entitled to cease supporting her in her own home, and instead to offer nursing home care – on the basis that although against her wishes, the latter was cheaper and would still meet her needs ([1996] 4 All ER 422, Court of Appeal).

R v NORTH AND EAST DEVON HEALTH AUTHORITY, ex p COUGHLAN

Closure of NHS unit for disabled people; promise of home for life; breach of human rights; abuse of power; judicial review

The health authority's decision to close a special residential unit for severely disabled people was successfully challenged, on the grounds that an explicit promise had been made, when the disabled people moved in some years earlier, that it would be a home for life. In the absence of the health authority being able to demonstrate an overriding reason of public interest for the closure, that closure represented an abuse of power by a public body, as well as a breach of article 8 of the *European Convention on Human Rights*, in that the residents would be deprived of their home ([1999] 2 CCLR 285, Court of Appeal).

R v NORTH DERBYSHIRE HEALTH AUTHORITY, ex p FISHER
Health authority not having regard to guidance about providing a service; unlawful policy

A case illustrating the importance of the NHS and local authorities properly taking account of guidance when deciding about service provision. The Department of Health had issued an executive letter about providing beta-interferon treatment for people with multiple sclerosis. The applicant in the case, who as a matter of policy had been denied such treatment by the health authority, successfully challenged this decision on the grounds that the authority had not properly taken account of the letter when formulating their policy. This failure to have proper regard to the letter – and if they were to depart from it, to provide clear reasons as to why – was unlawful, even though the letter itself did not include any of the 'badges of mandatory requirement' (such as the word 'shall'), but instead contained words such as 'ask' or 'suggest' (([1998] 8 MLR 327, High Court).

R v NORTH WEST LANCASHIRE HEALTH AUTHORITY, ex p G, A AND D
NHS decision-making; blanket policies; unlawfulness; gender reassignment surgery; healthcare rationing; judicial review

A significant case illustrating that even the NHS can be successfully challenged if it applies a blanket policy in the provision of services – whether or not manual handling related.

The Court of Appeal held that the health authority was *fettering its discretion* through application of what was in effect a blanket policy, in not providing gender reassignment surgery. Although the authority's policy in principle allowed exceptions to this policy in case of overriding clinical need, its approach meant that it would never recognise that there was any effective treatment for trans-sexualism – in which case provision for exceptions was meaningless ([1999] 2 CCLR 419, Court of Appeal).

R v NORTH YORKSHIRE COUNTY COUNCIL, ex p HARGREAVES
Community care; taking account of people's preferences but not necessarily following them; judicial review

A case illustrating that local authorities must at least take genuine account of people's preferences for community care services, even if they do not follow them.

The case concerned a woman with learning disabilities and her need for respite care. The local authority lost this case on two main grounds, including the fact that it had failed to take account of her preferences during its assessment under s.47 of the *NHS and Community Care Act 1990*. Although it was responsible for making the final decision about what services to provide, nevertheless in accordance with community care guidance, it had at least to take account of her preferences – even if, ultimately, it did not follow them ([1994] 26 BMLR 121, High Court).

R v SECRETARY OF STATE FOR SOCIAL SERVICES, ex p HINCKS
NHS decision-making; rationing; orthopaedic patients; resources; judicial review

A case illustrating the difficulty of challenging rationing by the NHS of services, whether or not manual handling related.

The case concerned patients who had been on a long waiting list for orthopaedic treatment; they claimed that there was a failure to provide a comprehensive health service and medical services under ss.1 and 3 of the *NHS Act 1977*. The court found that the *NHS Act 1977* did not impose absolute duties, since they were inevitably governed by the available resources; it could not be supposed that the NHS had to provide all the latest equipment or to provide everything that was asked for. The court also emphasised that patients should not be encouraged to think that such judicial review proceedings could enhance the standards of the NHS 'because any such encouragement would be based on a manifest illusion' ([1980] 1 BMLR 93, Court of Appeal).

RE 0
Human rights; proportional response of a local authority

A case demonstrating that the interference (whether or not manual handling related) by public bodies with people's right to respect for family and private life, under article 8 of the *European Convention on Human Rights* and the *Human Rights Act 1998*, should be proportionate to the need or problem identified. Thus, in all the circumstances of the case, the Court of Appeal ruled that a supervision order for a child, rather than the more drastic care order sought by the local authority, was the appropriate response ([2001] EWCA Civ 16; [2001]1 FCR 289, Court of Appeal).

REASONABLY PRACTICABLE

This is a key term in *health and safety at work legislation*, including the *MHOR 1992*. Legally, it entails a balancing of degree of risk against the cost necessary to remove or reduce that risk: see section 3 of the Overview to this book; *Edwards v National Coal Board*; and *Hawkes v Southwark London Borough Council*.

REDBRIDGE LONDON BOROUGH COUNCIL
Local government ombudsman; manual handling; community care; residential care; conflicting risk assessments; cost of care package; National Assistance Act 1948; Chronically Sick and Disabled Persons Act 1970; MHOR 1992

A particularly detailed *local government ombudsman* report concerning a dispute about whether a disabled person should live in the community in his own home (as he wished) or in a care home (against his wishes), and protracted disagreement about his manual handling needs. It illustrates a number of key issues involving manual handling and the provision of community care, not least the difficulties and complexity that sometimes arise:

(a)   **wishes and resources**: the extent to which a disabled person's wish to live in his own accommodation was consonant with the resources of the two local authorities concerned (an annual care package of up to £70,000 was at times being considered);

(b)   **choosing carers**: the wish and ability of the person to choose his own *carers*;

(c)   **manual handling:** the conflict between the man's wish to be handled manually, the residential home's insistence on use of a hoist, conflicting risk assessments, the training of carers, the person's wish to choose his own carers, and a dispute as to why the person wished to be handled only by women;

(d)   **contractual duty of care home to provide specified services:** the contractual obligation of the care home to provide the 24-hour care it was being paid by the council to provide, despite a breakdown in relationship between some of the staff and the disabled person;

(e)   **dispute about funding and the ordinary residence of the person:** a protracted dispute between two local authorities as to the ordinary residence of the person – first if he stayed in the care home (where he had been placed by Redbridge in another authority's area), and second if he moved into the community in that other authority's area. The Secretary of State was belatedly applied to for resolution of the dispute;

(f)   **Secretary of State's directions:** refusal of the Secretary of State, on the ordinary residence question, to issue specific directions as to what care should be provided by which authority;

(g)   **false expectations:** the misleading raising of the disabled person's hopes as a result of unauthorised and ultimately unfulfilled undertakings by particular staff.

In conclusion, the ombudsman found that there was maladministration on the following grounds.

Manual handling: maladministration. First, the council was aware of the complications surrounding lifting and handling from a previous placement but did not plan what to do if they recurred in the new placement; this was maladministration, although it was balanced by the fact that the man moved to the care home initially without the council's approval.

Second, for a substantial period of time the person did not receive an 'appropriate level of care' and so 'suffered considerably as a result'. His elderly parents, who undertook the caring tasks (instead of the care home staff), were put to a 'huge amount of stress, time and trouble that should not have been necessary'. However, the man contributed to the problem by behaving antagonistically to some of the care home staff; although this behaviour in turn might have been in part due to the frustration caused by his expectations which had been raised misleadingly by the council about moving into the community.

Third, although it was 'very difficult' for the council's officers to deal with these 'complex problems' at a distance (i.e. many miles away in the area of another local authority), this was no excuse, since the owners of the care home were acting on behalf of the council which had to 'take full responsibility for the ultimate failure to make appropriate provision'.

Last, there was a predominant medical view that use of a hoist could harm the man (in his thirties with a rare genetic disease which was progressively immobilising him) by further damaging his muscles. And despite the conflicting conclusions of expert lifting and handling assessments, there was a predominant view also that manual handling could be carried out safely if the right method was employed. However, the council did not deal with this issue effectively, particularly when a senior officer wrote to the man telling him that he would have to stay in bed for the time being. This was 'unacceptable', 'insensitive' and 'inappropriate', since the officer was not medically qualified and the man's general practitioner had stated that remaining in bed would be detrimental to his condition.

Home care package: maladministration. First, a decision about the man being able to live in the community in his own home had been made by an officer not authorised to do so; this led to a misleading offer of a community care package. Second, this offer was not rescinded in writing for a considerable time and then only in a letter less than frank about the failures that had occurred and without an apology. Third, there was delay in making clear that in any case the council was not empowered fully to support the home care package because, it was argued, s.2 of the *Chronically Sick and Disabled Persons Act 1970* – which contained a duty to provide such support – applied only to people ordinarily resident in the area of the authority, and not to people who had become ordinarily resident in another area.

All this resulted in (a) the person's expectations being 'unreasonably raised, somewhat dashed but then not clearly extinguished for a long time' and his subjection to great disappointment and stress; (b) the man's move from the care home being delayed unnecessarily for over two and a half years; (c) enormous time, trouble and expense on the part of himself and his relatives; and (d) a 'huge waste' of the council's own resources, particularly the time of its own officers.

Ordinary residence dispute. The council delayed in attempting to resolve the dispute as to the area of ordinary residence of the person both in relation to negotiating with the other council involved (12 months' delay) and then in relation to seeking a resolution by the Secretary of State (8 months' delay). This was maladministration, which 'significantly extended' the period of uncertainty for the person and caused him great frustration (1998: cases 95/C/1472 and 95/C/2543).

REGULATION OF CARE (SCOTLAND) ACT 2001
Coming into force during 2002, this Act will underpin in Scotland the regulation of care provided by local authorities and the independent sector – including manual handling related services and related equipment – in respect of, for example, care

homes, domiciliary care providers, and independent health services (whether run by local authorities, or voluntary or private organisations). For more detail, see *care homes* and *care agencies*; for England and Wales, see the *Care Standards Act 2000*.

REHABILITATION

Manual handling is sometimes an important part of rehabilitation, whereby therapists and other professionals attempt to restore physical function. However, rehabilitation sometimes raises questions about (a) how far it demands manual handling with risk; (b) what risks are acceptable; (c) what sort of employees, by profession or training, should be undertaking such manual handling; (d) the extent to which special (sometimes expensive) rehabilitation equipment can serve both patient need and staff safety; and (e) the extent to which specialist rehabilitation professionals, who traditionally have worked at higher risk, are in fact working safely.

Rehabilitation: health and safety. First is the health and safety issue: to what extent does the law allow staff to deliver rehabilitation involving manual handling, especially given the high incidence of back injury suffered by physiotherapists, who are professionals heavily engaged in rehabilitation (see under *physiotherapists*)?

The *MHOR 1992* clearly do not outlaw manual handling in rehabilitation, since they merely demand that employers either avoid risk if reasonably practicable or reduce the risk to the lowest level reasonably practicable. *Guidance* from the Health and Safety Commission makes the point that rehabilitation and maintaining mobility are situations in which staff – particularly physiotherapists, occupational therapists and their assistants – work at higher risk as part of specified care or treatment processes (HSC 1998, p.43).

Likewise, guidance from the Chartered Society of Physiotherapy points out that whilst chartered physiotherapists must minimise the risk of harm to those engaged in manual handling, their job is to enable the rehabilitation of patients (CSP 2002, p.4). This might mean (p.11) that the professional decisions of physiotherapists will not always accord with the different philosophy and approach contained in guidance issued by the Royal College of Nursing (RCN/NBPA 1997). It is also notable that the guidance for physiotherapists does not take a defensive stance by saying that physiotherapists should not delegate to, or give advice and guidance to, others – such as physiotherapy assistants, students, other professions, informal carers etc. – but that decisions to do this, and the manner of doing it, should be subject to the physiotherapist's overall risk assessment (p.26). In turn risk assessment is underpinned by the 'fundamental aim' of preventing harm or injury occurring to the handler, but also 'ensuring the best possible outcome for the patient' (CSP 2002, p.35).

The guidance also posits the drastic question of whether, in terms of the *MHOR 1992*, it is reasonably practicable for the physiotherapy profession to abandon its core skills and its aim of rehabilitating patients. It answers the question by stating that there is no judicial opinion or guidance on the point (p.11). Nor is there likely to be, since the courts generally take manual handling on a case by case basis, and are unlikely to set such a sweeping precedent.

However, a case such as *Stainton v Chorley and South Ribble NHS Trust* is perhaps informative in relation to this question. Although it was brought in negligence, it is likely in this author's view, that the court's fundamental reasoning would have been similar even had the *MHOR 1992* been in issue. The NHS Trust, through the actions of the physiotherapist, was held to be liable, when an occupational therapy assistant was injured assisting the physiotherapist to walk an obese patient. However, the liability was established, not because the judge ruled that manual handling with risk – for the benefit of the health of the patient – was not acceptable in principle, but essentially because he considered that (a) the physiotherapist's risk assessment was awry; (b) the occupational therapy assistant was only partially trained – and therefore (c) in all the circumstances, an acceptable level of risk had been exceeded.

Rehabilitation: rationing. Once a local policy in the NHS or a local authority establishes what manual handling is, in principle, permitted health and safety wise, there remains the question as to which patients or clients will actually receive rehabilitation (with any associated handling) and to what degree. This becomes a question of staffing, resources, eligibility criteria, local policies on rehabilitation, and ultimately the rationing of health and social care.

Intermediate care. It is true that central government issued *guidance* for England and Wales in 2001 about 'intermediate care', part of which is described as rehabilitation (HSC 2001/01), and any *guidance* about the importance of rehabilitation is welcome. However, a cautionary note is that (a) it is not law but only *guidance*; (b) the normal six weeks' duration of intermediate care imposes limits; and (c) the underlying reason for the policy is arguably to keep hospital beds clear of older people – and the policy could ironically result in damage to existing rehabilitation services, if managers conveniently confuse convalescence (in terms of spontaneous recovery) with more expensive rehabilitation (i.e. non-spontaneous recovery), and so divert funds away from the latter (see e.g. Grimley Evans and Tallis 2001).

RESOURCES

The seemingly eternal refrain from local authority social services departments and the NHS is that they have insufficient resources to meet everybody's needs either at all, or in the way in which they – or indeed clients or patients – would sometimes wish.

Health and safety at work legislation. First, as far as *health and safety at work legislation* is concerned, many if not all duties are qualified by the term 'reasonably practicable', for which the courts have developed a test consisting of a comparison of the level of risk against the cost of doing something about that risk. However, the implications of the test – applied mainly in the context of employees, but not always – are that in some circumstances, an argument resting on lack of resources will not avail an employer, if the risk is significant. See section 3 of the Overview.

Manual Handling in Health and Social Care

Negligence: employees. As far as the law of *negligence* goes, a similar balancing act will be carried out in respect of employees, such that in some circumstances, a lack of resources might not be an effective defence (see e.g. *Denton v South West Thames Regional Health Authority*), although the courts will of course consider the resource implications – for example, in replacing 76 beds all at one time to make manual handling easier (*Dewing v St. Luke's*); in not extending a duty of care in respect of particularly difficult patients to all disabled patients (*Fitzsimmons v Northumberland Health Authority*, Court of Appeal stage); and in understanding that hospitals did not have unlimited resources (*Moore v Norfolk Area Health Authority*).

Negligence: clients and patients. However, as far as clients and patients are concerned, when they sue in negligence for harm suffered through the provision or non-provision of NHS or local authority services, a defence based genuinely on a lack of resources might well succeed (e.g. *Kent v Griffiths*).

Judicial review: clients and patients. In judicial review cases, which can be brought to challenge NHS or local authority decisions (about assessments and service provision, including manual handling related), an argument based on lack of resources will generally mean that the NHS is immune from losing a case. Against local authority social services departments, such an argument will or will not succeed, depending on the stage of the decision-making process in question (see *patient and client need*).

RESTRAINT

The subject of physical restraint of patients and clients is beyond the scope of this book; however, where restraint is clearly justified in certain circumstances, then manual handling techniques become relevant and the *MHOR 1992* might apply. For instance, at the time of writing, the Department of Health has published draft guidance on the restraint of adults and children with learning disabilities or autism, which makes the point that staff who are expected to exercise physical intervention need specialised training on specific techniques (DH 2000, para 12). Guidance from the British Institute of Learning Disabilities and the National Autistic Society includes a chapter on staff safety in relation to physical interventions (Harris *et al.* 1996, p.53). Several cases involving restraint are included in this book (*Daws v Croydon London Borough Council; McLeod v Aberdeen City Council; Purvis v Buckinghamshire County Council*).

RISK ASSESSMENT

Suitable and sufficient risk assessments are explicitly demanded under both the *MHOR 1992* in respect of employees, and the *Management of Health and Safety at Work Regulations 1999* in respect of employees and non-employees (see discussion in the section 3 of the Overview, and under the entry *MHOR 1992: case law*).

ROTHERHAM METROPOLITAN BOROUGH COUNCIL
Local government ombudsman investigation; manual handling; delay in dealing with application for through-floor lift; carrying disabled child up and down stairs; maladministration

This was an investigation by the *local government ombudsman* illustrating, amongst other things, the manual handling implications for clients and *carers* of delay in dealing with applications for home adaptations.

It concerned a woman's application for a through-floor lift in order to help her care for her severely disabled son. The council was at fault in three respects. First, it had not been explained to the woman that her application for re-housing was not being actively considered because she had not been awarded any medical priority points; as a consequence she did not pursue the lift application for six months. Second, communication failure in the council meant that a message from the woman's social worker to a relevant officer was never received and caused a delay of two months. Third, the relevant officer did not process the application for five months owing to work pressure.

This all added up to a year's delay, during which the woman had to carry her growing disabled son up and down the stairs; this was injustice (1995: case 94/C/2287).

ROWE v SWANSEA CITY COUNCIL
Home care assistant; moving hoist; MHOR 1992

A senior home care assistant alleged injury when, helped by another care assistant in a client's home, she was moving a hoist in which the client was seated. She alleged that the cramped conditions required additional moves of the hoist; this rucked the carpet, which in turn meant that a wheel got stuck, so causing injury.

The claim failed. First, the plaintiff failed to prove that the accident had occurred as she claimed; instead the injury was attributed by the court to a constitutional back problem. Also, despite no formal risk assessment under the *MHOR 1992* having been carried out, informal assessments had been made by the council's disablement officer and by its manual handling coordinator. These assessments satisfied r.4 of the *MHOR 1992*. The plaintiff had also gone on an intensive five-day training course in manual handling ([2000] CL 00/April, County Court).

ROZARIO v POST OFFICE
Post office worker; lifting box; negligence case

A negligence case, falling into a category of cases involving what the courts view as relatively simple everyday tasks, and in which they shy away from imposing liability.

In October 1990, a man with previous back injuries was injured when he was lifting a box weighing 10.26kg. He was lifting it from below knee level, and twisting through ninety degrees in order to place the box on a rack. He had earlier in July of that year told his employers that he had trouble with his back, and been placed on light duties for nine days. Having then asked to go back to his former work, he was subsequently injured.

The Court of Appeal now found against the plaintiff, overruling the Recorder at first instance, and denying the argument that even experienced workers fall into bad habits and require more training and supervision. The employer's obligation was to take reasonable care to provide a safe *system of work* and to see that it was followed. Here the worker was experienced (he had worked for the Post Office for 15 years) and the task was simple; the *system of work* had not been such as to lead to foreseeable injury. Furthermore the employer was not obliged to request a medical certificate before agreeing to his return to normal work after the initial back trouble; nor to check and see that he was lifting correctly. That would have been 'a counsel of perfection with the benefit of hindsight' ([1997] PIQR 15, Court of Appeal).

SAFE SYSTEM OF WORK: see *system of work*

SALVAT v BASINGSTOKE AND NORTH HAMPSHIRE HEALTH AUTHORITY
State enrolled nurse; training; custom and practice; hoist available but never used; negligence case

In 1983, a state enrolled nurse aged 22 was lifting, with a student nurse, a patient weighing around fourteen stone, using the so-called 'drag lift'. The patient was 80 years old and had had one leg amputated. Each nurse placed one arm between one of the patient's arms and his body, and lifted using the power in each arm. The plaintiff wiped the patient's bottom and moved the patient away from the commode to his bed, about a foot away, and felt a sharp pain from her neck down to her arm. As they moved him, she suffered sharp pain in her arm.

Custom and practice not to use a hoist. The court heard evidence that the plaintiff had been taught a more suitable type of lift but that custom and practice at hospital was to use this unsafe drag lift (in respect of which, the Royal College of Nursing and Back Pain Association 1981 publication 'The handling of patients' was referred to). If the plaintiff had indeed picked up bad habits, then the court was not satisfied that there was adequate or suitable correction; and concluded also that although there was a hoist on the ward, it was kept in the bathroom and never used except for bathing. Yet for an exceptionally difficult patient such as the man in question, in terms of his age, incapacity and weight, a hoist should have been used. The judge also rejected the suggestion that the nurse had been contributorily negligent, since she was trying to do her job in the best possible way, and was not corrected; the employer was liable; damages amounted to £13,297 (1988, High Court, unreported).

SCHILIRO v PEPPERCORN CHILD CARE CENTRES
Childcare assistant; moving sand to sandpit; whether breach of health and safety legislation (Australia); negligence case

A negligence case, falling into a category of cases involving what the courts view as relatively simple everyday tasks, and in which they shy away from imposing liability.

Background. A 23-year-old child care assistant had formerly been employed as a nurse's aide, at which time she had suffered a minor back injury for which she had received treatment from a general practitioner and physiotherapist. Her current employer was unaware of any history of back problems, and her current full-time position involved caring for children aged three to five years old, including lifting them, and moving tables and play gym equipment. The judge at first instance had found that she had no difficulty doing all of this, despite her overweight and unathletic condition. On the particular day in question, a group leader was asked to move some spilt sand back into the sandpit. She responded that she had a lower back problem and so could not undertake this task. The assistant was then asked; she undertook the task and grumbled, but not to anybody in authority, because she claimed to have been concerned about losing her job had she refused. The judge found this to be an unreasonable view. She and another worker raked and shovelled the sand; she moved about eight loads in 25 minutes.

Low risk manual handling task. The Court of Appeal refused to overturn the judge's ruling in favour of the employer, and so dismissed the appeal, in respect of (a) the statutory duty 'to ensure the workplace health and safety of each of the employer's workers at work' (subject to a due diligence defence); and also (b) the common law of *negligence*. The court concluded:

> The employer demonstrated that it was willing to listen to any employee who did not wish to undertake the task, as this is precisely what it did with [the group leader]. The task was straightforward, ordinary and physically undemanding. It required the removal of a small quantity of sand over a short distance. It provided a suitable shovel and small wheelbarrow. It placed no pressure upon the employee to hurry or to accomplish the task within a particular time. It was a low risk manual task which was not susceptible to further consultations, inquiries or investigations… To find otherwise [than that the employer had discharged its obligations] would be to create an offence for failing formally to identify and manage trivial risks such as when an employee bends down to pick up a pen or reaches to take a book from the shelf and the employee suffers a consequential injury; it is notorious that sometimes serious back injuries are possible in such circumstances. The legislature could not intend such an unjust and unworldly outcome ([2000] QCA 18, Supreme Court of Queensland).

SCHOOLS

Staff working in schools might find themselves in situations where they are manually handling or sometimes restraining pupils – for instance, disabled pupils who need assistance, unruly pupils or pupils with behavioural difficulties. Injuries might be incurred and cases brought; for example, *Daws v Croydon Education Authority, McLeod v Aberdeen Council, Purvis v Buckinghamshire County Council*. School staff might also be injured pushing wheelchairs (Cassidy 2001) or moving tables (*Taylor v Glasgow City Council*).

Thus schools and education authorities need to consider their manual handling related duties toward staff under *health and safety at work legislation*, and also toward pupils (including those with special educational needs) under the *Education Act 1996, Education (Scotland) Act 1980*, and *Disability Discrimination Act 1995* (as amended by the Special Educational Needs and Disability Act 2001).

SCOTLAND

This book applies to Scotland as it does to England and Wales. The *health and safety at work legislation* applies directly, and so too does the common law of *negligence*; many Scottish manual handling cases are referred to in this book. As far as *welfare legislation* is concerned, the book includes the Scottish equivalents – for example, the *Social Work (Scotland) Act 1968*, the *NHS (Scotland) Act 1978* – to the legislation applying to England and Wales.

Where it is dealing with the same legislation or area of law, Scottish cases will be persuasive, but not binding, in England and Wales; and vice versa. In other words, the judges in each country can consider the other's case law, but are not bound to follow it. However, the exception to this is when a House of Lords case sets a precedent concerning any English and Welsh legislation (which is identical or very similar to that in Scotland); then that decision will be binding in Scotland. Such is the major community care rationing decision of the House of Lords in *R v Gloucestershire County Council, ex p Barry* about s.2 of the *Chronically Sick and Disabled Persons Act 1970* which – by means of the *Chronically Sick and Disabled Persons (Scotland) Act 1972* – applies equally to Scotland, as it does to England and Wales.

SEAMNER v NORTH EAST ESSEX HEALTH AUTHORITY
Nursing auxiliary; experienced but untrained; unsafe lift; negligence case

The plaintiff, a nursing auxiliary, suffered an accident in 1984 when she was 57 years old. At the time she worked two nights a week on a geriatric hospital ward. She had done this type of work for 17 years previously; in 1976 she had been off work for three months with a back injury; on her return to work she was advised to wear a surgical belt, which she did, and had since fully participated in her duties.

Injury. She was transferring a patient to the commode from the bed together with another nurse. Sometimes this patient was weight-bearing, sometimes not; however the safe assumption for nurses was to assume that she would not be. The plaintiff faced the patient sitting on the bed, and put her right arm through the patient's right armpit and placed her left hand part-way up the patient's back. The nurse similarly took the patient's other side. The patient flopped; the plaintiff felt a terrible pull in her back.

Hoist not required. The judge rejected the suggestion that the only appropriate method would have been to use a hoist, given that the patient was by no means over-weight and that her need for the commode could well have been urgent. The judge referred to the 1987 edition of 'The handling of patients' published by the Royal College of Nursing and Back Pain Association and considered the three different methods of transferring patients from bed to chair or to toilet. These were the cross-arm, shoulder and through-arm lifts. The judge had no hesitation in stating that the cross-arm lift which had been employed on this occasion was not suitable; the evidence was all one way on this.

Negligence of qualified nurse. The plaintiff, 'experienced though she was in the number of years she had worked, was untrained; she had never been instructed in lifting methods; she was wholly reliant upon her qualified colleague for deciding the method of work to be employed at any given time'. Yet the colleague had acted neg-ligently, by embarking on a lifting operation giving rise to a foreseeable risk of in-jury, not least to the plaintiff who already had a vulnerable back. Damages of £10,300 had already been agreed in the event of liability being established (1990, High Court, unreported).

SELF-EMPLOYED PERSONS
Duties imposed under the *MHOR 1992* on employers towards employees are im-posed on self-employed persons toward themselves; and the latter also have various duties under s.3 of the *Health and Safety at Work Act 1974*, r.3 of the *Management of Health and Safety at Work Regulations 1999*, r.2 of the *Lifting Operations and Lifting Equipment Regulations 1998*, and r.4 of the *Provision and Use of Work Equipment Regula-tions 1998*.

SHIRLEY v WIRRAL HEALTH AUTHORITY
Nurse; previous back injury; light duties; counter–instruction to lift heavy pa-tient; negligence case

A recently qualified state enrolled nurse had previously sustained a back injury and now returned to work. She was instructed by the ward sister to undertake light duties only. The ward sister went off duty and the staff nurse instructed the plaintiff to lift a 12-stone woman (who had had a recent abdominal operation) up the bed with an-other nurse. The so-called 'orthodox lift' was used. The patient yelped and experi-enced great pain; the other (young student) nurse let go; the plaintiff took the full weight.

Inexperience of student nurse. The court did not criticise the plaintiff's decision to use the orthodox lift in the particular circumstances, since 'she assessed in her mind that this patient, having had abdominal surgery, would be better assisted by means of the orthodox lift rather than the Australian lift'. The staff nurse either knew, or should have known, that the student nurse was inexperienced; and she had instructed the plaintiff to lift despite knowing what the ward sister had said only a matter of hours earlier. It was reasonably foreseeable that a patient, following an abdominal operation, would react in that way. The court rejected any suggestion of contributory negligence:

> The staff nurse, in a fairly hierarchical structure, issued that instruction also to the effect that a young inexperienced student nurse should be the assistant. In those circumstances, despite the fact that there may well have been adequate staff on duty on that ward for one or more of them to give assistance, I do not think the defendants have discharged the burden of satisfying me on the balance of probabilities that the plaintiff was negligent in failing to request or obtain such assistance. I think that that would be putting too high a burden on the plaintiff in the circumstances of this case and accordingly I reject all allegations of contributory negligence.

Damages were agreed at £14,000 (1993, County Court, unreported).

SKINNER v ABERDEEN CITY COUNCIL
Foreman road worker; lifting and laying pavement slabs; training and instruction; risk reduction under MHOR 1992; negligence case

A case demonstrating that under the *MHOR 1992*, the duty to provide training and instruction is a demanding one, even when the employee had been doing the job for ten years and was therefore experienced in the task which caused the injury.

The pursuer, aged 63 at the time of the accident, was employed by the council as foreman road worker in Aberdeen. His duties included lifting and laying slabs, in which tasks he was experienced. On the day in question he had been instructed to lift a number of paving slabs which had sunk, despite the fact that in his opinion it was too cold and frosty for this, since this made the slabs more difficult to raise. The council accepted this, but said that if there was serious risk to the public, then the task was unavoidable even in such conditions. He used two racking irons to lever slabs up; one of the slabs broke and he suffered injury.

The pursuer did not press the case in negligence, and the court found that avoidance of all risk under the *MHOR 1992* was not reasonably practicable. However, turning to the question of risk reduction, the court found that on the evidence the proper use of the racking irons would have been an oscillating motion, involving much less force, with a view to loosening and raising the slabs gradually. Therefore the pursuer would have benefited from training and information – but this he had not received in ten years of his employment. There was thus a breach of the *MHOR 1992*, and no contributory negligence, given this absence of instruction. Damages were agreed at £15,500 (2001, Outer House, Court of Session, Scotland, unreported).

SLATER v FIFE PRIMARY CARE NHS TRUST
Nursing auxiliary; whether arguable negligence case

A nursing auxiliary sought damages for exacerbation of a pre-existing back condition, after she had been moved from one ward to another where heavy duties were greater. The Trust sought to dismiss the action. The court found that there was an arguable case, because the employer knew about the back condition which had given rise to recent problems, and should also have been aware of the difference in duties on the two wards; the risk of injury was therefore foreseeable. The pursuer accepted that an objective risk of injury needed to be referred to; but this test was met by the defenders' own occupational health assessment which had endorsed the pursuer's concerns. The court held that the case should proceed (2000, Outer House, Court of Session, Scotland, unreported).

SMITH v SOUTH LANARKSHIRE COUNCIL
Independent living schemes; employment of care assistants by disabled people; identity of employer; local authority liability

A case of some relevance to the making of *community care direct payments* by local authorities, though not actually concerning such direct payments.

Organisation of the payments. A care assistant sought to bring a case against her employer for sex discrimination and breach of contract. A preliminary hearing took place to establish just who the employer really was: two people with learning disabilities, a voluntary organisation or the council.

The two persons with learning disabilities were in receipt of financial support from both the council and the Independent Living Fund, in order that they could employ the care assistant. In practice those monies were paid to the care assistant in effect by the local authority. The two disabled people received information and advice from the voluntary organisation. Despite apparent contracts for personal care between the two persons with learning disability and the care assistant, the employment tribunal held that the real employer remained the council, since it had in effect pulled all the strings – so that an action against the employer would in fact lie against the council, not the people with learning disabilities or the voluntary organisation:

> My evaluation of all the details suggests to me that the reality and substance of the arrangements is that the [council] were the employers of the applicant... I regard as particularly important the fact that the impetus for the [disabled persons] to live independently in the community came from the [council]; that the [disabled persons] had no experience and could not have had any experience of business affairs; that the responsibilities of an employer, and the consequences of an employer/employee relationship were never explained by the [council], nor did they take steps to ensure that an explanation was given by another person and properly understood by the [disabled persons]; that the funding for the wages of the applicant...and for Mr Sloan's [who was adviser in the voluntary organisation] salary...came from

the [council]; that in substance, the appointment of the applicant was that of the [council]; and that there was continuing communication between the [council] and Mr Sloan, not only in relation to the [disabled persons] but in regard to disabled people generally...

Looking to the circumstances as a whole, it appears to me that the control of the applicant came from the [council] and not from the [disabled persons] or the [voluntary organisation]. In my view the 'control' test is particularly apposite to the facts of this case. The form of the relationship is manifested by the written employment contract. The substance of the relationship, however, and the reality of matters, is manifested by the other circumstances to which I have adverted. In particular Mr Sloan was the person through which the [council] exercised control.

Appeal. The employment appeal tribunal upheld the original tribunal's decision but added some further observations. However, it should be borne in mind that these were not apparently made with the *community care direct payments* legislation in mind:

> **[Statutory context]** It is important to recognise that the position of the [council] is underpinned and dictated by the provisions of the Social Work (Scotland) Act and particularly section 12, which imposes the relevant statutory duty. We consider that to be highly important when considering the issue of control as between the local authority, the disabled parties and the carer. While it may not be determinative of the matter it does seem to us that the overall control of the way in which care is provided for disabled persons must always rest and never leave the role of the local authority. That role may be performed in a number of ways but always against a background of continuing responsibility.

> **[Disabled people as employers]** It does not therefore seem to us to be material that the physical control of the particular exercise in terms of assessment and management is being carried out by a third party, namely, Mr Sloan, nor do we consider [it] in general terms to be consistent with the local authority statutory duty to hand over control of the actions of the carer, including the right to dismiss, to the disabled persons to whom the services are being rendered in the first place, because of their needs. It is obviously highly desirable that when a care in the community scheme is being operated in relation to disabled people, the maximum amount of independence should be provided but [the fact that] that aim is being implemented in the maximum possible way does not depart from or detract from or even destroy the ultimate responsibility of the local authority to retain control of the whole operation...

> We would merely add that we would not for a moment seek to suggest that disabled persons cannot be an employer, particularly over someone caring for them. What is determinative of the present case, is that the provision of the

services is by a local authority under the obligations and terms of the Social Work Act and that dictates the whole background to this particular case. Privately funded care might well have met the possibility of a disabled person being the employer. (Employment Tribunal 1999, Employment Appeal Tribunal 2000, unreported)

SOCIAL WORK (SCOTLAND) ACT 1968

The Social Work (Scotland) Act 1968 contains community care duties in respect of adults. Section 12A contains a strong duty of assessment virtually identical to that applying to England and Wales under s.47 of the *NHS and Community Care Act 1990*. Other additions to s.12 cover *carers* and *community care direct payments*.

Once a Scottish local authority has carried out an assessment under s.12A and decided that services (including manual handling related services or equipment) under s.12 of the 1968 Act, or s.2 of the *Chronically Sick and Disabled Persons Act 1970*, are required for an individual, then it is under a duty to provide them within a reasonable time – and lack of resources will be no defence (see e.g. *MacGregor v South Lanarkshire Council*, and also *R v Gloucestershire County Council, ex p Barry*).

1. **Social Work (Scotland) Act 1968: promotion of social welfare assistance**. However s.12, which contains the main general duty to provide community care services, has no equivalent in England and Wales. It is a duty 'to promote social welfare by making available advice, guidance and assistance on such scale as may be appropriate for their area, and in that behalf to make arrangements and to provide or secure the provision of such facilities…as they may consider suitable and adequate, and such assistance may…be given in kind or in cash to, or in respect of, any relevant person'.

2. **Social Work (Scotland) Act 1968: relevant person**. The relevant person condition has to be satisfied twofold. First, he or she must be somebody in need who is not less than eighteen years of age. A person in need is someone who (a) needs care and attention arising from infirmity, youth or age, or (b) suffers from illness or mental disorder or is substantially handicapped by deformity or disability, or (c) needs care and attention arising from drug or alcohol dependency or from release from prison or other type of detention.

3. **Social Work (Scotland) Act 1968: other conditions of assistance**. Second, a relevant person is someone who requires 'assistance in kind or, in exceptional circumstances constituting an emergency, in cash, where the giving of assistance in either form would avoid the local authority being caused greater expense in the giving of assistance in another form, or where probable aggravation of the person's need would cause greater expense to the local authority on a later occasion'. In addition, before giving any assistance in cash to a relevant person, the local authority must have regard to the person's 'eligibility for receiving assistance from any other statutory body and, if he is so eligible to the availability to him of that assistance in his time of need'.

SOCIAL WORKERS

Local authorities need to consider the degree to which their social workers require information, warnings, instructions or training in the light of a case such as *Colclough v Staffordshire County Council*, in which a failure to provide instruction about manual handling to a social worker resulted in a successful compensation claim of over £200,000. See also *Watkins v Strathclyde Regional Council*, involving a social work assistant, and *Wiles v Bedfordshire County Council* concerning a residential child social worker.

SOMMERVILLE v LOTHIAN HEALTH BOARD

Nursing auxiliary; collapsing patient; adherence to care plan calling for mobility; evidence about training; negligence case

The pursuer was a nursing auxiliary who sustained an injury in 1991. At lunchtime on the ward, she was injured when escorting a patient back from the toilet. This patient was 72 years old, suffered from senile dementia and deafness, had a history of epileptic attacks (though none had been recorded since hospital admission), had osteo-arthritis of both knees, and was overweight (some 13 stone), liable to confusion and subject to unpredictable mood swings. Her care plan contained the aim of maintaining her mobility, in order to prevent complications with the osteo-arthritis. While escorting this patient back from the toilet the pursuer was injured when the patient became unsteady and collapsed.

Adherence to care plan: outweighing expert evidence. The pursuer's case was not however made out. First, the court accepted on the evidence that the patient had her two sticks with her, and thus it was never intended that the pursuer should handle or move her. Thus she was merely observing and escorting; this was the normal way in which the patient was mobilised. The court rejected the expert evidence from a nurse who had had wide experience of nursing and as an officer of the Royal College of Nursing, that two members of the nursing staff should have assisted the patient, even if the latter did have her sticks. Instead the court found that the senior nurse, who had requested that the pursuer escort the patient, had been entitled to rely on the care plan, and that 'greater weight should…be attached to the professional judgement of those who were concerned in the assessment'.

Training. As to training, the court found that although the evidence relied on by the employer to show that such training had been provided was not wholly satisfactory, nevertheless it was enough to satisfy the court that the pursuer had received an update about the lifting of patients, and that this had included a reminder of how to lower patients to the ground ((1994) SLT 1207, Outer House, Court of Session, Scotland).

SPECIAL MANUAL HANDLING SITUATIONS

Guidance identifies 'special situations' which call for special consideration and might involve manual handling with higher risk. For instance, *guidance* from the Health and Safety Commission lists ambulance staff, caring for people in their own homes, mobile blood transfusion services, maternity units, maintaining the mobility of patients and rehabilitation, babies and small children, and heavy patients (HSC 1998, pp.36–46). Royal College of Nursing and National Back Pain Association (now BackCare) guidance refers to, for instance, unconscious and deceased patients, the operating theatre, intensive care units, spinal injuries, nursing patients on the floor, pregnant women, podiatrists (e.g. leg lifting), very heavy patients, uncooperative patients, and so on (RCN/NBPA 1997, pp.181–197).

STAINTON v CHORLEY AND SOUTH RIBBLE NHS TRUST
Occupational therapy assistant; physiotherapist; walking a patient; negligence case

A 48-year-old occupational therapy assistant suffered a back injury when helping a physiotherapist to walk a 44-year-old patient at a day hospital unit. The patient weighed 12 stone and was obese. The policy of the physiotherapy department was to keep the patient as mobile as possible so she could manage better at home. The court found the Trust liable. The case is notable for the judicial attempt to identify the balance between staff safety and patient need in terms of what constituted an acceptable risk to staff.

The accident. The accident occurred when the patient needed to move to the dining area; the assistant and the physiotherapist helped her walk to the table. During the walk, the patient ceased to support herself and a chair had to be placed under her. Her movement downward caused a soft tissue injury to the assistant which required physiotherapy and meant she could not continue her work as an occupational therapy assistant. The plaintiff (the assistant) argued that the patient's condition by the date of the accident meant that a wheelchair should have been used; alternatively, she claimed that the support techniques she used were dangerous because of the employer's failure to instruct and/or supervise the plaintiff in the appropriate technique.

The drag lift. The court accepted that the 'drag lift' which had been used by the assistant both to raise the patient to a standing position and to walk her was unsound and potentially unsafe; however, the physiotherapist who was walking the patient on the other side had adopted a safe technique. In this respect, the plaintiff's expert referred to the 'Handling of patients: a guide for nurse managers', published by the Royal College of Nursing and Back Pain Association [as it was then].

Mobility and wheelchair use. The physiotherapist argued that although the patient could be unpredictable, nevertheless she had good days when she was more steady and could walk independently; furthermore, a bending of her head tended to

precede problems, and so through this observation, her keeling over could be anticipated.

Contrary to this view was evidence that her mobility and behaviour had become
more unpredictable by the date of the accident and this had been recorded in the patient's notes. The plaintiff's expert accepted that it was understandable that the
physiotherapists wished to keep the patient mobile, but that nevertheless by the date
in question a wheelchair should have been used for all longer distances. In fact, following the accident, the patient's notes read that a wheelchair should be used at all
times.

Conversely, the defendant's expert stated that it was quite inappropriate for the
patient to be confined to a wheelchair; that immobility could be life-threatening;
that a qualified physiotherapist should always support such a patient – but that it
would not be unusual for an unqualified member of staff to provide assistance to the
trained physiotherapist, provided that the assistant had received appropriate training.

The judge stated that on the evidence, the good day/bad day evaluation was no
longer a safe method of proceeding given the documented and continuing deterioration of the patient.

Balancing patient best interests and staff safety. The judge realised that 'the decision whether a wheelchair ought always to be used involved an awkward balance
between catering for the best interests of the patient so as to maximise mobility and
avoiding undue risk of physical risk injury to patient and staff by using a wheelchair'.
He concluded that trained physiotherapists would have been unlikely to suffer harm
in the circumstances; thus, were it the case that the patient could have been supported
by two trained physiotherapists, 'the balance of risk would not, in my judgement,
have placed upon the defendants a duty to require a wheelchair always to be used'.

Trained physiotherapists or untrained assistant? However, he found that 'an
entirely different consideration arises from the participation as supporters of members of staff who were not trained physiotherapists. In that case the physical risk to
such members of staff would be greater if they had not received walking training
equal to that given to physiotherapists'. Thus, in determining

> whether the presence of an occupational therapist, as distinct from a trained
> physiotherapist, materially increased the risk of physical injury to the point
> where it was sufficient to make it necessary to require a wheelchair always to
> be used in such cases, it is necessary to assume that, as was the case, the phys-
> iotherapist present was unable to supervise [i.e. because she could not see] the
> plaintiff's method of holding the patient and that the plaintiff had received
> no walking training.

In such circumstances there was a duty to use a wheelchair, since the judge accepted
the plaintiff's argument that she had not received the relevant walking training
(1998, High Court, unreported).

STARK v POST OFFICE
Maintenance of work equipment used at work; absolute obligation; maintenance system not enough; equipment must be in good repair; Provision and Use of Work Equipment Regulations 1992; negligence case

A case demonstrating the stringency of the duty to maintain equipment used at work in good working order and in good repair, under the *Provision and Use of Work Equipment Regulations 1992* (*PUWER 1992* – now *PUWER 1998*). Although involving a Post Office bicycle, the principle established in the case applies equally well to manual handling related equipment, as well as any other health or social care equipment used at work.

Bicycle accident. A postman suffered a serious accident when the stirrup, part of the front brake, broke in two and lodged in the front wheel. The wheel locked and the postman was thrown over the handlebars. The Post Office had a system of maintenance, part of which was to replace bicycles after 10 years unless it seemed that they had a few years of serviceable life left. This particular bicycle was in its fourteenth year of service.

No liability at first instance: competent inspection system. At first instance, the judge had found the Post Office liable neither in negligence nor for breach of statutory duty under *PUWER 1992*. This was because the defect would not and could not be discovered on any routine inspection, and even a 'perfectly rigorous examination' would not have revealed it. The judge considered that *PUWER 1992* imposed an obligation primarily to 'institute and carry out a system of maintenance to the very best of their ability and this the Post Office did'.

Strict liability imposed on appeal. The Court of Appeal now overturned this decision, agreeing on the *negligence* finding, since there was no suggestion of fault or carelessness on the part of the Post Office, but nevertheless finding a breach of statutory duty. This was because the duty under (what is now regulation 5 of *PUWER 1998*) was not just to have a system of maintenance, but actually to have equipment in an efficient state and in efficient working order; in other words it was an absolute obligation, and clearly the bicycle failed this test ([2000] PIQR P105, Court of Appeal).

STEWART v HIGHLAND HEALTH BOARD
Nurse; night shift; patient needing commode; inadequate staffing; training

The pursuer was working on a night shift in a female psycho-geriatric ward with some 30 patients. On the night of the accident there were three staff on the ward (the pursuer, a charge nurse, and an auxiliary nurse); however, the auxiliary was redeployed during the night to relieve other nurses elsewhere in hospital. The patient concerned was four inches higher than the pursuer, weighed fourteen to fifteen stone and needed a commode. The charge nurse and the pursuer assisted the patient onto the commode, then both had to leave to attend to another patient. The first patient tried to get up from the commode but had difficulty; the pursuer returned and decided to help the patient to her bed, concerned that otherwise the patient would be injured. Instead she was injured herself.

Changing approach to manual handling. The judge recognised from the evidence that

> there was a change to handling patients in the nursing profession beginning to emerge in the late 1970s and early 1980s. In brief this was that instead of regarding the physical safety and well-being of patients as paramount over the safety and well-being of nurses, nursing staff should be trained to bear in mind that in addition to their duty to care for their patients they also had a duty to themselves to maintain their own physical safety and well-being in order to continue caring for patients.

Three nurses required. Evidence was given that three nurses were required for the night shift on such a ward, and that two nurses were not enough. The evidence showed that a nurse of her training and experience would have tried to assist the patient and not allow her to fall to the floor. It would also have been clear that 'the nurses' devotion to their patients is such that two of them would simply soldier on doing the best they could and handling patients alone until the third nurse returned to the ward'. However, in the 'newer world', the nurse would have been trained to let the patient go to the floor in a controlled way, before summoning assistance. The employer was in breach of its duty to employ adequately trained, qualified and experienced staff. It was also breach of its duty to train the pursuer adequately; it knew or should have known that she had no training whatever in psycho-geriatric nursing and that the one-day course attended in 1981 was wholly inadequate. Thus liability was established (summarised in PMILL, December 1987, p.68, Sheriff's Court, Scotland).

STONE v COMMISSIONER OF POLICE FOR THE METROPOLIS
Stores officer; carrying stationery; no risk assessment; no training or warnings; no reduction of risk; cumulative strain; MHOR 1992

A case notable for the judge's acceptance that the injury claimed for had been caused by *cumulative strain* over an extended period of time.

The plaintiff worked as a divisional stores officer, taking delivery of stationery and transporting it to a storeroom. Neither trolley nor lift were available and she had to lift and carry stationery manually either to the basement or to the third floor. She spent an average of two hours a day doing this, carrying loads weighing at least 40lb. She received no training, was given no warnings about incorrect lifting, and her expressed concerns were not acted on. Following one particular day in October 1994, two years after beginning this work, the plaintiff suffered a back ache which did not disappear, as previously, after resting. She claimed that she was now permanently disabled and effectively unemployable.

Assessment of and reduction of risk. The court found that under the *MHOR 1992*, no risk assessment had been carried out, nor appropriate steps taken to reduce the risk of injury. Such steps should have included proper training, a proper system of assistance, provision of a trolley, and more and better-laid-out storage space. Had these steps been taken, the injury would probably have been avoided.

Common sense. The court did not hold the plaintiff responsible for her injuries: 'common sense was not a substitute for training and instruction and could not in any event warn of risks not readily apparent'.

Cumulative strain. The court found that 'the plaintiff's soft-tissue injury that caused her lower back pain and sciatica was likely not to have been caused by one specific incident but by a history of incidents where she was engaged in inappropriate manual handling'. Damages of some £325,000 were awarded ([2000] CL 00/1589, County Court).

STUDENTS
Students, for example of nursing or physiotherapy, are called on to carry out manual handling in their placements. The principles set out in this book clearly apply to such students – as the cases involving student nurses testify (listed in the At-a-glance list of cases (by occupation of claimant and by type of case) – at the beginning of this book). However, a key practical point made in guidance issued by the Chartered Society of Physiotherapy is that there must be clear contractual agreement between higher education institutions and the providers of student placements – and clarity about induction, manual handling training, manual handling responsibilities and so on (CSP 2002, p.36).

STUTHRIDGE v MERSEYSIDE METROPOLITAN AMBULANCE SERVICE
Ambulance worker; lifting stretcher; employer not applying mind to risk; negligence case

The plaintiff was an ambulance attendant, aged 34 years, weighing eight stone and five feet tall. In 1980, she was assisting a male ambulance driver weighing 12 stone and five foot nine inches tall to lift an 11-stone patient on a stretcher down six steps. Bending down, she picked up the rear of the stretcher; the load at her end was estimated at 120lb. Her induction training did not deal with safe handling of loads. The court would not transpose regulations applying to female labour in other industries but it was noteworthy that they set a limit of 65lb. The defendants were responsible at common law for her unnecessary exposure to risk; they did not apply their mind to the nature of the risk or even its existence. Damages of £8,500 were awarded (1986, unreported)

SUPERVISION

Supervision of employees is clearly a necessary part of a safe *system of work* in terms of manual handling, as well as other work activities; it is implicit in the *MHOR 1992*, and explicit in s.2 of the *Health and Safety at Work Act 1974*.

The courts have often considered the question of supervision. A momentary lapse on the part of a senior staff member involved in a lifting operation, which causes injury to a more junior member, might be classed as a failure in supervision (*Charnock v Capital Territory Health Commission*); likewise a failure to enforce the content of training (*Dickson v Lothian Health Board*), to correct bad lifting habits (*Salvat v Basingstoke and North Hampshire Health Authority*) or to consider how a particular type of lift ought to be carried out, given that the injured nurse had no experience of it (*McGowan v Harrow Health Authority*). When a physiotherapist could not see what a partly untrained occupational therapy assistant was doing this meant she was unable to supervise the latter (*Stainton v Chorley and South Ribble NHS Trust*). Ironically, even a manual handling trainer failed to supervise adequately the trainees on her course (*Beattie v West Dorset Health Authority*).

On the other hand, a potential breach of supervision duties will not avail an employee claimant or pursuer, unless the court believes better supervision would probably have prevented the injury (*Woolgar v West Surrey and North East Hampshire Health Authority*).

SWAIN v DENSO MARTIN
Removing roller; risk assessment; information about load; substantive duty of risk reduction and information provision; MHOR 1992

A case showing that the duty to reduce risk and to provide information is, in the final analysis, freestanding from the duty to carry out a risk assessment, under r.4 of the *MHOR 1992*. Hence the employer's argument – that the duty to reduce risk and to supply information did not arise in the absence of a prior risk assessment – failed.

Accident. An experienced production fitter was asked to replace the bearings on a conveyor roller. He removed the roller, expecting it to be hollow. In fact it was solid and weighed about 20kg. The unexpected weight crushed his hand when he removed the last of the bolts. At first instance, the judge held that in removing the roller, the plaintiff was in fact also carrying out a suitable and sufficient assessment under r.4(1)(b)(i) of the *MHOR 1992*, since he was the 'resident expert'. Thus, the employer could not have made any more of a sufficient and suitable assessment than it was already doing. The accident occurred before the assessment was complete, so the duty to perform r.4(1)(b)(ii) and (iii) – the taking of appropriate steps to reduce the risk of injury – never arose, because it was dependent on a completed risk assessment.

Adequate risk assessment. The Court of Appeal now held this to be an impossible view of the facts. The plaintiff had anyway asked for assistance, but none was available and he was told to go ahead on his own. The court was quite convinced that it was done as an urgent maintenance job, not as an assessment. The natural person to do the assessment would have been the firm's health and safety officer. Failing this, the plaintiff could have done it under the guidance of that officer, have had the task explained to him, have been given time to think about it, asked what assistance he required, and been given the opportunity to contact suppliers and if necessary to obtain manuals and specifications not available at this work place. This did not happen.

Consequences of failure to assess risk. Also the court could not accept that the three obligations under r.4 of the *MHOR 1992* – namely (i) risk assessment, (ii) taking appropriate steps to reduce risk and (iii) providing indications and information about load – were conjunctive (i.e. depended absolutely on each other), so that a conscientious employer who carried out (i) would face further obligations, whereas flouting the first obligation would relieve the employer of any further compliance. In fact:

> On the known facts of this case Denso Martin Ltd had a health and safety officer. The employer knew who had manufactured and supplied the conveyor in question. Any proper assessment by or on behalf of the employer would have been a systematic assessment under the control of either an outside consultant or the health and safety officer (even if part of the task was delegated to a person who was an experienced employee). The assessment would have considered whether repairs and non-routine maintenance for specialised plant and machinery should be carried out by the employer's staff, or by the manufacturer. The assessment would have had to consider what manual handling tasks were involved in repairs and non-routine maintenance. If no brochure or specification was available the assessment might have involved making inquiries of the manufacturer. If none of that had been possible (or none of that had disclosed the weight of the roller) then prudence would have dictated the assumption that it might be unexpectedly heavy. That assumption might have been communicated to those employees who need the information under Regulation 4(1)(b)(iii).

Liability was therefore established entailing damages of £2,040 ([2000] PIQR P129, Court of Appeal).

SYSTEM OF WORK

A safe system of work is legally and practically necessary where manual handling is concerned – as well, of course, as numerous other work activities and tasks. It is referred to in the *MHOR 1992*, in s.2 of the *Health and Safety at Work Act 1974*, and looked for by the courts in *negligence* cases as part of a common law duty of care. It is so fundamental a part of scrutiny by the courts, that it would be meaningless to list here the cases in which it has been considered. However, a number of the themes occurring in manual handling cases and identified in section 3 of the Overview of this book, are manifestations, or part, of a system of work, including *training, supervision, information,* provision of *equipment, employers* applying their mind to risk, and thought given to the protection of employees in various respects.

T (A MINOR) v SURREY COUNTY COUNCIL
Childminding adviser; careless information; negligence

A negligence case, illustrating how local authorities can be held liable for negligent provision of information, that leads directly to harm; in this case in respect of a child-minder who subsequently harmed the parent's baby ([1994] 4 All ER 577, High Court).

TAKING ACCOUNT OF ALL RELEVANT FACTORS

Taking account of all relevant factors is a ground on which the decision-making of public bodies such as the NHS and local authorities is challenged in *judicial review* cases by clients and patients. The courts will strike decisions down if the public body has not taken account of all relevant factors – such as *guidance* (*R v North Derbyshire Health Authority* concerning beta-interferon treatment), a residential home booklet referring to a 'home for life' (*R (Bodimeade) v Camden London Borough Council*) or medical information as part of a community care assessment (*R v Birmingham City Council, ex parte Killigrew* which also involved manual handling issues).

TAYLOR v GLASGOW CITY COUNCIL
Moving cupboard in school up stairs; school; information about its heaviest side; MHOR 1992

A case falling into a category of cases – whether in *negligence* or under the *MHOR 1992* – involving what the courts view as relatively simple everyday or factory tasks, and in which they shy away from imposing liability.

The pursuer claimed he had suffered a back injury through moving a cupboard (35kg in weight) up stairs in school, with two other employees, and that this was a breach of the *MHOR 1992*, because the employer had not provided precise information about the heaviest side of the cupboard. The action was dismissed; the pursuer had not shown that there was a risk of injury ([2000] SLT 670, Outer House, Court of Session, Scotland).

TIME LIMITS: see *limitation of actions*

TRAINING

In order to ensure both staff and patient/client safety, training is a key issue, and is well covered in legislation, as well as featuring significantly in manual handling cases in the courts.

Legislation. Duties in *health and safety at work legislation* to provide training are to be found, for instance, in s.2 of the *Health and Safety at Work Act 1974*, schedule 1 of the *MHOR 1992*, r.9 of the *Provision and Use of Work Equipment Regulations 1998*, and r.13

of the *Management of the Health and Safety at Work Regulations 1999*. Likewise in negligence case law, the question of training has loomed large.

Case law: inadequate training. Training has been considered by the courts in respect of training and: its simple absence (*Seamner v North East Essex Health Authority*) even after ten years of work (*Skinner v Aberdeen City Council*); its specificity and relevance to the risk facing employees when dealing with patient rehabilitation or mobility needs (*Bayley v Bloomsbury Health Authority; Brown v East Midlothian NHS Trust; Stainton v Chorley and South Ribble NHS Trust*) or when other particular tasks (*Watkinson v British Telecommunications*) are in issue.

Also covered has been misplaced reliance on a one-day course attended by a nurse on a psycho-geriatric ward (*Stewart v Highland Health Board*); absence altogether of manual handling as an element of induction training, and the overruling by his managers of a senior nurse manager who recognised the need for manual handling training (*Painter v Barnet Community Healthcare NHS Trust*); arrangement of training when the plaintiff was absent with a previous handling injury and not arranging an alternative for her (*Painter v Barnet Community Healthcare NHS Trust*); district nurses who are exposed to risk working alone in the community (*Hammond v Cornwall and Isles of Scilly Health Authority*); and the failure to train staff who were not injured in the accident but whose lack of training injured the plaintiff (*McCaffery v Datta*).

Yet other cases have involved inadequate time given to training videos (*Kelly v Forticrete Ltd*), incomplete training (*Stainton v Chorley and South Ribble NHS Trust*), training sessions delivered for nurses in the middle of the night (*Dickson v Lothian Health Board*), voluntary and unpaid training sessions for care assistants (*Hopkinson v Kent County Council*); the use of hoists (*Campbell v Dumfries and Galloway Health Board*), foster carers (*Beasley v Buckinghamshire County Council*), the handling and restraint of pupils in schools (e.g. *McLeod v Aberdeen City Council*), and even the duties of manual handling trainers themselves (*Beattie v West Dorset Health Authority*). Even if a long training course is not warranted for a social worker, information and instructions might be (*Colclough v Staffordshire County Council*).

Case law; adequate training or training not decisive of issue. Conversely, there might be sparse evidence as to what training should have been given – and even then the training might not have avoided the injury (*Daws v Croydon London Borough Council; Purvis v Buckinghamshire County Council*); the training might have been adequate in relation to the lift causing the injury (*Munrow v Plymouth Health Authority*); it might have been reasonable to conclude that the particular employee did not need training (*Woolgar v West Surrey and North East Hampshire Health Authority*); or the equipment, in the use of which training was lacking, might anyway not have been appropriate for the particular patient whose handling caused the accident (*Campbell v Dumfries and Galloway Health Board*). In another case a five-day training course in manual handling for a care assistant was deemed adequate (*Rowe v Swansea City Council*).

Guidance on training. Training gives rise to a number of questions and uncertainties concerning, for instance, its quality, length, frequency and the qualifications of the trainers (see e.g. HSC 1998, pp.32–34). Indeed, trainers can themselves be found legally liable (*Beattie v West Dorset Health Authority*). *Guidance* states that health care staff with no previous relevant experience or training might require three to five days of training with refresher courses at least once a year (HSC 1998, pp.32–33). More recently a set of basic training standards or guidelines has been suggested (*The Column 2001*).

Demonstration but not training? A distinction also needs to be drawn between training of other staff/employees and demonstration to individual patients or clients. For example, for the former but not the latter, professional guidance for occupational therapists demands that they should have 'necessary knowledge, experience and competence in the specialist subject of the handling of people and loads, and have required teaching skills. Competency should be gained by undertaking a validated and/or accredited post registration course' (COT 1995, p5).

UNDER-STAFFING

The courts sometimes consider issues of adequate staffing in manual handling cases involving injury to employees. For instance, they have considered whether a district nursing team was generally adequate for the local population and found that it was (*Channon v East Sussex Area Health Authority*), and found liability where a prevailing ethos arising from staff shortages meant that even experienced staff believed it their duty to perform unsafe lifting (*Forder v Norfolk Area Health Authority*), or where it was clear on the evidence that three, not two, nurses were required for the night shift (*Stewart v Highland Health Board*). Often, though, the consideration is of the number of nurses allocated to particular manual handling tasks (*Fitzsimmons v Northumberland Health Authority*).

UNREASONABLENESS

Unreasonableness is a ground on which the decision-making of public bodies such as the NHS and local authorities is challenged in *judicial review* cases by clients and patients. One application of the term involves the courts' striking down of decisions – whether or not relating to manual handling issues – if they represent a legal taking leave of senses, a departure from logic, or *irrationality*. For instance, the decision not to accept that a severely disabled boy was substantially and adversely affected in day-to-day activities was deemed irrational by the High Court (*R v Ealing London Borough Council, ex p C*); and at the High Court stage of *R v Gloucestershire County Council, ex p Barry*, the court stated that it would not be reasonable for a local authority to fail to assist disabled people at severe physical risk.

VICAR OF WRITTLE v ESSEX COUNTY COUNCIL
Social worker; failure to warn; negligence case

A negligence case illustrating that local authorities can be held liable for the negligent failure of professional employees to pass on information, in this instance a warning to head office about a client's fire-raising tendencies, with the result that the local church was set on fire ([1979] 77 LGR 656, High Court).

W v ESSEX COUNTY COUNCIL
Foster carers; whether contract with the local authority; negligence

A negligence case, the implications of which might suggest that the *MHOR 1992* will not specifically apply as between the local authority and the *foster carers* it makes arrangements with – although the courts do sometimes stretch the meaning of the word 'employee' when health and safety issues are in play.

The case, amongst other matters, confirmed that foster parents do not have enforceable contracts with the local authority, in respect of children fostered through arrangements under the *Children Act 1989*. However, the local authority still owed a potential duty of care negligence. The case involved the placement with the parents by the local authority of a child who had previously sexually abused other children, even though they had expressly asked not to foster such a child. The child subsequently abused the parents' natural children ([1998] 3 WLR 534, Court of Appeal).

WAKEFIELD v BASILDON AND THURROCK HEALTH AUTHORITY
Employee assisting epileptic employee; foreseeability of injury; magnitude of risk; reasonable steps

In 1989, a 50-year-old catering assistant in a hospital went to the assistance of a nursing auxiliary who had suffered an epileptic fit in the hospital and had fallen near a spring loaded door at the foot of some stairs. In trying to lift and roll the nursing auxiliary into a safe position, she suffered a prolapsed disc and was off work for 14 months. It was alleged that the employer was negligent in not previously dismissing the nursing auxiliary from employment on safety grounds. Both employees had been employed there for about 28 years.

The Court of Appeal now found no liability, overturning a County Court decision in favour of the plaintiff. It was foreseeable that she might have a fit and be assisted by another employee, but the court had to consider the likelihood of the plaintiff sustaining an injury and whether the extent of the risk demanded more action of the employer than had been taken over the years. First, nobody had sustained an injury over all those years when moving the nursing auxiliary; so the injury might have been possible, but not foreseeably likely. Second, such a risk could only have been removed by dismissing her. But because the risk of injury was slight, this would have been a draconian step. Further, following a fit in 1981, the auxiliary had been prescribed revised medication and there was no evidence that this was not effective. The court further pointed out that it would be repugnant to reach the conclusion that no employer could safely and without negligence employ a person with epilepsy (1990, Court of Appeal, unreported).

WALES
This book applies to Wales.

WARDLAW v FIFE HEALTH BOARD
District nurse; home visit; moving patient

A district nurse visited a patient with multiple sclerosis to provide general nursing care. The patient suffered spasms and was particularly uncooperative. Assistance involved washing, dressing, and moving the patient from bed to wheelchair. She followed the same pattern of moving the patient as previously, but this time the patient's legs gave way and as she fell she put her arms around the nurse's neck. Liability was admitted; the case now concerned a question of damages and the extent to which the pursuer could link the accident to the injuries now being claimed for; they were set at £11,500 ([2000] SCLR 840, Outer House, Court of Session, Scotland).

WARNINGS: see *instructions and information*

WARREN v HARLOW DISTRICT COUNCIL
Council worker; lifting buckets of water out of sink; MHOR 1992

The plaintiff was a 60-year-old woman, five foot five inches tall, with a pre-existing back problem. She suffered a further injury when lifting a bucket of water weighing 21lb out of a sink, the height of the lift being 52 inches. The injury occurred somewhere between removal of the bucket from the sink, resting it on the lip of the sink and then execution of a one-handed lift comprising a twisting and lowering motion.

Liability was established, since the risk was more than merely minimal or theoretical and called for a risk assessment. Such an assessment would have shown that it was reasonably practicable to avoid the lifting operation by means of a hose which could have filled the bucket whilst it was resting on the floor. Since the employer took no steps to avoid the lifting operation it was in breach of r.4 of the *MHOR 1992*. Damages of £7,900 were awarded ([1997] CL 2622, County Court).

WATKINS v STRATHCLYDE REGIONAL COUNCIL
Community social work assistant; moving furniture; Offices, Shops and Railway Premises Act 1963; negligence case

The pursuer, a community assistant in the social work department, sought damages arising from moving furniture (an 80lb desk) in an overcrowded social work office. The judge found liability in negligence, since once a new member of staff had started work, it was reasonably foreseeable that furniture would need rearranging and that injury would arise. The case under s.23 of the *Offices, Shops and Railway Premises Act 1963* (now obsolete) failed, because it could not be shown that the pursuer was actually 'required' to move the furniture, as s.23 of the Act demanded if a breach was to be found (1992, Outer House, Court of Session, Scotland).

WATKINSON v BRITISH TELECOMMUNICATIONS PLC
Handling reels of paper; lack of instruction; negligence case; Factories Act 1961

An older case, illustrating the enduring importance to the courts of instruction and training being given. The case was brought in common law *negligence* and under s.72 of the *Factories Act 1961* (now obsolete).

A storekeeper was injured while handling reels of paper weighing 220–245kg, rolling and turning them into position, without being given any training on how to do this. He succeeded in common law (the evidence showed that the duty of care was breached because there was a safe technique which could have been taught but had not been). Under s.72, the case was also made out, because the test was objective and related not just to the physical characteristics of the load, but also to the mechanical means available to move it, the particular employee, his skills and the training and supervision provided ((1996) SLT 72, Outer House, Court of Session, Scotland).

WELFARE LEGISLATION
Welfare legislation underlies the assessment and meeting of the needs of patients and clients. Logically it should perhaps be considered before *health and safety at work legislation*, since it is only when the NHS or local authorities undertake to meet people's needs that manual handling and other health and safety issues arise for staff. It can be seen that welfare legislation does not apply evenly as between the NHS and local authority social services departments; the latter have very much more to contend with. For the implications of this legislation, see section 6 of the Overview, and also under *patient and client need*.

NHS legislation. This includes the *NHS Act 1977* and *NHS (Scotland) Act 1978*.

Social services legislation. This includes the *NHS and Community Care Act 1990, National Assistance Act 1948, Chronically Sick and Disabled Persons Act 1970, Health Services and Public Health Act 1968, Community Care (Direct Payments) Act 1996, Carers (Recognition and Services Act 1995), Carers and Disabled Children Act 2000, Children Act 1989, Children (Scotland) Act 1995, Social Work (Scotland) Act 1968*.

Education legislation. This includes the *Education Act 1996* and the *Education (Scotland) Act 1980*.

Housing legislation. This includes the *Housing Grants, Construction and Regeneration Act 1996*, and the *Housing (Scotland) Act 1987*.

WELLS v WEST HERTFORDSHIRE HEALTH AUTHORITY
Midwife; pre-existing back problems; risk assessment; individual capability; MHOR 1992; negligence case

The plaintiff was a midwife with 28 years of experience; she was injured in November 1994 at the age of 50, when working in a hospital delivery suite. This involved heavy manual handling – for instance, where a mother had had an epidural, it would be difficult to move her around. The court accepted the strenuousness of the tasks, and that they were more strenuous than those tasks associated with home deliveries.

History of back problems communicated to employer. She had a long history of back complaints and disc prolapse. The court found that she had informed her managers about this and it did not accept the evidence of those managers to the contrary; yet they did not send her for assessment in the occupational health department.

Therefore, the requirement that she work in the delivery suite in November 1994 meant the employer was in breach of its common law duty of care in *negligence*.

No risk assessment of tasks or of individual. The *MHOR 1992* were also breached, since no risk assessment of either the delivery suite tasks or the plaintiff's individual capabilities had been carried out. The court referred to Health and Safety Executive *guidance*, which emphasised that particular consideration should be given to employees pregnant or recently pregnant or with a history of back problems – and also that significant findings of risk assessments should be recorded and kept readily accessible as long as relevant (guidance now to be found in HSE 1998, para 160).

Evidence of assessment. The judge was clearly not impressed by the evidence of any assessment under the *MHOR 1992*. One of the managers had said

> that assessment had been carried out...by a man known as 'Harry'. She did not know his surname. She told me that she had seen the document relating to that assessment. No document was produced [and the manager could not find it]... She told me that her recollection was that 'Harry' had recorded the risk as between 'moderate'or 'low'. It was not suggested by [the manager] nor is there any evidence to support the suggestion that the plaintiff's individual capability to work in the delivery suite was ever assessed.

Breach of duty was established.

Causation of injury: two weeks' cumulative injury. As a consequence of the breach of duty, the court held that the plaintiff suffered injury in delivery suite work. However, the judge noted that the plaintiff did not complain of a single incident but rather an 'accumulation of strain', and concluded that during that period of two weeks in November, she 'was asked to do work which caused her back condition to be exacerbated'.

Contributory negligence. On the evidence the injury had accelerated deterioration of the plaintiff's back by two years. There was no contributory negligence; it had been suggested that she should not have continued to 'soldier on' with the delivery suite work. However, the court regarded this 'as an unrealistic criticism of the plaintiff and is more typical of the view I have taken of her anxiety to do her job well and to serve her employers enthusiastically' ([2000] CL 00/2982, High Court).

WELSH v MATTHEW CLARK WHOLESALE LTD
Delivery driver; lifting kegs of beer; exacerbation of mild gastro-oesophageal reflux over period of years; cumulative injury; permanent impairment; MHOR 1992

The claimant was a delivery driver for a drinks depot. He maintained that a mild gastro-oesophageal reflux condition had been caused or substantially made worse by the lifting of heavy kegs and gas cylinders between 1992 and 1997 (when he was 35 years old), resulting in permanent impairment for that sort of work. In the County Court, the claimant won only limited damages, because the judge thought that even if the employer had not been in breach of its duty in causing the claimant to lift heavy kegs without assistance, nevertheless his final inability to do the job would have occurred anyway because of his constitutional weakness.

Appeal. He now appealed. He had done no really heavy work before June 1992, and the expert evidence suggested that a change at that time in working practices exacerbated what had previously been a mild and controlled reflux condition. The Court of Appeal accepted that but 'for the excessive lifting his symptoms would have stayed at the 1991 level, which did not interfere with his well-being or livelihood'. (Before 1992, he had done some occasional lifting of crates, but nothing as weighty as either the heavy or the light kegs from 1992 onwards.)

The employer had in fact admitted at the original trial breach of duty under the *MHOR 1992*, in respect of the lifting of all kegs, heavy or light; yet the judge's finding assumed that the breach was only in respect of heavy kegs. This was the basis on which he concluded that even if the claimant had been detailed to lift the lighter kegs, he would still have had the reflux problem and so been eventually unable to work.

Breaches of duty over time resulting in worse symptoms and permanent impairment. The Court of Appeal held that this was therefore the wrong approach; the full extent of the employer's admitted breach of duty should be taken into account. Thus, it concluded that 'the weight of the evidence supports the claimant's case that the defendant's admitted breaches of duty caused him significantly more severe and more prevalent symptoms while employed by them and that those breaches of duty further caused permanent impairment of his ability to work as a delivery driver'. The damages award should therefore reflect the extent to which the employer had conceded breach of duty. Because this would now include a loss of earnings award, the damages were increased from the original £5,080 to £37,605 ([2001] EWCA CIV 320, Court of Appeal).

WESTON v SOUTH COAST NURSING HOMES
Nurse; nursing home; time limits on bringing action; Limitation Act 1980

A case in which the courts decided not to exercise their discretion to extend the time limits for bringing a legal action.

A senior nurse was employed at a nursing home; she claimed to have suffered a back injury in 1991 when she tried to prevent a resident falling in the bathroom. Particulars of her claim included the employer's failure to provide a safe system of work, a non-slip floor surface in the bathroom, and adequate night lighting in the bathroom. The action had been dismissed at first instance because it was brought out of time; the judge had noted particularly that she had visited her own GP six times and been referred to a consultant who diagnosed a chronic strain in the lower lumbar region, yet still she had delayed bringing the case. The judge had s.14(2) of the *Limitation Act 1980* in mind (concerning the point in time when a claimant gains requisite knowledge for bringing a claim).

As to s.33 of the 1980 Act and the court's discretion to waive the time limits in an individual case, the Court of Appeal also approved the judge's balancing act in favour of the defendant, who would have suffered a greater degree of prejudice had the case been allowed to proceed (1997, Court of Appeal, unreported).

WILD v UNITED PARCEL SERVICES
Moving pallet; reliability of evidence; MHOR 1992; negligence case

The plaintiff fell off a curtain-sided truck in 1993, when trying to move a pallet on the truck; he claimed that he had to use a hook to try to move it. At first instance, the Recorder took a dim view of the two accounts of the accident given originally by the plaintiff which made no mention of the hook, and concluded that he was in fact using a pallet truck. The Court of Appeal now would not interfere with the Recorder's finding that there was no negligence or breach of statutory duty (1998, Court of Appeal, unreported).

WILES v BEDFORDSHIRE COUNTY COUNCIL
Residential social worker; disabled girl falling; taking manual handling operations as a whole; breach of MHOR 1992

A residential social worker took a disabled girl to the lavatory at a respite residential care home. She regularly looked after the girl, who weighed 29.5kg (about 4.5 stone), and often took her to the lavatory on her own. The girl used an electric wheelchair, could weight-bear for short periods of time, but could not walk. Her upper limbs were prone to occasional involuntary spasm. On this occasion, the plaintiff lifted her out of the wheelchair in the lavatory, so the girl could lean against a support bar, while the plaintiff crouched down to remove her underclothes. At this point, the girl threw out her hands unexpectedly and fell backwards against the plaintiff, causing a back injury.

The plaintiff brought the case in negligence and under the *MHOR 1992*, claiming that the task should have been designated as a two-person job, and that there should have been another member of staff in the home to help her carry out the task. Following the accident, the council instructed staff to use a hoist, used by two staff, in order to take the girl to the lavatory.

The judge found liability. First, he concluded that the *MHOR 1992* applied, even though the plaintiff was not actually handling a load at the precise moment of injury, since the whole task of taking the girl to the lavatory should be considered a manual handling operation. Second, the task involved a risk of injury, so r.4 of the *MHOR 1992* applied. Third, there was a breach of r.4 because the council failed to avoid the need for the plaintiff to carry out the operation, and failed to make a proper assessment or take steps to reduce the risk of injury. The fact that the plaintiff had carried out the task previously was no defence, and there was no contributory negligence ([2001] CL 01/June, County Court).

WILLIAMS v GWENT HEALTH AUTHORITY
Nurse; moving patient from bed to chair; system of work; negligence case

A negligence case illustrating the importance of employers having safe *systems of work* for manual handling based on up-to-date knowledge of the subject.

Accident. The plaintiff was a state enrolled nurse (SEN) employed at a small hospital housing 29 patients. She sustained a back injury when moving, together with another SEN, a patient from bed to chair. The patient was partially paralysed and weighed over 12 stone; the plaintiff nurse weighed less than eight stone. She and another nurse were performing a 'drag lift' which involved placing one arm under each of the patient's armpits and resting the other on the bed, and then lifting and turning the woman onto the chair near the bottom of the bed. The woman made an unexpected movement during this manoeuvre.

Evidence as to patient's weight-bearing capacity. The crucial issue was whether the patient was weight-bearing, since if she was not, even the employer accepted that the 'drag lift' was negligent. The court accepted the plaintiff's evidence, that the patient could not bear weight, against that of the matron and ward sister who maintained the opposite.

Thus the health authority was found liable in negligence for an unsafe *system of work*. In the light of agreed statistics relating to lifting accidents in the hospital, within the area of the health authority and nationally, there was a foreseeable risk of injury to nurses involved in handling patients. In the circumstances of this case, the method of lifting used by the plaintiff and her colleague was unsafe, imposing extra strain on the spine. Evidence to this effect was derived from the Royal College of Nursing's 'Handling of patients: a guide for nurse managers', which stated that the 'shoulder' or 'Australian' lift was preferred. The plaintiff was not responsible for an unsafe *system of work* and was following the system in operation; she was not to blame for this (1982, High Court, unreported).

WILSON v BRITISH RAILWAYS BOARD
Railway employee; lifting bag of gravel; no evidence from employer as to reasonable practicability; MHOR 1992

A railway employee suffered injury in 1995 when lifting a 50–60lb bag of gravel some five feet above ground level, in order to throw it into a compactor. He had thought of it as if it was like lifting his two-year-old daughter; but he felt its weight and, having already suffered discomfort that day, he asked a supervisor if he could leave the bag and get help later. The supervisor said it was contrary to policy to leave things lying near the compactor. In the absence of evidence supporting a defence under r.4 of the *MHOR 1992*, the judge found breach of statutory duty. Damages were set at £4,400 (1998, Outer House, Court of Session, Scotland).

WOODS v BARRY CLAYMAN CONCERTS
Dancer; instructions; MHOR 1992

A case illustrating the potential scope of the *MHOR 1992*, and also potential implications of their over-strict application.

The plaintiff was an exceptionally talented young Irish dancer who claimed that he had been injured through a failure to instruct and train him in lifting movements in dance. On the evidence the court rejected the claim – the most important point being that the plaintiff could not identify anything relating to lifting which he was not aware of. This suggested that he had been taught all there was to be taught. The judge accepted that his lifting inexperience had been taken into account, and that he was adequately supervised – not least since the instructor was the dance captain throughout and actually danced with the plaintiff. Also rejected was the suggestion that training and instruction should have been given early in the day and not at its end when the plaintiff was tired from rehearsal.

Liberal interpretation of what is reasonably practicable. The judge also pointed out that the *MHOR 1992* could scarcely be interpreted so strictly as to make lifting in dancing a criminal offence; thus a liberal interpretation of what was reasonably practicable was required. In any case, the judge also concluded that any injury the plaintiff had suffered was not caused by lifting (as opposed e.g. simply to movement) – and certainly not by incorrect lifting technique (1998, High Court, unreported).

WOOLGAR v WEST SURREY AND NORTH EAST HAMPSHIRE HEALTH AUTHORITY
Staff nurse; lifting patient; nurse's own judgement; negligence case

A *negligence* case illustrating that there is a point at which the courts will attribute the cause of an accident to employees, even in the 'altruistic' context of health care.

The plaintiff was a 27-year-old staff nurse who suffered a back injury when lifting a patient on a geriatric ward in 1985. The patient was elderly, obese, suffering from a degree of senile dementia and incontinent. She weighed about 15 stone. She could be uncooperative and difficult but did not appear to have been so on the day in question. She was sitting in a high-backed chair and needed to be washed because of her incontinence. The plaintiff and a student nurse lifted her to a standing position; during this operation, the plaintiff injured her back.

Type of lift used. The lift used was akin to but not the same as the 'drag lift', and was common practice in the hospital, so long as the patient was weight-bearing – in which case it was more of an 'assisted stand'. Although evidence was given that a 'waistband or belt lift' should have been used on such a patient, the court found that in 1985, a competent ward sister would not have insisted on such a lift. However, the evidence was that if the patient was not weight-bearing then the lift used by the plaintiff should not have been used. Thus, what went wrong was that the plaintiff either used excessive force or allowed excessive weight to bear on her forearm.

Training. When the plaintiff started work at the hospital, she was asked whether she felt she needed any further training in lifting techniques, and she replied that she did not think it was necessary, being so newly qualified. It was therefore decided, reasonably in the court's view, that as she was recently qualified, and had worked in an elderly care ward in her training, that she could be expected to be competent in lifting techniques and certainly aware of problems. Thus, any necessary instruction or reminders about techniques would be given by staff on the ward. In addition, she was also told prior to the accident that if a patient was too heavy or difficult, she should call for assistance from the porter and not lift if she did not feel capable of doing so.

Nurse's own judgement. The Court of Appeal now agreed with the judge at first instance, that in the end

> the method to be adopted by a nurse must be a matter for her individual judgement, particularly in the case of a trained nurse. Only she will know what pressure or force she is having to apply in any given situation. If she judges that the force required is so large that assistance is required or another method must be adopted she must take the appropriate steps either to obtain assistance or to work out and adopt another method.

Supervision. Furthermore, the plaintiff had not proved that 'observation by the ward sister would have shown that what she was doing was placing a strain upon her which she should not have been asked to bear or called for intervention requiring her to adopt another practice' ((1993) TLR 8 November 1993, Court of Appeal).

WRIGHT v FIFE HEALTH BOARD
Nursing auxiliary; moving patient up bed; orthodox lift; national guidance not followed; conflicting expert evidence on lifts; negligence case

The pursuer sought damages for an injury alleged to have been sustained in 1985, while working as a nursing auxiliary in a hospital. The incident involved moving a ten-stone patient up her bed. The patient was a dead weight and had to be handled carefully because of the pain she was in. She could not weight-bear and had no power in her arms.

Training. The pursuer claimed to have received no relevant training, but the court preferred the evidence of the employer that she had indeed been taught lifting techniques.

Orthodox lift and expert evidence. The lift used by the pursuer had been the 'orthodox lift'. The judge heard detailed expert evidence about different lifts – hearing, for instance, that the 'Australian lift' had limitations if the patient was not cooperative, and that the 'draw sheet' lift risked causing pressure sores and also relied on some cooperation, as well as the patient being able to sit up. Indeed one of the witnesses, if she had still been teaching, would have continued to teach the 'orthodox lift'. The judge preferred this evidence to that of the pursuer's expert who had been involved in the publication in 1981 by the Royal College of Nursing and National Back Pain Association of 'The handling of patients'. Both the 1981 edition and the 2nd edition in 1987 had discouraged the 'orthodox lift' (more strongly in the 1987 edition). The judge found that the employer's expert witnesses had greater experience of practical nursing problems than the pursuer's ergonomic expert. The judge concluded that if trained in manual handling techniques, staff could apply safe lifting principles to the 'orthodox lift'. Thus the employer could not reasonably have foreseen the risk to the employee (1992, Outer House, Court of Session, Scotland).

WYATT v HILLINGDON LONDON BOROUGH COUNCIL
Home care; local authority social services; hypothetical dropping of woman by home carer; negligence case

A woman with disseminated sclerosis sought damages for negligence and breach of statutory duty against the local authority in relation to the provision of home help, practical assistance in the home and the provision of an invalid bed. The court dismissed the case for breach of statutory duty out of hand. Likewise, the negligence case failed, since the nature of the provision she was complaining about came under a statutory duty in the *Chronically Sick and Disabled Persons Act 1970* and *National Assistance Act 1948*. However, the court noted that a claim in *negligence* might have been possible if, for instance, the home help had dropped the woman and injured her, or if the bed provided by the local authority had been defective, collapsed and caused injury ([1978] 76 LGR 727, Court of Appeal).

X v BEDFORDSHIRE COUNTY COUNCIL

[1995] 2 AC 633 (House of Lords): see *Z v United Kingdom*

YOUNG v SALFORD HEALTH AUTHORITY

Student nurse; pulling back young person from edge of play mat; negligence case

This was an appeal against a High Court decision in favour of the plaintiff, a student nurse, working at Manchester Royal Children's Office. She claimed that she suffered injury when she attempted to pull back into a safer position a severely mentally retarded 15 to16-year-old patient who was playing on a thick mattress-like play mat and who was near the edge of it. Reviewing the evidence, the Court of Appeal did not find the plaintiff's evidence convincing, but nevertheless was not prepared to interfere with the finding of the trial judge, even though it doubted it would have reached the same decision (1996, Court of Appeal, unreported).

Z v UNITED KINGDOM

Human rights; abuse and neglect of children; prolonged failure of social services to intervene; breach of European Convention; inhuman and degrading treatment

An example of a breach of article 3 of the European Convention on Human Rights, in terms of inhuman and degrading treatment, and illustrating the fairly extreme circumstances necessary to found such a breach. (See *European Convention on Human Rights* for possible manual handling implications.)

Background. A family was first referred to social services in 1987 by a health visitor over concerns about the four young children. Over the next four years many referrals were made by neighbours, a family member, general practitioner, head teacher, social worker, and police officers. Reports included reference to the children being locked out of the house, the children being dirty, filthy rooms including used nappies and sanitary towels in a cupboard, scavenging for food in bins, urine-soaked mattresses, broken beds, being hit with a poker, screaming, bruising, defecation in the bedrooms and excrement smeared on the windows, and so on. Finally, in 1992 the children were eventually taken into care after the mother had demanded it, because otherwise she would batter them. Between 1987 and 1992, during which time no steps had been taken to remove the children, there had been something in the order of eleven meetings of professionals, and a case conference.

Inhuman and degrading treatment. In 1993, the Official Solicitor, acting for the children, commenced proceedings against the local authority, seeking damages for breach of statutory duty (under child care legislation) and in *negligence*. The case went all the way to the House of Lords where, essentially on public policy grounds, it was held that the local authority and its social workers owed no duty of care in such circumstances (*X v Bedfordshire County Council*). The case was subsequently taken to the European Court of Human Rights, which found a breach of article 3, given that there was no dispute that the neglect and abuse suffered had reached the threshold of in-human and degrading treatment; that the local authority had a statutory duty to pro-tect the children; that for four and a half years the children had been subjected to horrific experiences and appalling neglect; and that over an extended period they had suffered physical and psychological injury directly attributable to a crime of vio-lence. The court acknowledged the difficult and sensitive decisions facing social ser-vices, and the importance of respecting and preserving family life; but the present case left no doubt about the failure of the system to protect the children from serious, long-term neglect and abuse. Damages of some £350,000 were awarded ([2001] 2 FCR 246, European Court of Human Rights).

REFERENCES

ACPIN (2001) Association of Chartered Physiotherapists in Neurology. *Guidance on manual handling in treatment: ACPIN manual handling working party 2001*. London: ACPIN.

APCP (undated) Graham, J., Hurran, C. and Mackenzie, M. *Paediatric manual handling: guidance for paediatric physiotherapists*. London: Association of Paediatric Chartered Physiotherapists.

Audit Commission (2000) *Fully equipped: the provision of equipment to older or disabled people by the NHS and social services in England and Wales*. London: Audit Commission.

BackCare (1999) *Safer handling of people in the community*. Teddington: BackCare.

Cassidy, S. (2001) 'Record payouts for assaults and accidents in class.' *The Independent*, 12th May 2001, p.13.

CHI (2000) Commission for Health Improvement. *Investigation into the North Lakeland NHS Trust: Report to the Secretary of State for Health*. London: CHI.

CNA (1997) Carers' National Association. *In on the Act? Social services' experience of the first year of the Carers Act*. London: CNA.

Conneeley, A.L. (1998) 'The impact of the Manual Handling Operations Regulations 1992 on the use of hoists in the home: the patient's perspective.' *British Journal of Occupational Therapy*, January 1998; 61(1), pp.17–21.

COT (1995) College of Occupational Therapists. *Manual Handling Operations Regulations 1992 and their application within occupational therapy: guidelines*. London: COT.

COT (2000) College of Occupational Therapists. *Code of ethics and professional conduct for occupational therapists*. London: COT.

CSP (2002) Chartered Society of Physiotherapy. *Guidance on manual handling for chartered physiotherapists*. London: CSP.

CSP, COT and RCN (1997) Chartered Society of Physiotherapy; College of Occupational Therapists; Royal College of Nursing. 'Partnership in the manual handling of patients.' *British Journal of Occupational Therapy*, September 1997; 60(9), p.406.

Cunningham, S. (2000) *Disability, oppression and public policy: disabled people and the professionals' interpretation of the Manual Handling Operations Regulations 1992*. Keighley: Sue Cunningham.

Cunningham, S. (2001) 'The downside of lifting.' *Therapy Weekly*, 5th April 2001, p.6.

DH (2000) Department of Health. *Draft guidance on the use of physical interventions for staff working with children and adults with learning disability and/or autism*. London: DH.

DH (2001a) Department of Health. *Practitioner's guide to carers' assessments under the Carers and Disabled Children Act 2000*. London: DH.

DH (2001b) Department of Health. *Care Homes for Older People: national minimum standards*. London: DH.

DH (2001c) Department of Health (Draft/consultation document) *Fair access to care services.* London: DH.

DH (2001d) Department of Health. *Domiciliary care: national minimum standards, consultation document.* London: DH.

Ellis, R. (2000) '£800,000 for nurse who tried to lift 12 stone patient.' *The Express,* 15th February 2000, p.22.

George, M. (2001) 'A precarious package.' *Community Care,* 5–11 April 2001, pp.30–1.

Glendinning, C., Halliwell, S., Jacobs, S., Rummery, K. and Tyrer, J. (2000) *Buying independence: using direct payments to integrate health and social services.* Bristol: Policy Press.

Grimley Evans, J. and Tallis, R.C. (2001) 'A new beginning for care for elderly people? Not if the psychopathology of this national service framework gets in the way.' *British Medical Journal,* 7 April 2001, vol.322, pp.807–8.

Harris, H., Allen, D., Cornick, M., Jefferson, A. and Mills, R. (1996) *Physical interventions: a policy framework.* Kidderminster: British Institute of Learning Disabilities (and National Autistic Society).

Hasler (2000) 'Lifting debate: users must come first.' *Community Care,* 29th June, p.16.

Hayes, D. (2001) 'Woman receives £37,000 damages for injuries from restraining pupils.' *The Independent,* 17th April 2001, p.4.

Henwood, M. (1998) *Ignored and invisible? Carers' experience of the NHS.* London: Carers National Association.

Henwood, M. (2001) *Future imperfect? Report of the King's Fund Care and Support Inquiry.* London: King's Fund.

Hignett, S. (2001) 'Manual handling risk assessments in occupational therapy.' *British Journal of Occupational Therapy,* February 2001; 64(2), pp.81–86.

HSC 2001/01; LAC(2001)1. Department of Health. *Intermediate care.* London: DH.

HSC 2001/008; LAC(2001)13. Department of Health. *Community equipment services.* London: DH.

HSC 2001/15; LAC(2001)18. Department of Health. *Continuing care: NHS and local councils' responsibilities.* London: DH.

HSC 2001/17; LAC(2001)26. Department of Health. *Guidance on free nursing care in nursing homes.* London: DH.

HSC (1998) Health and Safety Commission. *Manual handling in the health services.* Sudbury: HSE Books.

HSC (1998a) Health and Safety Commission. *Safe use of work equipment: approved code of practice and guidance.* Sudbury: HSE Books.

HSC (1998b) Health and Safety Commission. *Safe use of lifting equipment: approved code of practice and guidance.* Sudbury: HSE Books.

HSE (1998) Health and Safety Executive. *Manual handling: Manual Handling Operations Regulations 1992, guidance on regulations.* Sudbury: HSE.

HSE (2001) Health and Safety Executive (Draft/consultation document) *Handling home care: practical solutions to manual handling in home care situations.* Chelmsford: HSE.

HSE NIGM 7/F/1998/2 (1998) Health and Safety Executive. *Roles and responsibilities of parties involved in community care.* Chelmsford: HSE.

HSE SIM 7/1999/18 (1999) Health and Safety Executive. *Application of the Provision and Use of Work Equipment Regulations 1998 (PUWER) and the Lifting Operations and Lifting Equipment Regulations 1998 (LOLER) to equipment in health services and social care.* Chelmsford: HSE.

HSO (2001) Health Service Ombudsman. HC 278–I. *Investigations completed August–November 2000, part I: summaries of investigations completed.* London: Stationery Office.

Hurwitz, B. (1998) *Clinical guidelines and the law.* Abingdon: Radcliffe Medical Press.

Jones and Lenehan (2000) *Effect of the Manual Handling Regulations on family based short break services.* Bristol: Shared Care Network.

Kelly, D. (2001) 'Backs are a sore point for Scots workers.' *Evening Times* (Glasgow), 20th September 2001, p.16 (advice column).

Kelso, P. (2000) 'He only wanted to end his wife's pain. He ended up in court, at 84.' *The Guardian*, 7th June 2000, p.1.

LAC(92)27 (1992) Department of Health. *National Assistance Act 1948 (Choice of Accommodation) Directions 1992.* London: DH.

Mandelstam, M. (1997) *Equipment for Older or Disabled People and the Law.* London: Jessica Kingsley Publishers.

McGuire, T., Moody, J., Hanson, M. and Tigar, F. (1996) 'A study into clients' attitudes towards mechanical aids.' *Nursing Standard*, 23rd October 1996; 11(5), pp.35–38.

MDA DB9801 (1998) Medical Devices Agency. *Medical device and equipment management for hospital and community-based organisations.* London: MDA.

MDA DB9801 Supplement1 (1999) Medical Devices Agency. *Checks and tests for newly delivered medical devices.* London: MDA.

MDA DB (2000)2 Medical Devices Agency. *Medical devices and equipment management: repair and maintenance provision.* London: MDA.

MDA HN2000(11) (2000) Medical Devices Agency. *Hoskins Healthcare 'Rondo' variable height couch: risk of collapse.* London: MDA.

MDA SN9627 (1996) Medical Devices Agency. *Patient hoist: Arjo Ambulift – sudden dropping of jib arm.* London: MDA.

MDA SN9637 (1996) Medical Devices Agency. *Transfer and lifting equipment: problems associated with moving patients.* London: MDA.

MDA SN9705 (1997) Medical Devices Agency. *Pisces bath lifter: Huntleigh Community Care.* London: MDA.

MDA SN9817 (1998) Medical Devices Agency. *Oxford Major electric and hydraulic patient hoists.* London: MDA.

MDA SN9828 (1998) Medical Devices Agency. *Maxilift patient hoists.* London: MDA.

MDA SN9829 (1998) Medical Devices Agency. *Patient hoist slings: plastic sling attachment clips.* London: MDA.

MDA SN9832 (1998) Medical Devices Agency. *Self-lift chair: the Caithness, Cairngorm and Clansman.* London: MDA.

MDA SN9838 (1998) Medical Devices Agency. *Chiltern Wispa mobile patient hoist (also badged as Homecraft Maxi/Midi/Dual models).* London: MDA.

MDA SN9929 (1999) Medical Devices Agency. *Patient lifting and transfer devices: sling, strap and clip failures.* London: MDA.

MDA SN9938 (1999) Medical Devices Agency. *Patient lifting and transfer devices: Arjo strap stretchers.* London: MDA.

MDA SN2001(21) (2001) Medical Devices Agency. *Ferno Mk 1, Mobyle carry chair: risk of frame collapse due to failure of pivot pins.* London: MDA.

MDD HN9418 (1994) Medical Devices Directorate. *Patient hoists: band slings, risk of fatal or serious injury.* London: MDD.

Oliveck, M. (1998) 'Lifts and hoists: strategy for parents.' *Therapy Weekly,* 16th July 1998, pp.6–8.

Parkinson, J. (1999) 'Risk is part of life.' *Disability Now,* August 1999, p.12.

RCN (2001) Royal College of Nursing; BackCare; Arjo Ltd. *Changing practice, improving health: an integrated back injury prevention programme for nursing and care homes.* London: RCN.

RCN/NBPA (1997) Royal College of Nursing; National Back Pain Association. *Guide to the handling of patients.* 4th edition. Teddington: NBPA.

Resuscitation Council (UK) (2001) *Guidance for safer handling during resuscitation in hospitals.* London: Resuscitation Council.

Royal College of Midwives (1999) *Handle with care: a midwife's guide to preventing back injury.* 2nd edition. London: RCM.

SAB8914. Department of Health; Scottish Home and Health Department; Welsh Office; Department of Health and Social Services (Northern Ireland). *Patient lifting devices: sling, harness and strap failures.* London: DH

Scottish Executive (2000) *Community care: a joint future.* Edinburgh: Scottish Executive.

SIB 8403 (1984) Department of Health and Social Security; Scottish Home and Health Department; Welsh Office; Department of Health and Social Services (Northern Ireland). Safety Information Bulletin. *Patient lifting hoists/slings.* London: DHSS, SHHD, WO, DHSS(NI).

Snell, J. (1995) 'Raising awareness.' *Nursing Times,* 2nd August 1995; 91(31), pp.20–21.

SO (1996) Scottish Office. *Children and young persons with special educational needs: assessment and recording.* Edinburgh: SO.

SO (2001) Stationery Office. *Special Educational Needs and Disability Act 2001: explanatory notes.* London: SO.

SSI (2001) Social Services Inspectorate (Woods, G.) *Safe enough? Inspection of health authority registration and inspection units, 2000.* London: DH.

The Column (2001) 'Manual handling: training guidelines.' *The Column,* August 2001, pp.12–13.

Therapy Weekly (2001) 'Care staff accused of blocking beds.' News. *Therapy Weekly,* 9th August 2001, p.3.

UKCC (1998) United Kingdom Central Council for Nursing, Midwifery and Health Visiting. *Guidelines for records and record keeping.* London: UKCC.

Williams, K. (1996) 'Handle with care.' *Nursing Standard,* 3rd April 1996; 10(28), pp.26–7.

Winchcombe, M. (1998) *Community equipment services: why should we care? A guide to good practice in disability equipment services.* London: Disabled Living Centres Council.

Zindani, G. (1998) *Manual handling: law and litigation.* London: CLT Professional Publishing.